One third of human cancers have a hormonal basis. Breast cancer, the most common cancer of women, is increasing in incidence in many countries, as, in epidemic proportions, is prostate cancer, which, in the United States, has just become the most common cancer of men. Concurrently, the development of molecular biology has led to a refinement of the definition of hormones to include the complex interaction between tumour cells and both locally and distantly secreted factors.

This volume in the series Cancer: Clinical Science in Practice considers the many aspects of hormonally dependent cancer, including the molecular basis for the autocrine and paracrine regulation of cancer, preventive strategies in limiting the epidemic of hormonally related cancers, and new treatment approaches.

Up-to-date and authoritative, volumes in this series are intended for a wide audience of clinicians and researchers with an interest in the application of biomedical science to the understanding and management of cancer.

MOLECULAR ENDOCRINOLOGY OF CANCER

CANCER: CLINICAL SCIENCE IN PRACTICE

General Editor

Professor Karol Sikora

Department of Clinical Oncology
Royal Postgraduate Medical School
Hammersmith Hospital, London

A series of authoritative review volumes intended for a wide audience of clinicians and researchers with an interest in the application of biomedical science to the understanding and management of cancer.

Also in this series

Cell Therapy: Stem cell transplantation, gene therapy, and cellular immunotherapy
Edited by George Morstyn and William P. Sheridan

Tumor Immunology
Edited by A. G. Dalgleish and M. J. Browning

MOLECULAR ENDOCRINOLOGY OF CANCER

Edited by
Jonathan Waxman
Royal Postgraduate Medical School
Hammersmith Hospital, London

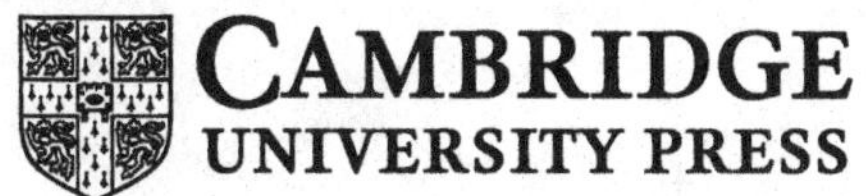

CAMBRIDGE UNIVERSITY PRESS
Cambridge, New York, Melbourne, Madrid, Cape Town, Singapore,
São Paulo, Delhi, Dubai, Tokyo, Mexico City

Cambridge University Press
The Edinburgh Building, Cambridge CB2 8RU, UK

Published in the United States of America by Cambridge University Press, New York

www.cambridge.org
Information on this title: www.cambridge.org/9780521159494

First published 1996
First paperback edition 2011

A catalogue record for this publication is available from the British Library

Library of Congress Cataloguing in Publication Data

Molecular endocrinology of cancer / edited by Jonathan Waxman.
p. cm. (Cancer. clinical science in practice)
Includes index.
ISBN 0-521-46067-0 (hardback)
1. Cancer-Endocrine aspects. 2. Endocrine glands-Cancer.
I. Waxman, Jonathan. II. Series.
[DNLM: 1. Neoplasms-physiopathology. 2. Neoplasms-therapy.
3. Hormones. 4. Endocrinology. QZ 200 M718332 1996]
RC262.M662 1996
616.99'4-dc20
DNLM/DLC
for Library of Congress 95-39973 CIP

ISBN 978-0-521-46067-5 Hardback
ISBN 978-0-521-15949-4 Paperback

Contents

Contributors

Lorraine Anderson
MRC Reproductive Biology Unit
Centre for Reproductive Biology
Edinburgh, UK

Bradley A. Arrick
Department of Medicine
Dartmouth Medical School
Hanover, New Hampshire

Donald M. Black
The Beatson Institute for Cancer Research
Bearsden, Glasgow, UK

Steven Bloom
Department of Endocrinology
Royal Postgraduate Medical School
Hammersmith Hospital
London, UK

Peter Boyle
Division of Epidemiology and Biostatistics
Istituto Europeo di Oncologia
Milan, Italy

Arthur E. Broadus
Department of Internal Medicine and Cellular and Molecular Physiology
Yale University School of Medicine
New Haven, Connecticut

Robert Clarke
Vincent T. Lombardi Cancer Center
Georgetown University Medical Center
Washington, D.C.

Rik Derynck
Departments of Growth, Development and Anatomy
Programs in Cell Biology and Developmental Biology
University of California, San Francisco
San Francisco, California

Robert B. Dickson
Vincent T. Lombardi Cancer Center
Georgetown University Medical Center
Washington, D.C.

Karin A. Eidne
MRC Reproductive Biology Unit
Centre for Reproductive Biology
Edinburgh, UK

Audrey D. Goddard
Department of Molecular Biology
Genetech Inc.
South San Francisco, California

W. J. Gullick
ICRF Oncology Unit
Imperial Cancer Research Fund
Hammersmith Hospital
London, UK

Terry Hamblin
The Royal Bournemouth Hospital
East Bournemouth, Dorset, UK

Peter Hammond
Department of Endocrinology
Royal Postgraduate Medical School
Hammersmith Hospital
London, UK

Pita Enriquez Harris
Department of Biochemistry
University of Oxford
Oxford, UK

John K. Heath
Department of Biochemistry
University of Oxford
Oxford, UK

Patrick Maisonneuve
Division of Epidemiology and Biostatistics
Istituto Europeo di Oncologia
Milan, Italy

Carole B. Miller
The Johns Hopkins Oncology Center
Division of Hematology
Department of Medicine
The Johns Hopkins School of Medicine
Baltimore, Maryland

Hardev Pandha
Department of Clinical Oncology
Hammersmith Hospital
London, UK

T. Rajkumar
ICRF Oncology Unit
Imperial Cancer Research Fund
Hammersmith Hospital
London, UK

Enrique Rozengurt
Growth Regulation Laboratory
Imperial Cancer Research Fund
London, UK

Michael J. Seckl
Imperial Cancer Research Fund
London, UK

Jerry L. Spivak
The Johns Hopkins Oncology Center
Division of Hematology
Department of Medicine
The Johns Hopkins School of Medicine
Baltimore, Maryland

Andrew Stubbs
Department of Clinical Oncology
Hammersmith Hospital
London, UK

Jonathan Waxman
Department of Clinical Oncology
Hammersmith Hospital
London, UK

John J. Wysolmerski
Departments of Internal Medicine and Cellular and Molecular Physiology
Yale University School of Medicine
New Haven, Connecticut

PART I

The Regulation of Cancer

1

The Type 1 Growth Factor Receptor Family, Their Ligands and Their Role in Human Cancers

T. RAJKUMAR AND W. J. GULLICK

INTRODUCTION

Peptide and polypeptide growth factors, unlike classical hormones, are produced in a variety of tissues throughout the body. These bind to their cell surface receptors and thereby initiate a cascade of intracellular events culminating in either a positive or a negative growth signal. Growth factors can act by an autocrine, juxtacrine paracrine or endocrine process (Figure 1.1). Autocrine action is due to the secretion by a cell of growth factors for which it possesses receptors. Juxtacrine stimulation occurs when one cell possessing cell surface bound growth factors interacts with an adjacent cell possessing receptors. Paracrine action is defined as the release of soluble factors by cells that diffuse to and act upon adjacent or closely located cells. In the final case of endocrine stimulation, growth factors may act on distant sites very much like a classical hormone; for instance, epidermal growth factor (EGF) produced in mice in the submandibular gland has been shown by sialadenectomy to stimulate spermatogenesis.

General Characteristics of the EGF Ligand Family

The EGF family of growth factors are among the most studied of this class of molecules (Prigent and Lemoine, 1992). Several of these, in addition to displaying a role in normal development and wound repair, have been implicated in malignant transformation of cells (Aaronson, 1991). All the members of the EGF family of ligands, whether they bind to the EGF receptor or another receptor, have six cysteine residues that occur with a conserved spacing. Table 1.1 shows

AUTOCRINE

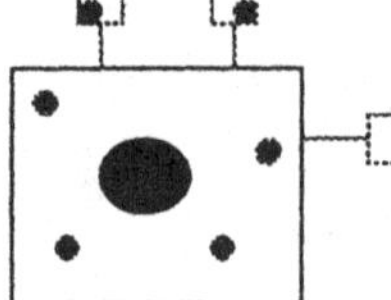

JUXTACRINE

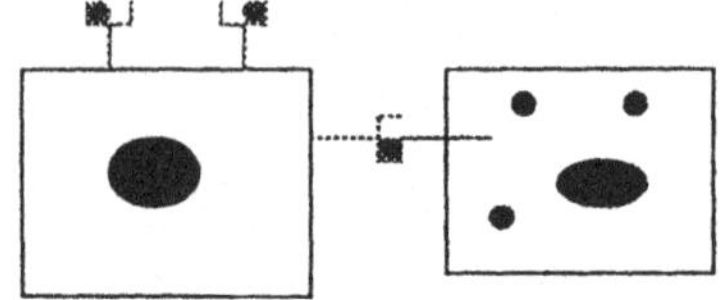

PARACRINE

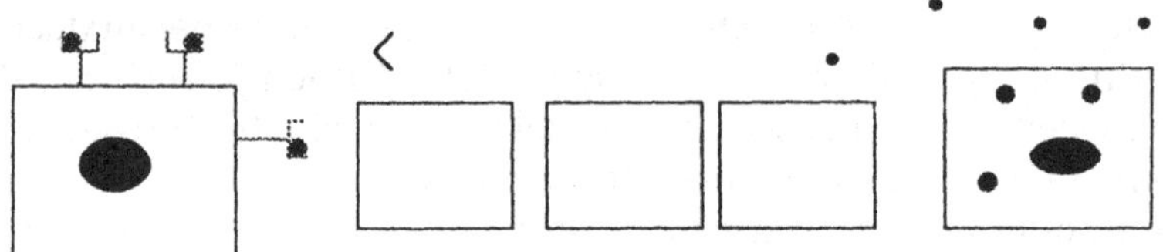

ENDOCRINE

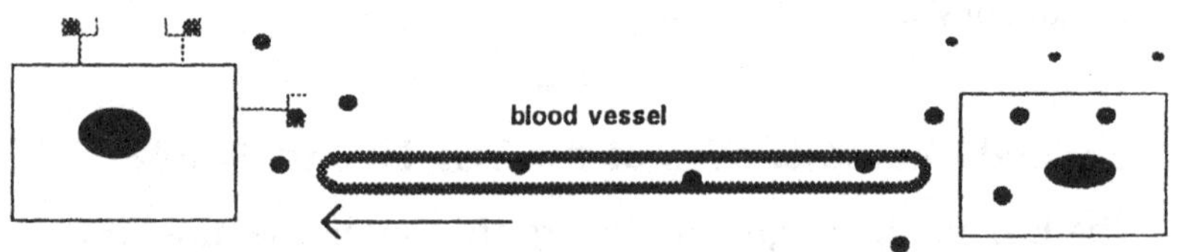

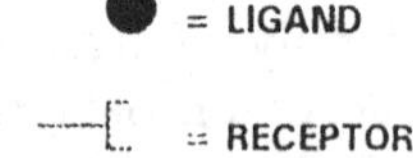

Figure 1.1 Mechanisms of action of growth factors.

Table 1.1. Currently Known Members of the EGF Ligand Family

Ligands	Receptors
EGF, TGF-α, amphiregulin (AR), heparin binding EGF, betacellulin, viral growth factors	EGFR
?	c-*erb*B2
Heregulin/NDF/GGF/ARIA	c-*erb*B3
Heregulin/NDF/GGF/ARIA	c-*erb*B4
Cripto	?

the currently known members of the family with their receptors. We will now review briefly the properties of the ligands and receptors identified thus far in this family. Several reviews have also been published on specific members of the family.

EGF

The 53 amino acid form of human EGF is derived by proteolytic cleavage from a 1,217 amino acid precursor. Thirty-seven of the 53 amino acids are homologous with mouse EGF and 14 of the 16 amino acids that differ could have resulted from single base pair changes. In fact, most members of this family have been found to be fairly well conserved in amino acid sequence during evolution. The EGF gene has been localized to chromosome 4q2.5, which transcribes an mRNA of 4.75 kb. In the adult human, EGF is produced by the submandibular salivary gland, gastric epithelium, Brunner's glands in the duodenum, pancreas, kidney, sweat glands (especially the apocrine glands), breast, thyroid gland, pituitary gland and the nervous system. EGF expression is also induced in areas of gastric, pancreatic or intestinal epithelium surrounding sites of chronic inflammation, necrosis or ulceration (Browne, 1991). In addition to existing in a secreted form, the EGF protein precursor is membrane bound, occurs widely and appears to be functional by a juxtacrine mechanism.

EGF induces its effect on cells through the EGF receptor, which undergoes tyrosine autophosphorylation and phosphorylates other proteins such as phospholipase C-II on specific tyrosine residues, which in turn leads to their activation and relocation to the cell membrane. The phosphorylated enzyme then activates the inositol phosphate pathway, leading to stimulation of protein kinase C. In addition, other pathways are also stimulated. The nature of the second messenger systems utilized by individual type 1 growth factor receptors is currently a topic of much research. It is clear that not all the receptors activate the same pathways providing a mechanism for their specificity of action. Later events following receptor activation include increased protein synthesis, inhibition of protein catabolism and increased synthesis of the c-*fos* and the c-*myc* gene products. EGF by itself is often not effective in inducing cell division but requires the presence of other factors such as insulin-like growth factor type 1 (IGF-1) or platelet-derived growth factor (PDGF), suggesting that more than one intracellular signalling pathway needs to be activated to stimulate mitogenesis.

Addition of EGF to cells in culture leads to down-regulation of expression of the receptor protein; however, somewhat paradoxically, EGF has been shown to stimulate EGF receptor synthesis by inducing increased mRNA transcription. EGF can induce proliferative responses in cancer cells. Increased EGF levels have, for instance, been reported in high-grade brain tumours (glioblastoma multiforme), which also tend to have a high incidence of gene amplification of EGFR receptor, suggesting the possibility of an autocrine loop in these tumours. However, the incidence of increased expression of EGF in human cancers is much less frequent and reliably documented than some other ligands of this family.

Transforming Growth Factor Alpha (TGF-α)

TGF-α shares structural similarity with EGF in both its precursor (consisting of 160 amino acids) and mature forms (50 amino acids) (Derynck, 1992). TGF-α binds to the EGFR with high affinity and generally produces the same effects on the target cells as EGF itself. Some reports have suggested, however, that TGF-α is half as potent as EGF at the same concentration. In addition, the two ligands display different abilities to bind to the EGF receptor at high and low pH values, although it is not clear if this is physiologically significant. TGF-α differs in its distribution in that it seems to be one of the main ligands for the EGF receptor during foetal development when the levels of EGF are either very low or absent. In adults, it is expressed very widely and its distribution includes keratinocytes, bronchus, intestine, renal tubule, pituitary and decidua. Most notably, however, its production is enhanced in some transformed cells. The proliferation of squamous cell carcinoma cell lines has been found to be sustained by a TGF-α autocrine pathway with the growth factor produced constitutively while its receptors are simultaneously overexpressed. Similar pathways have been demonstrated in high-grade brain tumours and breast carcinomas.

Apart from its direct effect on tumour cells, it has been reported that TGF-α as well as EGF can also promote bone resorption leading to hypercalcemia of malignancy, although TGF-α appeared to be ten times as potent as EGF. Another important property of this class of ligands first demonstrated with TGF-α is that they can induce angiogenesis, suggesting a second function in tumourigenesis.

One of the most compelling pieces of evidence for the transforming capabilities of TGF-α is the demonstration that transgenic mice expressing TGF-α in breast cells develop adenocarcinomas in the post-lactational mammary gland. Expression in other transgenic mouse strains leads to cancers developing in the liver and pancreas.

Amphiregulin

Amphiregulin is the third member of the family to be identified. The gene for amphiregulin is located on the long arm of chromosome 4 (4q13-4q21), which is transcribed into a 1.4-kb mRNA. The mRNA is translated to yield a precursor with 252 amino acids that is then cleaved to yield a mature peptide of either 78 or 84 amino acids. The mature peptide has structural homology with EGF (43% sequence identity) and the other EGF-like ligands, conserving all six cysteine residues. High levels of mRNA have been detected in human ovary and placenta; intermediate levels were seen in pancreas, colon, lung, breast, cardiac muscle, spleen, kidney and testis; it was absent or at very low levels in adrenal, parathyroid, thymus, prostate, epidermis, duodenum, brain and liver. The distribution of the amphiregulin protein has not, however, yet been studied in detail.

Amphiregulin binds to EGF receptor with a reportedly lower affinity than EGF and apparently has some different biological properties. It also inhibits the growth of tumour cell lines derived from different sites (A431cells, breast tumour cell lines HTB 132 and 26, the ovarian adenoma cell line HTB 75 and the neuroblastoma cell line HTB 10). It was, however, found to stimulate growth of several fibroblast cell lines, the pituitary tumour cell line CRL7386 and the ovarian carcinoma cell line HTB 77. Amphiregulin did not have any significant effect on the growth of other tumour cell lines such as the breast tumour cell line MCF-7, the lung carcinoma cell line A 549, the squamous carcinoma of the larynx Hep 2 and the colon carcinoma cell line H3347. One possible factor explaining these early observations is that amphiregulin can inhibit cell growth at low concentrations but will stimulate division at higher levels. In ovarian tumour cell lines (3/6) and surface epithelial cell lines (2/3), it inhibited growth at picomolar concentrations but stimulated their growth at nanomolar levels.

Amphiregulin has a unique pattern of expression in human colon, being expressed in the cytoplasm and nucleus of terminally differentiated, nonproliferative surface columnar and secretory epithelial cells of the mucosa but not in the proliferative epithelial cells of the crypts. In a series of colonic tumours, 50% showed moderate levels of amphiregulin expression, with a greater proportion (71%) of positivity being observed in well-differentiated tumours than in poorly differentiated tumours (18%). A colon carcinoma cell line, GEO, was found to secrete amphiregulin and co-express EGFR, thereby completing the autocrine loop.

In breast cancer cell lines, amphiregulin was found at high levels in ER positive cell lines, MCF-7, ZR75-1 and T47D and was absent or expressed at low levels in SKBR 3, MDA MB 231, MDA MB 468 and Hs 578T. Amphiregulin mRNA was found to be increased after oestradiol treatment of oestrogen-responsive MCF-7 cells. Amphiregulin protein detected by immunostaining was predominantly cytoplasmic, but nuclear and occasional nucleolar staining was also observed in some of the cells.

Similar immunocytochemistry of ovarian cancer cells revealed the protein to be localized to the nucleus of all the cells. However, in the carcinoma cell lines, the nuclear staining was concentrated in the nucleolus but was diffuse in the nucleus of the normal surface epithelial cells.

Keratinocyte autocrine factor (KAF), secreted by human keratinocytes, has been shown to be structurally, immunologically and biologically identical to amphiregulin.

Heparin Binding EGF Like Growth Factor

Heparin binding EGF like growth factor was purified from the conditioned medium of a human histiocytic cell line. The protein is encoded by a 2.5-kb mRNA and appears to be synthesized as a membrane-bound precursor of 208 amino acids that is then cleaved to release a mature protein of about 75 amino acids. The growth factor has one of the putative nuclear targeting sequences found in amphiregulin. Heparin binding EGF like growth factor binds to smooth muscle cells with a greater affinity than EGF and has been found to be mitogenic to keratinocytes. The growth factor has been postulated to play a role in wound healing. Recently the gene structure and chromosomal location (chromosomes) of the human heparin binding EGF like growth factor have been reported.

Betacellulin

Betacellulin is another recent addition to the EGF family of ligands. It is a 32-kDa glycoprotein first identified in the conditioned medium of cell lines derived from mouse pancreatic β cell tumours. Betacellulin binds to and stimulates tyrosine phosphorylation of the EGF receptor. It has been shown to be a potent mitogen for vascular smooth muscle cells and retinal pigment epithelial cells, suggesting a role in the vascular complications of diabetes.

Viral Growth Factors

Pox viruses including vaccinia virus, Shope fibroma virus, myxoma virus and molluscum contagiosum synthesize and release EGF-like peptides from cells they infect. Vaccinia virus growth factor has been purified and found to have structural homology with EGF. Vaccinia virus growth factor binds to EGF receptor and activates its kinase and stimulates mitogenesis. However, the exact role of these factors in the pathogenicity of the viruses is unknown, as it has been reported that vaccinia virus can infect cells without EGF receptor as efficiently as cells with high levels of them. Other reports, however, have contradicted this, suggesting that very high levels of EGF ($>10^{-8}$ M) or antibodies to the EGF receptor can inhibit infection of cells, perhaps by inhibiting viral particle binding.

Heregulin/Neu Differentiation Factor (NDF)

Heregulin is the human homologue of the murine Neu differentiation factor (NDF). The gene for heregulin is located on the short arm of chromosome 8 (8p12-p21). The mature protein is expressed in at least ten forms due to differential splicing; however, each form contains a region structurally similar to the other members of the EGF family. The factors do not bind to EGF receptors nor c-*erb*B2 but bind to c-*erb*B4 and c-*erb*B3. Heregulin/NDF related factors derived from alternate gene splicing during transcription have been identified as acetylcholine receptor inducing factor (ARIA) and glial growth factor (GGF). The expression pattern of NDF mRNA has been examined in adult rat tissues. The highest levels of NDF were detected in the spinal cord, followed by lung, brain, ovary and stomach. Low levels were seen in kidney, skin and heart but expression was undetectable in the liver, spleen and placenta.

Heregulin/NDF has been shown to induce tyrosine phosphorylation of c-*erb*B4/HER4 in a series of human tumour cell lines derived from breast, colon and neuronal tissue but not in ovarian tumour cells lacking the receptor. Heterodimerization of c-*erb*B4 and c-*erb*B2 has been demonstrated, following stimulation with heregulin, in cells expressing both the receptors. Heregulin was found to be growth stimulatory for mammary tumour cell lines at low concentrations but inhibitory at higher levels. NDF, however, was shown to induce differentiation of mammary tumour cells to milk-producing nondividing cells. The exact interactions between the heregulin/NDF isoforms and individual members of the type 1 receptor family are currently a rapidly evolving area. Clarification of this will help in interpreting the biological activity of this complex ligand famiy.

Cripto

Cripto is a human gene encoding a protein similar in sequence to EGF, and in particular to EGF's six conserved cysteine residues. It differs substantially in not possessing an A loop structure and in not being synthesized in a membrane-bound form. No receptors have yet been identified for cripto. Expression of cripto in certain cell types can promote their growth in soft agar and leads mouse NOG8 mammary epithelial cells to form tumours in nude mice. In this, however, it resembles TGF-α which in cells with low or moderate levels of EGF receptors produces the same behaviour.

Several authors have now examined cripto mRNA and protein expression in different tumour types. Cripto has been reported to be expressed in 79% of colon tumours with almost equal incidence between well-differentiated and poorly differentiated tumours. In one study 60% of adenomas and 12% of the noninvolved normal colon samples adjacent to tumours were positive but none of the nine normal colon samples showed expression. This suggests that cripto could be evaluated as a potential marker for colonic tumourigenesis. Seventy-five percent of a series of breast tumours were found to overexpress cripto protein as determined by immunohistochemistry. The staining was predominantly in the cytoplasm, with some specimens showing membrane staining. The stroma and the adjacent uninvolved breast epithelium were negative. Cripto was found to be expressed in all the seven breast cancer cell lines studied and oestradiol failed to modify the expression of cripto in MCF-7 cells. Overexpression of cripto has also been reported in gastric carcinomas.

EGF RECEPTOR FAMILY

Growth factor receptors with tyrosine kinase activity have been classified into nine different families based on the structure of the extracellular domain, their kinase domain and the nature of their ligand.

The type 1 family includes the EGF receptor, c-*erb*B2/HER2/*neu*, c-*erb*B3/HER3 and c-*erb*B4/HER4 (Table 1.1). The members of the type 1 family have a common structure which features an extracellular domain, a transmembrane region, a kinase domain and a carboxyterminal tail. The extracellular domain has ligand-binding sites flanked by two cysteine-rich regions which presumably contribute to structural integrity. Among the receptors, EGF receptor, c-*erb*B2 and c-*erb*B4 bear greater structural homology in their kinase domain than they do with c-*erb*B3. The kinase domain of c-*erb*B3 protein has two nonconservative amino-acid replacements, histidine replacing glutamic acid at position 740 and asparagine replacing aspartic acid at 815. However, the c-*erb*B3 protein has been shown to possess weak stimulatable kinase activity in some systems.

Many excellent reviews have been published describing the signalling mechanisms of the various receptors and their regulation by other proteins. Here we will briefly review the mechanism by which these receptors have been found to be activated and the occurrence of these changes in particular tumour types.

EGF Receptor

The EGF receptor gene located on chromosome 7q21 is transcribed into mRNAs of 6 and 10 kb which are then translated into a 135-kDa receptor protein which is then modified by *N*-linked glycosylation to the 170-kDa mature form (Gullick and Waterfield, 1987). Overexpression of EGFR in the presence of an activating ligand has been found to transform immortalized fibroblasts in vitro. Gene amplification of EGF receptor occurs in about 40% of glioblastoma multiforme, 10–20% of head and neck carcinomas, 8–14% of oesophageal tumours, 3% of gastric tumours and 2% of breast tumours (Gullick, 1991). Overexpression due to altered transcriptional control occurs in a much larger percentage of tumours and is described in 30% of breast, 35% of gastric, and 30–80% of bladder cancers. Overexpression of EGFR in breast tumours has generally been shown to be associated with an ER-negative phenotype and in some reports with short disease free interval and overall survival (Gullick, 1991).

Tyrosine kinase growth factor receptors may be activated by mutation as well as overexpression. In glioblastoma multiforme, not only has the gene been subjected to amplification but it is also often rearranged, resulting in a truncated EGFR lacking part of the extracellular domain. This mutated form of the receptor does not bind EGF but may be constitutively active.

c-*erb*B2

The c-*erb*B2/HER2/*neu* receptor protein has been found to be expressed widely in the normal foetus and the placenta. In adults, it is expressed on gastrointestinal, genitourinary, respiratory tracts and breast epithelial tissue. The gene is located on chromosome 17q21, and transcribed into a 4.5-kb mRNA which then is translated into a 185-kDa glycoprotein. Overexpression can be due to gene amplification or transcriptional deregulation as with the EGF receptor (Lofts and Gullick, 1992). In breast carcinomas, gene ampification occurs in about 20% of cases and is associated with a poor disease-free interval and overall survival in node-positive tumours. In node-negative tumours some studies have shown an asssociation with poor prognosis while others observed no significant effect.

Experimental studies have shown that overexpression of c-*erb*B2 in an ER-positive MCF-7 cell line leads to resistance to tamoxifen, although the parent cell line was still sensitive. Molecular cross-talk between EGF receptor and c-*erb*B2 has been shown to occur in the breast tumour cell line SKBR3, with EGF receptor inducing tyrosine phosphorylation of c-*erb*B2 following stimulation with EGF. c-*erb*B2 is also overexpressed in 20 to 30% of ovarian carcinomas, although perhaps less than half of these are due to gene amplification. Overexpression has been associated with a poor prognosis in this group of turnovers. Overexpression is also seen in 20% of gastric and pancreatic cancers, 30% of bladder carcinomas and 10% of endometrial carcinomas.

c-*erb*B3

c-*erb*B3 protein has a distinct pattern in adult human tissues and is expressed primarily in the terminally differentiated tissues of the gastrointestinal tract, skin, bladder urothelium, distal and proximal renal tubules of the kidney, CNS neurons and spinal ganglion cells. The gene is located in the long arm of chromosome 12 (12q13). The glycosylated protein has a molecular weight of 180 kDa and is derived from a 6.2-kb mRNA.

Although overexpression of c-*erb*B3 has been reported in breast, pancreatic, gastric and colonic carcinomas, no evidence of gene amplification has yet been reported.

c-*erb*B4

The fourth and recent addition to the type 1 family of tyrosine kinase growth factor receptors has a molecular weight of 180 kDa.

The 6.0-kb c-*erb*B4 mRNA has been detected at high levels in brain, skeletal muscle, pituitary, parathyroid, heart, breast, kidney and testis. It has been shown to be activated by a factor first described as heparin-binding breast cancer differentiating factor, and subsequently shown to be heregulin/NDF (Plowman et al., 1993a,b).

FUTURE DEVELOPMENTS

The type 1 growth factor receptor family has a primary role in cancer and perhaps holds the key to new treatments for malignant disease.

Therapeutic strategies aimed at interfering with the ligand-receptor loop are being evaluated. These include growth factor antagonists, monoclonal antibodies to the receptors and growth factors either used as independent molecules or conjugated to toxins, drugs or radioisotopes, receptor dimerization inhibitors, tyrosine kinase inhibitors, antisense oligonucleotides and transcriptional inhibitors.

REFERENCES

Aaronson, S.A. (1991) Growth factors and cancer. *Science*, **254**, 1146–1153.

Browne C.A. (1991) Epidermal growth factor and transforming growth factor a. *Bailliere's Clinical Endocrinology and Metabolism*, **5**, 553–9.

Derynck R. (1992) The physiology of transforming growth factorα *Advances in Cancer Research*, **58**, 27–52.

Gullick W.J. (1990) Growth factors and oncogenes in breast cancer. In *Progress in growth factor research*, Vol. 2, pp. 1–13. Pergamon Press.

Gullick W.J. (1991) Prevalence of aberrant expression of the epidermal growth factor receptor in human cancers. In *British Medical Bulletin*, 1st ed. Vol. 47,1, The British Council, 87–98.

Gullick W.J., & Waterfield M.D. (1987) Epidermal growth factor and its receptor. In A.D. Strosberg (Ed.) *The molecular biology of receptors techniques and applications of receptor research*, Ellis Horwood.

Lofts F.J.. & Gullick W.J. (1992) c-erbB2 amplification and overexpression in human tumours. *In*, R.B. Dickson & M. E. Lippman (Eds.) *Genes oncogenes and hormones: advances in cellular and molecular biology of breast cancer*, 1st ed. Vol. pp. 161–79. Kluwer Academic Publishers, Norwell,

Plowman G.D., Culouscou J.M., Whitney G.S., Green J.M., Carlton G.W., Foy L., Neubauer M.G. & Shoyab M. (1993a) Ligand specific activation of HER4/p180erbB4, a fourth member of the epidermal growth factor receptor family. *Proceedings of the National Academy of Science, U.S.A.* **90**, 1746–50.

Plowman G.D., Green J.M., Culouscou J.M., Carlton G.W., Rothwell V.M. & Buckley S. (1993b) Heregulin induces tyrosine phosphorylation of HER4/ p.180erbB4. *Nature*, **366**, 473–5.

Prigent S.A. & Lemoine N.R. (1992) The type 1 (EGFR related) family of growth factor receptors and their ligands. *Progress in Growth Factor Research*, **4**, 1–24.

2

The Fibroblast Growth Factor Family and Their Receptors

PITA ENRIQUEZ HARRIS AND JOHN K. HEATH

INTRODUCTION

The fibroblast growth factors (FGFs) are a family of nine structurally similar polypeptides that also have the common property of interacting with heparin. They induce the multiplication of a wide variety of cell types in vitro and in vivo and exhibit pleiotropic effects on cell migration, differentiation and gene expression. The FGFs exert their biological function as a result of binding to a family of FGF receptors (FGFRs) of the tyrosine kinase class. The FGFRs are subject to alternate splicing to produce mature receptors that exhibit specific affinities for different FGF family members. FGFs also interact with heparan sulphate containing proteoglycans (HSPGs). Increasing evidence indicates that the physical association of FGFs with HSPGs is a necessary requirement for cell signalling mediated by FGFRs.

A considerable body of indirect evidence implicates the FGF family in both the aetiology and biology of different types of tumours. The evidence includes the expression of FGF genes in tumour cells, gene amplification of specific FGFs in certain human tumours, the well-characterized effects of FGFs on cell function in vitro as well as the demonstrated oncogenicity of FGFs in rodent tumour models.

THE FGF FAMILY OF LIGANDS

The FGF family of proteins have together been isolated from a wide range of sources but, in mammals, are encoded by nine distinct genes, *FGFs* 1 through 9.

Probably the most abundant FGFs, and the first to be identified and characterized at the molecular level, are the so-called prototype

FGFs, FGF-1 (acidic FGF) and FGF-2 (basic FGF). They were purified as proteins from a variety of tissues by virtue of the mitogenic action on fibroblast cells in vitro (hence the origin of the name 'fibroblast growth factor'), sequenced and then cloned (Burgess & MacCaig, 1989).

Additional members of the FGF family have been identified in recent years. A key feature in the discovery of at least some of these genes was their ability to induce tumourigenic behaviour in target cells either in vivo or in vitro. FGF-3 (previously known as *int*-2) was first identified as a gene located near frequent sites of provirus insertion in mouse mammary tumours induced by murine mammary tumour virus. In many cases the FGF-3 gene was found to be transcriptionally active in the virally induced tumours. The isolation of cDNAs encoding FGF-4, FGF-5 and FGF-6 was, directly or indirectly, based upon screening for DNA sequences able to transform NIH3T3 cells in vitro. The FGF-4 gene (previously known as *hst*-1 or *k*FGF), isolated as a transforming oncogene from Kaposi's sarcoma and human stomach tumour DNAs encodes a 206 amino acid polypeptide with 40% homology to human FGF-2 (Delli-Bovi et al., 1987; Yoshida et al., 1987). The gene for FGF-6 was cloned by virtue of its homology to FGF-4 (Marics et al., 1989) using cross hybridization with an FGF-4 probe and proved to be 80% identical to FGF-4 and about 40% similar to FGF-2. FGF-6 was also identified by cross-hybridization as *hst*-2 (Iida et al., 1992). FGF-5 was also isolated, from the DNA of an osteosarcoma-derived cell line, as a transforming oncogene for NIH3T3 cells in vitro (Zhan et al., 1987, 1988) and is also about 40% related to FGF-2, although more distantly related to FGF-4 and FGF-6.

The remaining three family members were all identified by their mitogenic effects on specific cell types. FGF-7 (originally KGF) was isolated from keratinocytes (Finch et al., 1989). It is a 197-residue polypeptide, with 30% homology to FGF-2. The eighth member of the family, androgen-induced growth factor (AIGF) was isolated and cloned from a mouse mammary carcinoma cell line which requires androgen for growth stimulation (Tanaka et al., 1992). The AIGF cDNA encodes 215 amino acid protein with 30 to 40% homology to the FGF family. FGF-9, also known as glia-acting factor (GAF), was purified from a human glioma cell line (Miyamoto et al., 1993). FGF-9/GAF is a 208 amino acid polypeptide with around 30% homology to other members of the FGF family.

A comparison of the amino acid sequences of the nine members of the FGF ligand family is shown in Figure 2.1. The main sequence homologies occur around a core region of 120 residues. There are only 11 amino acid residues conserved amongst all members of the FGF family,

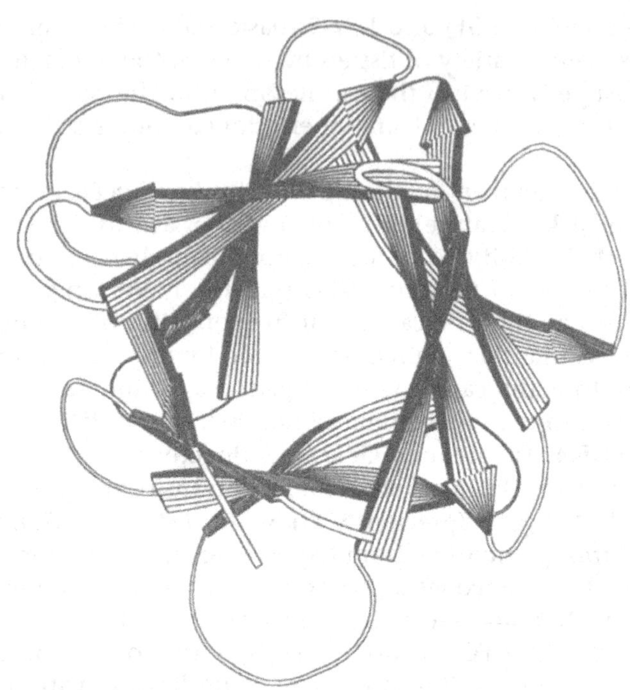

Figure 2.1 A comparison of the amino acid sequences of the eight members of the fibroblast growth factor family. Regions of full-sequence homology are highlighted in black and regions that contain similar types of amino acids are highlighted in grey.

although similarities between individual pairs of the family (such as FGF-4 and FGF-6) can be high. One notable feature is the presence in FGF-3 of 12 amino acid sequence (residues 145–157), the 'bridge' region which appears as an insertion into the main body of the sequence.

THREE-DIMENSIONAL STRUCTURE OF FGF

The three-dimensional structure of both FGF-1 and FGF-2 has been determined by X-ray crystallographic techniques (Zhu et al., 1991). The two molecules exhibit very similar structures and are composed of twelve antiparallel β strands woven into a molecule with approximate three-fold symmetry (see Figure 2.2). The molecular design of FGFs 1 and 2 is similar to interleukin-1, which is distantly related by sequence to the FGF family (Gimenez Gallego et al., 1985). The 'bridge' region of FGF-3 has been predicted from this structure to form an exposed loop on the surface of the molecule between two

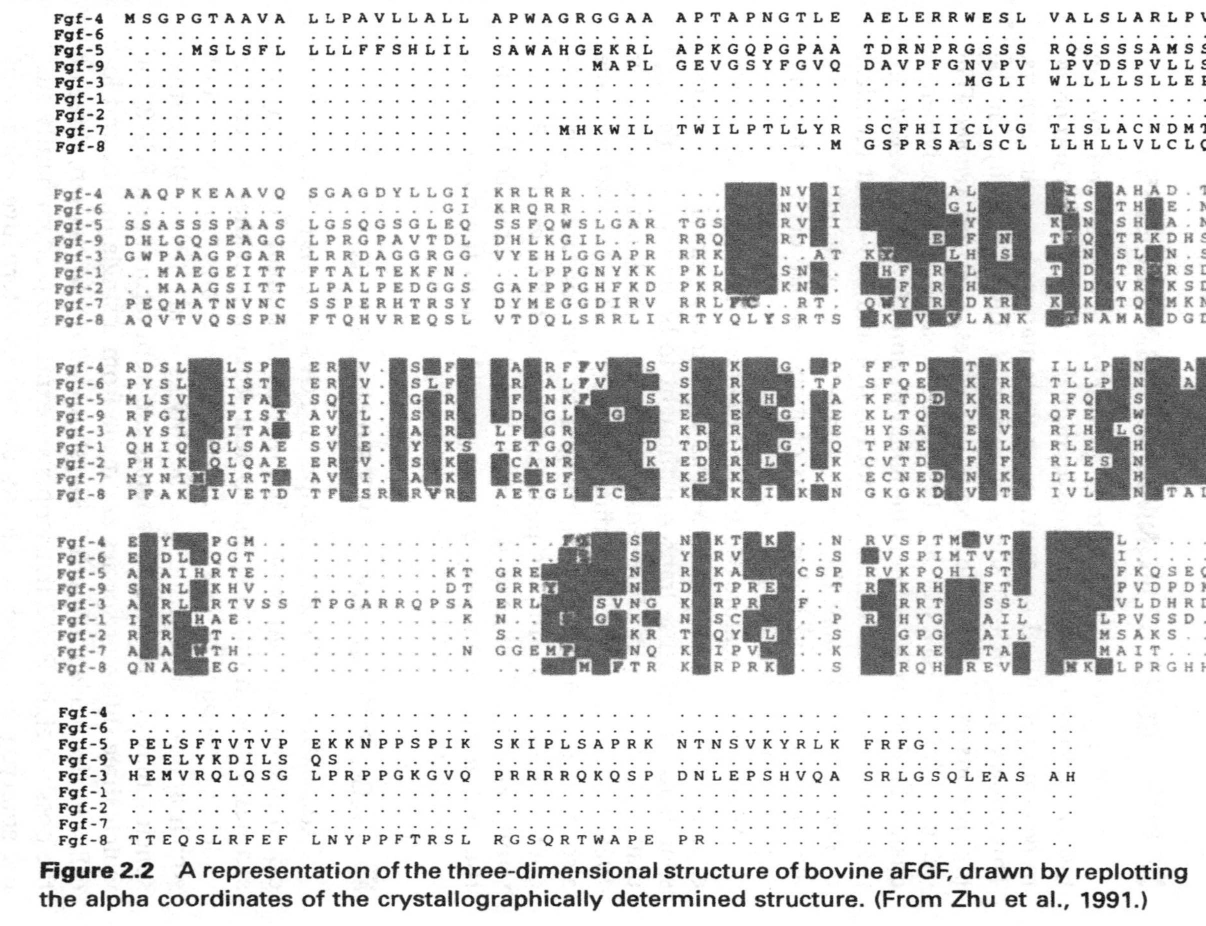

Figure 2.2 A representation of the three-dimensional structure of bovine aFGF, drawn by replotting the alpha coordinates of the crystallographically determined structure. (From Zhu et al., 1991.)

adjacent β strands. These two strands (β10 and β11) have also been implicated in heparin binding, suggesting (see below) that this region of the molecule may have some role to play in receptor recognition.

FGF GENES IN NONMAMMALIAN SPECIES

The *Xenopus* and chick homologues of FGF-2 (XbFGF and chicken bFGF) have been isolated by cross-hybridization techniques and prove to be almost identical in sequence to their mammalian counterparts. This shows that at least some members of the FGF family can be highly conserved over wide species differences. A second *Xenopus* FGF (termed XeFGF; Isaacs et al., 1992) was isolated using polymerase chain reaction (PCR) primers designed to amplify FGF-4. XeFGF appears, however to be similar to both FGF-4 and FGF-6 but identical to neither. XeFGF may therefore represent an 'ancestral' FGF from which the FGF-4 and FGF-6 genes of mammals are derived by gene duplication and sequence divergence.

An interesting feature of XbFGF is the existence of a 1.5-kb mRNA expressed during *Xenopus* oogenesis and embryogenesis that corresponds to an antisense transcript thought to be involved in the regulation of stability of bFGF sense transcripts (Kimelman & Kirschner 1989, Volk et al., 1989). Eight different chicken FGF-2 transcripts have also been detected during embryogenesis, two of which bear a sequence homology with the previously isolated *Xenopus* FGF-2 antisense transcript (Zuniga et al., 1993). It is therefore possible that antisense transcripts may play a more general role in the maintenance of mRNA levels of FGFs.

PROCESSING OF FGF TRANSCRIPTS

Alternatively spliced transcripts of FGFs-1, -2 and -3 have been discovered to date. At least four isoforms of human FGF-1 may be synthesized, with differing amino acid sequences at their N-termini which are encoded by one of four alternative exons, the selection of which appears to be tissue specific (Myers et al., 1993). Alternative splicing may also be used to generate different forms of rat FGF-2, for which three different species are made from a single mRNA and localize to the nucleus (Powell & Klagsbrun, 1991). In chicken, three of the possible eight FGF-2 transcripts are expressed predominantly during embryogenesis and are clearly derived by alternative splicing of the first coding exon (Zuniga et al., 1993). FGF-3 transcripts may also differ at their 3′ ends and in at least one case described, the translated products may also differ (Acland et al., 1990).

SECRETION AND SUBCELLULAR TARGETING OF FGFs

An important distinction between the prototype FGFs, FGF-1 and FGF-2 and the remaining family members is the lack of a conventional signal peptide in newly synthesized forms of FGFs 1 and 2. It is, indeed, now clear that FGF-1 and FGF-2 proteins are not synthesized in association with the endoplasmic reticulum (Paterno et al., 1989) and are not normally secreted from cells but need to be released by some form of cell lysis or apoptosis. The newest member of the family, FGF-9, also appears to lack a typical signal sequence (Miyamoto et al., 1993) but can be detected exclusively in the culture supernatant of the human glioma cell line from which it derives and in the medium of COS cells transfected with FGF-9 cDNA.

The observation that FGFs with proven oncogenic potential (FGFs 3, 4, 5, and 6) and FGF-7 and FGF-8 are secreted suggests that the ability to mediate cell transformation is markedly dependent upon secretion. Transfection of NIH3T3 cells with FGF-2 expression vectors does not result in cell transformation; however, addition of a secretion signal sequence to the FGF-2 cDNA greatly increases the transforming potential of such vectors (Rogelj et al., 1988). However, FGFs 1, 2 and 9 are detectable in the extracellular matrix, or medium in the case of FGF-9 and are presumably released by some alternative pathway (Jackson et al., 1992). Unusually, FGF-3 possesses a structural feature in its N-terminus that confers upon it the property of its retention in the Golgi complex (Kiefer et al., 1993). This may be a mechanism to ensure slow and controlled release of the mature FGF-3 into the extra cellular matrix.

Several laboratories have reported detection of FGF in the nuclei of a variety of cell types (Bouche et al., 1987; Tessler & Neufeld, 1990; Sano et al., 1990; Dell'Era et al., 1991; Speir et al., 1991; Brigstock et al., 1991; and Bugler et al., 1991). Nuclear translocation of FGFs has its basis in a sequence rich in basic amino acids that is similar to nuclear translocation sequences of other nuclear proteins (Dang & Lee, 1989). A mutant of FGF-1 that lacked this sequence retains heparin-binding ability but fails to induce mitogenesis, the property of which can be rescued by the addition of a histone nuclear translocation sequence (Imamura et al., 1990).

There is, however, evidence that this NLS is not actually required for translocation of FGF-1 to the nucleus (Zhan et al., 1992, Cao et al., 1993). FGF-2, which is translated in three different forms (Prats et al., 1989), may be localized to the nucleus only if translation initiates at a CUG codon that lies upstream of the AUG codon (Bugler et al.,

1991). Similarly, FGF-3 isoforms initiated at an upstream CUG start site also yield a protein which is translated to the nucleus (Acland et al., 1990). In the case of FGF-2, the nuclear localization signal lies between the CUG and AUG codons (Bugler et al., 1991). This suggests a translational control of nuclear localization of FGFs 2 and 3.

In early embryos of *Xenopus*, immunocytochemical analysis shows nuclear localization of bFGF during mesoderm induction (Shiurba et al., 1991). However, although overexpressed bFGF accumulates in the nuclei of blastulae, formation of mesoderm did not follow unless a secretion signal was engineered onto the bFGF construct (Thompson & Slack, 1992), suggesting that bFGF is unlikely to be involved directly in mesoderm induction.

FGFs are known to have some effects on gene transcription and it has been demonstrated that in the case of the repression of myogenesis by FGF, the inhibitory effects of FGF on muscle transcription are mediated indirectly by FGF-induced phosphorylation of myogenic helix-loop-helix transcription factors in their DNA-binding domains (Li et al., 1992). The possibility of translocation of FGFs to the nucleus has raised the question of whether FGFs might also directly effect gene transcription and it has been suggested that this is indeed possible, at least in vitro (Nakanishi et al., 1992).

EXPRESSION PATTERNS

Information concerning the sites of expression of the more recently cloned FGF genes has been gathered using RNA in situ hybridization and immunohistochemical techniques. FGFs 1 and 2 are widely expressed in both foetal and adult tissues (see reviews by MacCaig & Burgess, 1989; Goldfarb, 1990). FGFs 3, 4 and 5, on the other hand, are predominantly expressed during gastrulation and later embryogenesis (Wilkinson et al., 1988, 1989; Haub & Goldfarb, 1991; Niswander & Martin, 1992). FGF-6 expression appears to be restricted to developing skeletal muscle (deLapeyriere et al., 1993). FGF-7 is expressed in the dermis but not the epidermis of skin and also in other adult tissues; for example, kidney, colon, ileum and muscle as well as various sites of the midgestation embryo including heart and muscle (P. Lonai, personal communication). The expression patterns of the newest members of the FGF family are less well understood, although FGF-9 expression can be detected by Northern blot analysis of adult brain and kidney tissues. Taken together these data show that each FGF family member exhibits specific domains of expression in both the embryo and adult. It is also notable that the expression of some FGFs appear, in normal development, to be confined to the embryonic phases of life; their 'reactivation' in pathological adult tissues may accordingly be significant.

FGFs AND HEPARIN

A characteristic biochemical feature of the FGF family is that they exhibit a high affinity for polysulphated carbohydrate heparin. Indeed, the discovery of this property provided a key breakthrough in the first purification of FGFs 1 and 2. It is now very clear that this diagnostic feature of the FGFs has considerable significance for their biological function.

Affinity chromatography of chemically and enzymatically cleaved fibroblast-derived heparan sulphates on immobilized FGF-1 has permitted the identification of a core carbohydrate sequence with equivalent affinity for FGF-1 as the parent molecule. This is a heptasaccharide that is rich in sulphated iduronic acid and glucosamine residues (Turnbull et al., 1992). Specific basic amino acids of the FGF have been implicated in the binding of heparin, using chemical modification (Harper & Lobb, 1988) and peptide-binding studies (Baird et al., 1988). The same regions have been shown directly to have affinity for anions from the X-ray crystallographic studies of human FGF-1 and bovine FGF-2 (Zhu et al., 1991).

It is clear, therefore, that the high affinity exhibited towards heparan-containing glycoproteins by FGFs results from high-affinity association with specific polysaccharide sequences. These FGF-binding sequences, in vivo, form part of the polysaccharide chains of the family of heparan sulphate containing proteoglycans (Gallagher & Turnbull, 1992). This association between FGFs and specific sugar sequences in HSPGs has been substantiated by the parallel demonstration that FGFs bind to 'low-affinity' receptors on the cell surface which, in most cases, turn out to be HSPGs such as syndecan-1 (Saunders et al., 1989; Kiefer et al., 1991). The characteristic feature of the association between FGFs and low-affinity HSPG receptors is that binding can be blocked in the presence of soluble heparin. In addition, FGF can be released from low-affinity receptors by treatment of the target cells with heparanase (reviewed by Klagsbrun, 1990).

The ability of heparin-degrading enzymes to release cell surface bound FGF has led to the suggestion that cellular heparanases may release FGF sequestered by HSPGs in the ECM (Klagsbrun, 1990). The FGF may associate with the ECM in order to regulate its activity in vivo. For example, release of ECM-bound FGF in a biologically active form may occur by displacement or by degradation by heparin and heparanases produced by platelets and macrophages at local sites of injury or inflammation.

A comparison of the dissociation constants for FGF-2 bound to its low-affinity receptors (HSPGs) on CHO cells shows that FGF-2 dissociates rapidly from HSPGs (half-time of 0.5 minute). This suggests that where HSPGs bind FGFs in close proximity to FGFRs, degradative enzymes need not be required to release FGF, since the dissociation from HSPGs occurs rapidly enough to allow FGF to bind to unoccupied receptors by laws of mass action. Proteoglycans that act as low-affinity receptors for FGF may also provide an alternative route for internalization of the FGFs. CHO cells that lack significant numbers of FGF receptors will internalize exogenously added FGF-2 as effectively as do such CHO cells when transfected with tyrosine kinase FGF receptor expression vectors (Roghani & Moscatelli, 1992). Interestingly, there is some evidence that the intracellular fate of FGF actually depends on the route of internalization. In one study, FGF-2 was conjugated to saporin, a ribosome-inactivating protein that is cytotoxic in the cytoplasm but for which cells lack receptors. Cells expressing both HSPGs and FGF receptors were killed upon exposure to this FGF:saporin conjugate, but another cell line that expressed only the proteoglycan was resistant to the toxic effects of saporin even though the conjugate was internalized (Reiland & Rapraeger, 1993).

Finally, an intriguing recent observation suggests that HSPG may also play a key role in developmental regulation of cellular responses to FGF by switching the binding specificity of a cell population from one FGF to another during development of neurons (Nurcombe et al., 1993). This study demonstrates that neuroepithelial cells switch expression from FGF-2 to FGF-1 at around embryonic day 11. This switch is accompanied by a change in the binding specificity of the neuroepithelial HSPG from FGF-2 to FGF-1. FGF-2 is thought to play a role in regulation of neural precursor cell division (Bartlett et al., 1988; Murphy et al., 1990), whilst FGF-1 is associated in large amounts with neuronal development and specifically with neural populations and so is probably more important for neural development. By linking synthesis of FGF-1 by the neural precursor cells to synthesis of a differentially glycosylated HSPG species, the response of these cells to the new FGF is ensured.

FIBROBLAST GROWTH FACTOR RECEPTORS OF THE TYROSINE KINASE CLASS

Whilst FGFs associate with the extracellular matrix and cell surface via association with 'low-affinity' HSPG receptors, the intracellular signalling mediated by FGFs is mediated by a second, 'high-affinity' group of receptors of the tyrosine kinase class. To date there are four genes known that code for the family of high-affinity growth factor receptors FGFR1–4. The first to be identified, previously known as *flg*, was cloned by its homology to the *fms* proto-oncogene (Ruta et al., 1989). It only became apparent that *flg* encoded a transmembrane FGF receptor when amino acid sequences of peptides from an affinity purified receptor for FGF-1 were identified as being present in *flg* (Lee et al., 1989). It was similarly discovered that the murine *bek* (bacterially expressed kinase) gene (Kornbluth et al., 1988) encoded a variant of another FGF receptor (FGFR2). The latter gene was also found to encode other variants, namely human K-*sam* gene (Hattori et al., 1990) and the receptor for keratinocyte growth factor (Miki et al., 1991). A third human receptor gene (FGFR3) was cloned from the chronic myelogenous leukemia cell line K562 by its homology to the chicken v-*sea* gene, a receptorlike tyrosine kinase (Keegan et al., 1991). The gene for FGFR4 was initially cloned as a fragment by PCR amplification of poly(A) RNA from K562 cells (Partenen et al., 1990) and the fragment then used as a probe to obtain the cDNA from another human cell line (Partenen et al., 1991). Following the initial isolation of cDNA clones of chicken FGFR1 (*flg* – Lee et al., 1989), the gene was also found in other species including humans, mouse (Safran et al., 1990), *Xenopus* (Musci et al., 1990) and *Drosophila* (breathless – Glazer & Shilo, 1991).

All four FGF receptors so far discovered share a common general domain structure comprising the signal sequence and three immunoglobulinlike domains with a run of acidic amino acids between the first and second immunoglobulin domains. Then a transmembrane domain is followed by a cytoplasmic domain that comprises two tyrosine kinase (TK) domains with an insert of variable size between these two TK domains. Variant forms of *flg* transcripts have also been predicted from the discovery of shorter *flg* cDNAs. The existence of both membrane-bound and secreted forms of FGFR1 is implied, since deletions can occur in either the extracellular, cytoplasmic or transmembrane domains. All of the isoforms of FGFR1 that are found can be predicted from the gene structure of FGFR1 (Johnson et al., 1991). Selection of polyadenylation sites in the extracellular domain may result in transcripts coding for secreted forms of FGFR1. Alternative usage of splice sites determines the composition of the third immunoglobulin domain or splicing out of the transmembrane domain. Splice site selection may also result in FGFR transcript variants with either a deletion of an Arg-Met amino acid pair just after the acidic box or a Thr-Val pair at the juxtamembrane region (Yayon & Givol, 1992; Jaye et al., 1992; Johnson & Williams, 1993).

LIGAND BINDING TO FGF RECEPTORS

At the time of writing, there are more known FGF-like polypeptide mitogens than known potential receptors for these molecules. It is possible, even likely, that more of both types of molecule remain to be discovered. However, it has been clear from the outset that some of the FGF ligands probably share the same receptors. Early studies demonstrated that FGFR1 isoforms containing both Ig domains II and III were able to bind both FGF-1 and FGF-2 with kDa's in the range of approximately 50 pM (Dionne et al., 1990; Johnson et al., 1990). FGFR2 isoform *bek* was similarly shown to bind FGF-1 and FGF-2 with high affinity whilst the KGF receptor, an N-terminal immunoglobulin domain truncated and splice variant of FGFR2, bound FGF-7 and FGF-2 but not FGFR-2 (Miki et al., 1992; Yayon et al., 1992). It was clear then that not only were the first two FGFRs to be cloned highly cross-reactive with their polypeptide ligands, but also that the ligand specificity depended upon sequences in the second and/or third immunoglobulin domain.

The isolation and cloning of two more genes for FGF receptors revealed that both FGFR3 and FGFR4 were able to bind FGF-1 with high affinity (Keegan et al., 1991; Partenen et al., 1991). In addition, human FGFR3 responds to both FGF-1 and FGF-2 as measured by the ability to cause Ca^{2+} efflux when expressed in *Xenopus* oocytes (Keegan et al., 1991). Interestingly, mouse FGFR3 shows very low affinity for or biological response to FGF-2 (Ornitz & Leder, 1992). Other FGF ligands have also been investigated; for example, binding of FGF-4 to murine FGFR3 results in biological activity, whereas FGF-3 elicits no response (Ornitz & Leder, 1992). The same study demonstrates that both FGF-4 and FGF-5 bind to murine FGFR1 as measured by mitogenic response of cells expressing FGFR1 but result in less proliferation than when cells are stimulated with FGF-2 or FGF-1. Recombinant human FGF-5 expressed in *Escherichia coli,* although not glycosylated, is biologically active and has been shown from competition binding studies to bind both FGFR1 and FGFR2 with molecular weight of between 0.5 and 1.5 nM (Clements et al., 1993). FGF-6 has been shown to bind to FGFR4 (Vainikka et al., 1992), which also binds FGF-1 and to a lesser degree FGF-4. Comprehensive studies of binding for all combinations of receptors and FGF ligands remain to be completed. The chief importance of the results of such investigations is that all cells that express FGF receptors bind and respond mitogenically to more than one FGF ligand. It should be remembered, however, that these are in vitro studies and the biological significance of any of the results may only begin to be understood when it is seen whether or not a given FGF receptor and one of its known potential ligands are temporally and spatially co-expressed. The existence of various possible isoforms of FGFR1, FGFR2 and FGFR3 further complicates the issue (Avivi et al., 1993).

THE LIGAND-BINDING SITE

An understanding of the ligand binding site will provide the rationale required to design agonists or antagonists to the FGF receptors and for construction of homogous recombinants of the FGFR gene that might be used to knock out production of functional protein in mice using gene targeting in embryonic stem cells.

Initial clues to the location of the ligand-binding site were discovered by examination of the binding specificities in two isoforms of both FGFR1 (Werner et al., 1992) and FGFR2 (Yayon et al., 1992; Miki et al., 1992). As previously discussed, it was known from the structure of the FGFR1 gene that the third immunoglobulin domain of the FGF receptor could vary in its C-terminal half, being coded for by one of two potential exons, IIIb or IIIc (Figure 2.3). Translation of

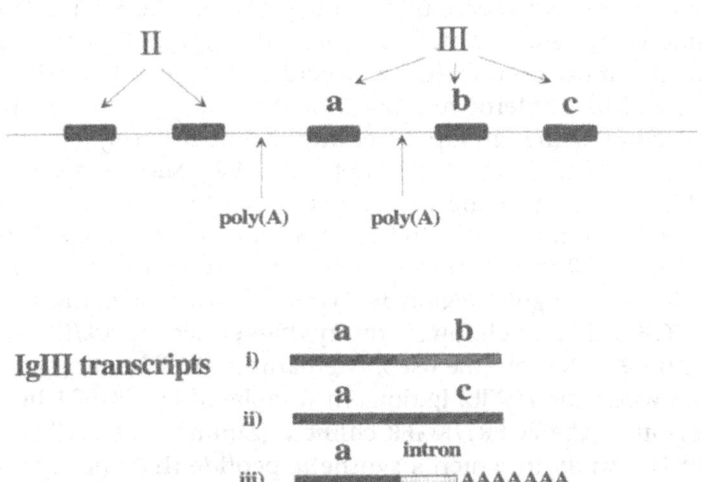

Figure 2.3 A schematic representation of the potential RNA transcripts that can be generated from the IgIII region of the gene for FGF receptor 1. Alternative splicing of the primary transcript can produce two forms of IgIII, whereas use of the polyadenylation site between exons a and b will result in a transcript that consists only of the extracellular components of the receptor. FGFR2 and FGFR3 can also undergo alternative splicing of the primary transcript to yield two forms of the IgIII domain.

FGFR1 isoforms possessing either exon resulted in proteins able to bind FGF-1 with similar affinity, whilst the binding affinity for FGF-2 was much lower for the IIIb isoform (Werner et al., 1992). The IIIb exon of FGFR1 is highly homologous to the corresponding region of the keratinocyte growth factor receptor, known to be a splice variant of FGFR2. The fact that the only major structural difference between KGFR and the *bek* form of FGFR2 lies within the third immunoglobulin domain implies that in this case also, binding specificity would be determined by the choice of the IIIb or IIIc exon. That this is indeed the case was demonstrated by construction of chimeric *bek*/KGFR molecules in which the *bek* variable region (C-terminal half of the third Ig domain) was replaced by a 50 amino acid sequence from the corresponding region of KGFR. This *bek*/KGFR was shown to bind FGF-7 but had lost the ability to bind FGF-2, a high-affinity ligand for the *bek* form of FGF (Yayon et al., 1992). Yet another form of FGFR2 exists in which the IIIb exon sequence is present and confers the ability to bind FGF-1 with high affinity but not FGF-2 (Dell & Williams, 1992). This form (FGFR2-IIIb) is identical to KGFR in the third Ig domain and so is likely also to bind FGF-7. These studies imply that the ligand-binding site comprises sequences coded for by the C-terminal half (approximately 50 amino acids) of the third Ig domain.

More recently, evidence from mutagenesis of the FGFR as well as from studies of peptide antagonists to FGF suggests that the ligand-binding site must be formed by structures inherent in both Ig domains II and III. Cysteine residues thought to be involved in the tertiary structure of the Ig loops were mutated in either Ig loop II or III of FGFR1 isoforms a and b (Hou et al., 1992). Such a mutation in either loop resulted in the loss of ligand-binding activity. A similar conclusion is drawn from studies of a chimeric molecule between FGFR1 and KGFR in which the specific binding motif from KGFR replaces the homologous region in FGFR1. In this case, the chimera bound KGF with a much lower affinity than either the *bek*/KGFR molecule or the KGFR molecule itself. High-affinity KGF binding was only achieved when the FGFR2 Ig domain II replaced the FGFR1 homologous region in the FGFR1/KGFR chimera (Zimmer et al., 1993). Also relevant is a study in which a synthetic peptide that corresponds to the amino acid sequence in the third Ig domain of KGFR is shown to be antagonistic to KGF, blocking KGF-induced mitogenic activity as well as the interaction between the KGF ligand and its receptor (Bottaro et al., 1993). Binding of KGF to the KGF receptor, however, is more efficient than binding of KGF to the peptide antagonist, suggesting that this peptide lacks residues contributed elsewhere in the KGFR ligand binding site that confer a high affinity for KGF. Again the implication is that sequences in the third Ig domain are not enough to constitute a high-affinity ligand binding site.

DIVERSITY OF LIGAND BINDING

The genes for FGFR1and FGFR2 and more recently FGFR3 (Werner et al., 1993; Avivi et al., 1993) possess two variable exons in the region coding for the C-terminal half of the third Ig domain. The choice of exon will largely determine the ligand-binding specificity for such molecules. Exon IIIb appears to specify preferential binding to FGF-1 and also in KGFR, to FGF-7. FGFR1-, 2- and 3-encoded receptors containing the IIIc coded sequences will bind FGF-2 as well as FGF-1. The exon IIIb from FGFR3, however, shows little homology to either that in FGFR1 or FGFR2 (Avivi et al., 1993) and so it will be interesting to see which ligand is favoured by the IIIb form of FGFR3. Thus, alternative splicing of transcripts of FGFR1, -2 and -3 constitutes one major mechanism of creation of ligand-binding diversity.

Broadly then, there appear to be at least two potential mechanisms to generate receptors with diverse specificities for ligands. Furthermore, there are indications that the alternative splicing mechanism is probably also under developmental control, with expression of the IIIb isoform being associated mainly with a differentiated cell phenotype. Different splice variants of FGFR2 and FGFR3 are expressed in different compartments of skin tissue, with IIIc isoforms found in both dermis and epidermis but IIIb isoforms in epidermis only (Werner et al., 1992; Werner et al., 1993). There is also evidence that only upon differentiation do murine EC and ES cells express significant quantities of the IIIb isoforms of FGFR2 and FGFR3 (McDonald & Heath, 1993). Intriguingly, as epithelial cells become malignant and stroma-independent, exclusive expression of the IIIb isoform of FGFR2 is switched to that of the IIIc isoform (Yan et al., 1993). The switch over to production of FGFR2-IIIc is followed by increased expression by the malignant epithelial cells of FGF-2, which is in fact the ligand for the FGFR2-IIIc isoform. These observations suggest that FGF-2 that is switched on during malignant transformation may act in an autocrine fashion to direct a switch to expression of its own receptor.

TYROSINE KINASE FGFRs AND HSPGs COOPERATE IN SIGNAL TRANSDUCTION

The relationship between the HSPG class of FGF receptors and the tyrosine kinase class of receptor is intimate: heparin or HSPGs have been shown to be required for the interactions between the FGF and its high-affinity tyrosine kinase receptor and consequential cellular signalling. This has been convincingly demonstrated in experiments in which CHO cells deficient in HSPG production were transfected with murine FGF receptor cDNA. These cells do not bind FGF-2 unless heparin or heparan sulfate is added to the media (Yayon et al., 1991). A cell line that is dependent on both heparin and FGF for growth has been used to show that when transfected with the human FGF receptor (*flg*) the mitogenic activity of these cells has an absolute requirement for heparin and a dose-dependent requirement for FGF (Ornitz et al., 1992). Thus association between FGFs and HSPGs appears to be a necessary prerequisite for tyrosine kinase receptor function.

The nature of the interaction between heparin in the form of HSPGs, FGF and the tyrosine kinase FGF receptor has been the subject of some discussion (Klagsbrun & Baird, 1991). Previous suggestions have included models in which heparin binding to FGF modifies it in some way, perhaps inducing oligomerization (Ornitz et al., 1992), in order that binding of FGF to the FGF receptor takes place. However, it has been recently observed that heparin and also HSPGs may interact independently of the FGF ligand with a specific domain in the N-terminal region of the extracellular domain of the transmembrane tyrosine kinase FGF receptor and that this association with heparin is actually required for binding of FGF (Kan et al., 1993). This would corroborate models of a trimolecular complex in which low-affinity HSPG receptors bind FGFs and then effectively present the FGF to the tyrosine kinase FGF receptor (Figure 2.4). This presentation would take the form of a direct interaction of both the oligosaccharide and peptide moieties in the FGF:heparan sulfate complex with the extracellular domain of the tyrosine kinase FGF receptor.

This model has some important implications for the manipulation of FGF action, since it strongly implies that agents which modify the association between FGFs and HSPGs or between HSPGs and tyrosine kinase receptors may be able to modify the action of FGFs in vivo.

FGF RECEPTOR MEDIATED SIGNAL TRANSDUCTION

Analysis of the mechanism of FGF receptor mediated signal transduction has been strongly influenced by an understanding of the mechanisms employed by other receptor tyrosine kinases such as platelet-derived growth factor receptor, epidermal growth factor receptor, colony-stimulating factor receptor and the insulin receptor

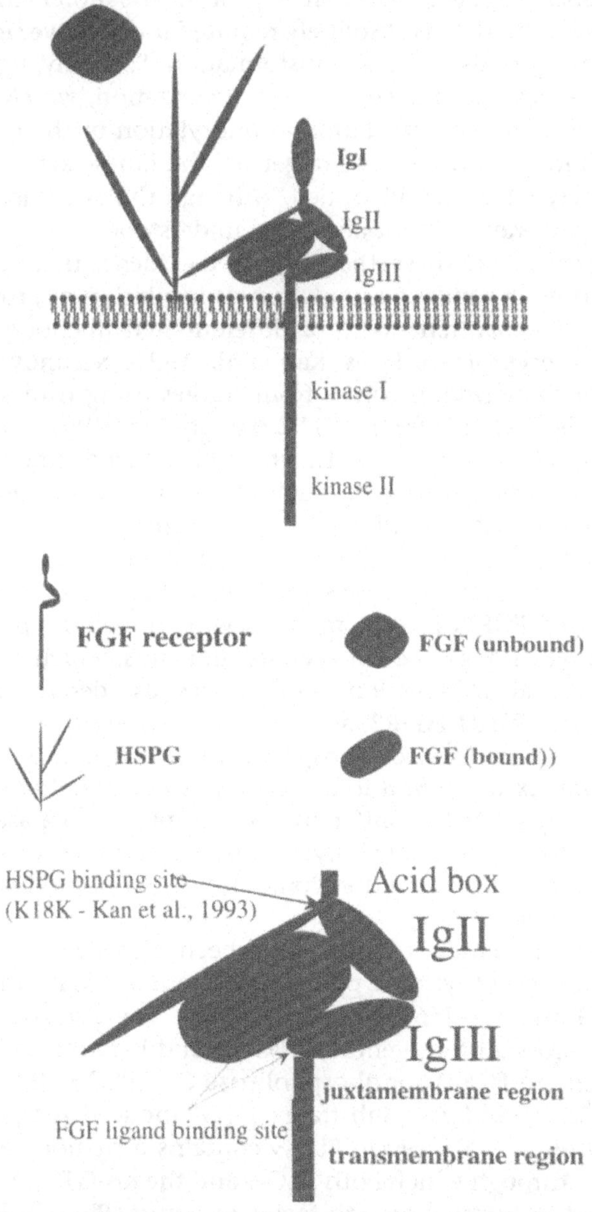

Figure 2.4 (A) A schematic representation of the trimolecular interaction between the FGF ligand, HSPG and the high-affinity FGF receptor. Each participant in this complex has a specific binding site for the other two components. (B) Detail of the binding interactions. Both the IgII and IgIII domains of the FGFR are involved in the formation of the FGF-binding site. IgII also has a specific binding site for HSPG.

(Ullrich & Schlessinger, 1990). Firstly, for all the aforementioned receptors, ligand binding is absolutely required for effective signal transduction, mitogenesis and cell transformation. Secondly, ligand binding is also known to induce receptor dimerization, which facilitates the activation and tyrosine autophosphorylation of the cytoplasmic domain. Thirdly, some cellular targets of the kinase activity of most receptors may have been identified, although the exact details of the signalling pathway may not always be understood.

Taking the first of these, there is indeed evidence that ligand binding elicits dose-dependent stimulation or inhibition of growth or alternatively the maintenance of a differentiated phenotype in cells that display receptors for FGFs (Kan et al., 1991). Secondly, evidence for receptor dimerization comes from studies using truncated forms of FGFR1 (Ueno et al., 1992), FGFR2 (Bellot et al., 1991) and *Xenopus* FGF receptor (Amaya et al., 1991), which have demonstrated that isoforms of the receptor that lack much of the cytoplasmic domain will inhibit signal transduction by wild-type receptors in cells expressing DNA encoding both the truncated and wild-type forms of the receptors. These results are interpreted to mean that the cytoplasmic region-truncated FGFRs form complexes with the wild-type receptors by interacting through the extracellular domains, which are then incapable of signal transduction. Both studies also demonstrated that heterodimeric (FGFR1:FGFR2) as well as homodimeric (FGFR1:FGFR1) complexes may be formed. Phosphorylation of the receptor in the dimeric complex was found to be accomplished by either transphosphorylation between two different FGF receptors (a kinase negative *bek* mutant would be phosphorylated by *flg* and vice versa) or else intermolecular phosphorylation could occur in a homodimeric complex (Bellot et al., 1991)

Two tyrosine kinase residues have been identified as the major intracellular sites for tyrosine phosphorylation: in FGFR1 and -2 these are Tyr 653 and Tyr 766 (Hou et al., 1992). The Tyr 766 residue is conserved across all four genes for FGFRs and is found to be part of a binding site in FGFR1 for phospholipase C-γ (PLC-γ) (Mohammadi et al., 1991), a candidate substrate of FGF-induced receptor kinase activity (Burgess et al., 1990). PLC-γ contains a *src*-homologous domain (SH2), through which both PLC-γ and the *ras*-GTPase activating protein bind to tyrosine growth factor receptors. Phospholipases are known to be required for phosphatidylinositol hydrolysis, which is a key event in the Ca^{2+} signalling pathway. It is significant, however, that whilst mutation of this Tyr 766 residue to phenylalanine abolishes the binding to PLC-γ and also the resultant hydrolysis of phosphatidylinositol (Mohammedi et al., 1992; Peters et al., 1992), this mutated Tyr 766–Phe mutant may still phosphorylate itself and other cellular proteins as well as stimulating DNA synthesis. These observations suggest that PLC-γ is not involved in the FGF-induced mitogenesis or possibly that an alternative signalling pathway may become available in the absence of a funcional PLC-γ.

Interestingly, although PLC-γ binds to a region that includes a highly conserved Tyr residue, PLC-γ is by no means a substrate for all FGFRs. FGFR4 shows very little affinity for PLC-γ and phosphorylates PLC-γ poorly (Vainikka et al., 1992). This is consistent with the observation that PLC-γ binding to the FGFR is not a requirement for FGF-induced mitogenicity. *raf*-1 kinase is also a candidate signalling molecule in FGF cell-mediated cell responses. Phosphorylation occurs when cells expressing *raf*-1 kinase are exposed to FGF (Morrison et al., 1988). More recently it has been observed that FGF stimulates mesoderm induction in explants of *Xenopus* which are injected with a dominant negative *raf*-1 kinase mutant (MacNicol et al., 1993). This implies that *raf*-1 kinase mediates signalling by FGF receptors during mesoderm induction. Several questions remain to be answered on the subject of FGF receptor-mediated signal transduction. The signalling pathway must be elucidated as well as the precise nature and significance of any interactions with downstream phosphorylation substrates. It is also possible that different FGF receptors may operate through distinct signalling pathways.

FGFs AND CANCER

It will be seen from the foregoing that the FGFs represent a diverse group of mitogenic agents with wide-ranging expression in vivo and a diversity of actions in vitro. There is clear evidence that expression of at least some of the FGF family and in particular those with functional secretory signal sequences such as FGF-4 and FGF-5 can induce malignant transformation of responsive target cells. It is possible that FGFs might be used as prognostic markers for those cancers that secrete FGFs. For example, the detection of FGF-2 in the urine of patients with renal cell carcinoma (Chodak et al., 1988) has led to the demonstration that serum levels of FGF-2 correlate relatively well with tumour stage or grade in patients with this cancer (Fujimoto et al., 1991).

EXPRESSION OF FGF IN TUMOUR CELLS

High and inappropriate expression of FGFs is often associated with an increasingly malignant phenotype and many types of tumour are known to produce FGF. Such tumours include pituitary adenomas (Li et al., 1992) and prostate cancer (Matuo et al., 1992; Nakamoto et al., 1992), which produce FGF-2. Bladder carcinoma (Ravery et al., 1992) produces FGF-1 and FGF-5 (Zhan et al., 1988). Kaposi's sarcoma lesions (Huang et al., 1993) and human breast cancers (Liscia et al., 1988) produce FGF-3 whilst stomach tumours produce FGF-4 (Yoshida et al., 1988). In addition, at least three of the FGFs have been identified as oncogenes. *Int-2*/FGF-3 was known as a cellular gene that co-amplified with the mouse mammary tumour virus (MMTV) but has been identified as a member of the FGF family (Dickson & Peters, 1987). FGF-4 and FGF-5 have been cloned by their ability to transform NIH3T3 cells (Yoshida et al., 1987; Iida et al., 1992).

A ROLE FOR FGFs IN MALIGNANT CONVERSION AND PROGRESSION?

This production by tumours of FGFs led to the suggestion that FGFs may exert an autocrine or paracrine effect on malignant cells. The observation that some of the FGFs have transforming potential implies that FGFs may be involved in the creation of a malignant phenotype. Furthermore, the metastatic potential of a tumour is largely determined by its ability to migrate, proliferate and neovascularize, forming blood vessels in situ. The initiation of this process, angiogenesis, by the stimulation of endothelial cell proliferation is known to be directed by FGFs (Thompson et al., 1988). These observations taken together strongly suggest a key role for FGFs in the initiation, progression and spread of cancer.

Control of Cell Growth

One mechanism by which FGFs may act to influence a cell's progression towards malignancy is by exerting autocrine control over the growth of cells expressing FGFs and their receptors. In addition to its oncogenic action, FGF-4 also acts as a mitogen. Thus NIH3T3 cells supplied with the FGF-4 protein acquire a phenotype indistinguishable from those transformed by the FGF-4 oncogene (Delli Bovi et al., 1987). These FGF-4 transformed cells also acquire the ability to grow in serum-free medium (Delli Bovi et al., 1988). Also, antibodies raised against FGF-4 will cause the transformed phenotype to revert (Talarico & Basilico, 1991). These findings have been interpreted to suggest that constitutive expression of FGF-4 and perhaps, in an analagous manner, also the other oncogenic FGFs result in cell transformation due to the extracellular stimulation of the FGF receptor.

Generally, the ability of a cell to secrete the FGFs encoded by transfected DNA is a requirement for transformation of such cells. FGFs 1 and 2, which lack signal sequences, have limited oncogenic potential as measured by their ability to induce foci when transfected as cDNAs. The addition of a signal peptide to cDNA encoding FGF-1 (Jouanneau et al., 1991; Forough et al., 1993) or FGF-2 (Rogelj et al., 1988) confers a high transforming potential. Following transfection of NIH3T3 cells with FGF-3, which has a signal sequence, the ligand is detected in the extracellular matrix around the cells (Kiefer et al., 1991). The frequency of transformation by FGF-3 is, however, much lower than that for FGF-4 or FGF-5 (Goldfarb et al., 1991). Analysis of the intracellular processing of FGF-3 reveals that its secretion is impaired due to its unusually long retention in the Golgi complex (Kiefer et al., 1993), which may account for the apparent lower oncogenicity of FGF-3.

That FGF must be presented extracellularly to the receptor rather than intracellularly along the secretion pathway has been shown by deletion of the FGF-4 signal sequence, which reduces its ability to transform NIH3T3 cells. The same study shows that addition of a KDEL Golgi retention signal causes intracellular accumulation of the FGF-4 mutant and again a much lower ability to induce foci in NIH3T3 cells (Talarico & Basilico, 1991). The oncogenic potential of FGF-4 in vivo has been examined using a recombinant mouse retrovirus containing cDNA encoding FGF-4. This construct exhibited very low tumourigenicity in nude mice: only one highly undifferentiated fibrosarcoma was induced 7 months after transfection (Talarico et al., 1993). Upon closer examination it was found that the retrovirus which had induced this tumour was now highly tumourigenic in both nude and immunocompetent mice and was the product of an in vivo recombination between the helper virus with which the mouse had been co-infected. The recombination event had generated a fusion protein FGF-4 and a retroviral envelope protein. This protein retained all the transforming properties of FGF-4. It is not clear why the in vivo recombinant virus that expressed a mutant form of FGF-4 is so much more tumourigenic than that which expressed the unrearranged FGF-4.

Other evidence that FGF-mediated autocrine control of cell growth contributes to malignancy comes from the malignant progression of epithelial cells (Yan et al., 1993). Activation of FGF-2, FGF-3 and FGF-5 genes occurred during the progression to malignancy. In addition, increased expression of the isoform of FGFR-2 which is a receptor for FGF-2 was observed. Therefore, it is feasible that FGF-2 may be acting to increase the malignancy of cells by up-regulating production of its own receptor. However, it cannot be certain that if indeed such up-regulation occurs it is due to an autocrine rather than a paracrine action of the FGF ligand. This is a general caveat of the argument for the involvement of an autocrine mechanism. Co-expression of an FGF ligand and its receptor by a cell is an absolute requirement for autocrine stimulation of growth. Documentation of such co-expression exists for human colon tumour cells (New & Yeoman, 1992) and also for cells from an invasive bladder carcinoma (Allen & Maher, 1993) but has not thus far proved to be widespread.

The evidence summarized above might suggest some involvement of FGFs in malignancy by means of autocrine-induced growth. This is far from demonstrating that FGFs provide the key switch to malignancy. Autocrine/paracrine effects of growth factors may occur in cells already on the path to malignancy mediated by other agents. There might be several other reasons for the production of FGFs by tumour cells and although the in vitro results certainly suggest that autocrine growth stimulation is possible, it remains to be convincingly demonstrated that a population of normal cells can become malignant, remain malignant and form tumours in vivo due solely to an FGF that is produced by those cells and in which a functional receptor is co-expressed.

It may be the case that FGF acts as a progression factor rather than a transforming factor. Evidence for this comes from a study in which FGF-1 was used to transfect two different rat cell lines. One of the lines used was already slightly tumourigenic whilst the other was not at all. FGF-1 transfection was shown to transform the cell line that possessed characteristics of partial transformation whilst the control cell line retained its nontumourigenic phenotype (Takahashi, Fukumoto et al., 1992). Furthermore, immunohistochemical determinations of FGF-2 in human gliomas demonstrate a correlation of levels of FGF-2 transcripts with the degree of malignancy, whilst FGF-2 was undetectable in normal brain tissues (Takahashi, Hoshimaro et al., 1992).

FGF GENE AMPLIFICATION IN TUMOURS

Tumour cells can be genetically very unstable and processes such as amplification, mutation and gene translocation events occur at a much higher frequency than in a normal cell. These events may result in the activation of genes or oncogenes that might direct the expression of the malignant or metastatic properties. Genes encoding FGFs and their receptors may be amplified in some tumour cell lines. For example, the FGF-3 gene is amplified in primary breast tumours (Lidereau et al., 1988) and epithelial ovarian cancer (Rosen et al., 1993) and the adjacent FGF-4 gene is also found to be amplified in a variety of tissues, although this has not been correlated with increased levels of expression (Adelaide et al., 1988; Theillet et al., 1989; Yoshida et al., 1988). The K-*sam* gene has been isolated as an amplified sequence from a stomach cancer cell line (Nakatami et al., 1986). However, where the sequence of the amplified gene has been examined, these genes have so far been found to encode unaltered forms of the proteins (Meyer & Dudley, 1992; Hattori et al., 1990). It is possible that in both cases the FGF or FGFR genes have been adventitiously amplified as a result of inclusion in an amplicon that includes another gene which is the target for amplification in these tumours. Thus, although gene amplification itself may sometimes correlate statistically with the aggressiveness of the cancer (Rosen et al., 1993), the exact relevance of such FGF-related amplification events to human carcinogenesis is as yet unclear.

An examination of FGF amplification in tumours can sometimes be used to predict prognosis. Thus the degree of amplification of the FGF-3 gene in breast and ovarian tumours has been shown to correlate with the aggressiveness of the cancer, although no correlation with overall survival was observed (Lidereau et al., 1988; Rosen et al., 1993).

FGFs AND METASTASIS

As the malignancy of the cell increases, metastasis, may occur and it is probable that the action of the FGF family of factors may have an important role in either inducing or facilitating metastatic behaviour in a number of tumour cell systems.

There is circumstantial evidence that associates increased FGF expression and the metastatic phenotype of murine mammary tumours (Murakami et al., 1990). Furthermore, the metastatic potential of FGF-expressing cells has been directly demonstrated in experimental systems. NIH3T3 cells transfected with FGF that are injected into athymic nude mice may become metastatic (Damen et al., 1991). In another study MCF-7 breast cancer cells transfected with FGF-4 become tumourigenic and also metastatic when injected into ovariectomized or tamoxifen-treated nude mice (McLeskey et al., 1993). How then might expression of FGF increase the metastatic potential of a cell?

One possibility is that FGF transformation of a cell results in the increased motility of the cell, which then acquires a more invasive phenotype. Time-lapse video microscopy has been used to show increased cell locomotion in NIH3T3 fibroblasts transfected with cDNAs encoding FGF-2 or FGF-4 (Taylor et al., 1993). Additionally metastasis may involve the altered secretion of enzymes and their inhibitors, such as heparanase, which leads to enhanced degradation of extracellular matrix components in the immediate environment thus facilitating migration and invasion of the tumourigenic cells. It is important to note that the induction of matrix-degrading enzymes, such as collagenase and stromolysin, by FGFs is a well documented feature of normal fibroblastic cells cultured in vitro (Edwards et al., 1987). It is entirely possible, therefore, that FGFs, expressed by primary tumours, can also act to facilitate metastatic invasion by induction of matrix-degrading enzymes in the nonmalignant stromal cells surrounding the original tumour (Figure 2.5).

It has already been discussed that FGFs may be sequestered, bound to HSPGs in the extracellular matrix. FGFs might therefore be re-

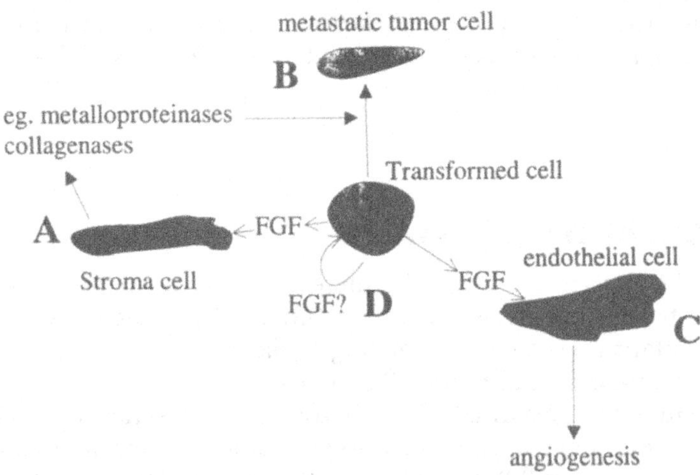

Figure 2.5 Summary of the modes by which FGFs are thought to contribute to the conversion of a cell to malignancy and progression of a tumour to metastasis. (A) FGFs can stimulate nonmalignant stromal cells to increase production of matrix degrading metalloproteinases and collagenases, thereby facilitating metastatic invasion of the tissue by nearby transformed cells. (B) FGF-transformed cells secrete FGF and can become metastatic after exposure to FGFs. (C) The action of FGFs on endothelial cells can initiate angiogenesis. (D) FGF secreted by transformed cells may exert an autocrine stimulatory effect on cell transformation.

leased, as a result of breakdown of matrix components with associated effects on surrounding stromal cells. As metastatic tumour cells are borne in the blood to sites distant from the location of the tumourigenic event, they must invade both the endothelial cell layer as well as the subendothelial basement membranes in order to establish neovascularization. Enzymatic and mechanical destruction of the surrounding extravascularization tissues takes place. The endothelial basement membrane of subendothelial matrix is composed largely of proteoglycans, approximately 90% of which are HSPGs. It is therefore not surprising that metastatic tumour cells possess the ability to both solubilize and degrade these glycoproteins, possibly by secretion of heparan-degrading enzymes (Kramer et al., 1982).

FGFs AND ANGIOGENESIS

Whether or not FGFs alter the properties of a transformed cell and thus predispose it to metastasis, it is clear that a metastatic tumour depends on successful neovascularization for its establishment. One of the characteristics of the FGF-transformed phenotype of NIH3T3 cells is its ability to form a well-vascularized tumour in nude mice and indeed a hallmark feature of FGF-1 and FGF-2 is their mitogenic action on endothelial cells of both capillary and main vessels (Burgess & Macaig, 1989). The formation of blood vessels in situ involves the orderly migration, proliferation and also differentiation of vascular cells. There is good direct evidence that FGF-stimulated cell proliferation is involved in the initiation of angiogenesis as shown by the following experiment. Commercial gelatin sponges impregnated with FGF-1 were placed directly in neck and peritoneal cavities of a rat, resulting in in situ, FGF-1 dependent neovascularization after 1 week (Thompson et al., 1988). The concentrations of FGF-1 used were physiologically relevant (i.e., close to the molecular weight for the FGF-1 receptor).

More recently, DNA liposome conjugates containing an expression vector encoding a secreted form of FGF-1 have been used to transfer FGF-1 directly into porcine arteries. Expression of FGF-1 induced intimal thickening and the formation of new capillaries in these expanded intima (Nabel et al., 1993). Analysis of tissue sections from the new blood vessels in the expanded intima suggests that mitotic activity is induced by FGF-1 in the wall of the vessel. These angiogenic effects of FGF-1 might be mediated directly on endothelial cells or perhaps indirectly through the induction of other endogenous growth factors.

FGF-BASED THERAPIES FOR CANCER

FGF expression and action are involved in a variety of facets of tumourigenesis including not only local growth of the tumour but its ability to undergo metastasis and induce neovascularization. This leads to possible therapeutic approaches based upon the inhibition or manipulation of FGF action.

FGFs – Toxin Conjugates

Tumour cells that produce FGFs will establish neovascularized masses and may then metastasize to establish colonies at other sites. Once cancer has progressed to this stage it becomes very difficult to arrest. It has been argued that one of the most important stages of cancer progression on which to focus therapeutic intervention is that of angiogenesis (Kerbel et al., 1991). It therefore follows that cells which express and secrete FGFs, which initiate angiogenesis, should be targeted for destruction. The principal strategy so far used to specifically destroy cancer cells is that which employs recombinant toxins; these molecules consist of a cell surface ligand, which will permit internalization of the molecule plus a cytotoxic compound (Pastan & FitzGerald, 1991).

Chimeric toxins composed of FGF fused to a cytotoxin have been shown to be active and to elicit cytotoxic and antiangiogenic effects on target cells. Chimeras that link FGF-1 to mutant forms of the *Pseudomonas* exotoxin (PE) and FGF-2 to the plant toxin saporin are toxic to a variety of tumour cell lines that express FGF receptors (Siegall et al., 1991; Lappi et al., 1990, 1991). Rat microvascular endothelial cells that are cultured in a three-dimensional collagen gel and treated with an FGF1-PE chimeric protein differ from control cells in their viability and ability to respond with angiogenesis to transforming growth factor β (Merwin et al., 1992). Moreover, these cytotoxic effects are also seen in vivo. FGF-2 saporin mitotoxin injected into mice bearing tumours derived from various human cancer cell lines elicits reductions in tumour volume and, in some cases, complete tumour regression (Beitz et al., 1992).

FGF Antagonists As Therapeutic Agents

A more complete understanding of the interaction between FGF, HSPGs and the FGF receptor molecules and also of the FGF signalling pathway will allow design of specific FGF antagonists that might prove useful in cancer treatments. Two molecules presently known to act as FGF inhibitors are suramin and pentosan polysulfate (PPS). Both are polysulfated and may therefore behave as heparin analogues, inhibiting binding of FGFs and other growth factors to their receptors. PPS shows selective inhibition of FGF-4 induced proliferation in mice that have FGF-4 expressing tumour xenografts. The inhibitory effects were shown to be reversible in vitro by adding excess FGF-4 to a cell line derived from the same tumour (Wellstein et al., 1991). Suramin, a polysulfated naphthylurea, has also been used to inhibit proliferation of mouse mammary cancer cells induced by FGF-1, FGF-2 and AIGF (FGF-8), to decrease the number of binding sites and to reduce the number of FGFR1 transcripts (Kasayama et al., 1993). Another possible FGF antagonist is medroxyprogesterone acetate, an anticancer, antiangiogenic steroid drug that may exert its effects through inhibition of FGFs (Fujimoto et al., 1989).

FGF-BASED BIOLOGICAL MODELS OF CANCER

Cell and animal models of breast cancer and prostatic hypertrophy have recently been developed. These include a transgenic mouse that overexpresses the FGF-3 gene, and under the control of the MMTV promoter produces an epithelial benign prostatic hyperplasia that is hormonally sensitive (Tutrone et al., 1993). In addition, a human breast cancer cell line transfected with both FGF-4 and *lacZ* genes shows rapid growth and spontaneous metastasis in ovariectomized and tamoxifen-treated nude mice with the advantage that the metastatic cells can be traced by whole organ staining for beta-galactosidase activity (Kurebayashi et al., 1993). Such models should prove particularly useful in testing any potential FGF antagonists for cytotoxic, antiangiogenic and antimetastatic activity.

CONCLUSIONS

The nature of the involvement of FGFs in cell transformation remains incompletely understood. Whilst some members of this polypeptide family clearly have oncogenic effects on certain cell lines, the lack of understanding of the process by which FGFs transmit intracellular signals makes it difficult to interpret many of these effects. However, the importance of FGFs to the biology of a tumour cell is undeniable. The angiogenic properties of FGFs are perhaps more important than any transforming ability and highlight an interesting and promising area of future research into potential therapeutic agents. An advantage of using drugs that specifically interfere with

FGF action on cells would be that such drugs might be used to prevent secondary spread of the types of cancers with which FGFs are mostly associated, namely the solid, endothelial tumours for which at the moment there are very few specific treatments.

REFERENCES

Acland P., Dixon M., Peters G. & Dickson C. (1990) Subcellular fate of the *int-*2 oncoprotein is determined by choice of initiation codon. *Nature,* **343**, 662–5.

Adelaide J., Mattei M.G., Marics I., Raybaud F., Planche J., De Lapeyriere O. & Birnbaum D. (1988) Chromosomal localization of the *hst* oncogene and its co-amplification with the *int*.2 oncogene in a human melanoma. *Oncogene,* **2**, 413–16.

Allen L.E. & Maher P.A. (1993) Expression of basic fibroblast growth factor and its receptor in an invasive bladder carcinoma cell line. *Journal of Cellular Physiology,* **155**, 368–75.

Amaya E., Musci T.J. & Kirschner M.W. (1991) Expression of a dominant negative mutant of the FGF receptor disrupts mesoderm formation in *Xenopus* embryos. *Cell,* **66**, 257–70.

Avivi A., Yayon A. & Givol D. (1993) A novel form of FGF receptor-3 using an alternative exon in the immunoglobulin domain III. *FEBS Letters,* **3**, 249–52.

Baird A., Schubert D., Ling N. & Guillemin R. (1988) Receptor- and heparin-binding domains of basic fibroblast growth factor. *Proceedings of the National Academy of Sciences of the United States of America,* **85**, 2324–8.

Bartlett P.F., Bailey K. & Bernard O. (1988) Immortalization of mouse neural precursor cells by the c-*myc* oncogene. *Proceedings of the National Academy of Sciences of the United States of America* , **85**(9), 3255–9.

Beitz J.G., Davol P., Clark J.W., Kato J., Medina M., Frackelton A.R., Jr., Lappi D.A., Baird A. & Calabresi P. (1992) Antitumor activity of basic fibroblast growth factor-saporin mitotoxin in vitro and in vivo. *Cancer Research,* **52**, 227–30.

Bellot F., Crumley G., Kaplow J.M., Schlessinger J., Jaye M. & Dionne C.A. (1991) Ligand-induced transphosphorylation between different FGF receptors. *EMBO Journal,* **10**, 2849–54.

Bottaro D.P., Fortney E., Rubin J.S. & Aaronson S.A. (1993) A keratinocyte growth factor receptor-derived peptide antagonist identifies part of the ligand binding site. *Journal of Biological Chemistry,* **268**, 9180–3.

Bouche G., Gas N., Prats H., Baldin V., Tauber J.P., Teissie J. & Amalric F. (1987) Basic fibroblast growth factor enters the nucleolus and stimulates the transcription of ribosomal genes in ABAE cells undergoing G0——G1 transition. *Proceedings of the National Academy of the Sciences of the United States of America,* **84**, 6770–4.

Brigstock D.R., Sasse J. & Klagsbrun M. (1991) Subcellular distribution of basic fibroblast growth factor in human hepatoma cells. *Growth Factors,* **4**, 189–96.

Bugler B., Amalric F. & Prats H. (1991) Alternative initiation of translation determines cytoplasmic or nuclear localization of basic fibroblast growth factor. *Molecular and Cellular Biology,* **11**, 573–7.

Burgess W.H., Dionne C.A., Kaplow J., Mudd R., Friesel R., Zilberstein A., Schlessinger J. & Jaye M. (1990) Characterization and cDNA cloning of phospholipase C-gamma, a major substrate for heparin-binding growth factor 1 (acidic fibroblast growth factor)-activated tyrosine kinase. *Molecular and Cellular Biology*, **10**, 4770–7.

Burgess W.H. & Maciag T. (1989) The heparin-binding (fibroblast) growth factor family of proteins. *Annual Review of Biochemistry*, **58**, 575–606.

Cao Y., Ekstrom M. & Pettersson R.F. (1993) Characterization of the nuclear translocation of acidic fibroblast growth factor. *Journal of Cell Science*, **104**, 77–87.

Chodak G.W., Hospelhorn V., Judge S.M., Mayforth R., Koeppen H. & Sasse J. (1988) Increased levels of fibroblast growth factor-like activity in urine from patients with bladder or kidney cancer. *Cancer Research*, **48**, 2083–8.

Clements D.A., Wang J.K., Dionne C.A. & Goldfarb M. (1993) Activation of fibroblast growth factor (FGF) receptors by recombinant human FGF-5. *Oncogene*, **8**, 1311–16.

Crumley G.R., Howk R., Ravera M.W. & Jaye M. (1989) Multiple polyadenylation sites downstream from the human aFGF gene encoding acidic fibroblast growth factor. *Gene*, **85**, 489–97.

Damen J.E., Greenberg A.H. & Wright J.A. (1991) Transformation and amplification of the K-*fgf* proto-oncogene in NIH-3T3 cells, and induction of metastatic potential. *Biochimica et Biophysica Acta*, **1097**, 103–10.

Dang C.V. & Lee W.M. (1989) Nuclear and nucleolar targeting sequences of c-*erb*-A, c-*myb*, N-*myc*, p53, HSP70, and HIV tat proteins. *Journal of Biological Chemistry*, **264**, 18019–23.

deLapeyriere O., Ollendorff V., Planche J., Ott M., Pizette S., Coullier F. & Birnbaum D. (1993) Expression of the FGF-6 gene is restricted to developing skeletal muscle in the mouse embryo. *Development*, **118**, 601–11.

Dell'Era P., Presta M. & Ragnotti G. (1991) Nuclear localization of endogenous basic fibroblast growth factor in cultured endothelial cells. *Experimental Cell Research*, **192**, 505–10.

Dell K.R. & Williams L.T. (1992) A novel form of fibroblast growth factor receptor 2. Alternative splicing of the third immunoglobulin-like domain confers ligand binding specificity. *Journal of Biological Chemistry*, **267**, 21225–9.

Delli Bovi P., Curatola A.M., Newman K.M., Sato Y., Moscatelli D., Hewick R.M., Rifkin D.B. & Basilico C. (1988) Processing, secretion, and biological properties of a novel growth factor of the fibroblast growth factor family with oncogenic potential. *Molecular and Cellular Biology*, **8**, 2933–41.

Delli Bovi P., Curatola A.M., Kern F.G., Greco A., Ittmann M. & Basilico C. (1987) An oncogene isolated by transfection of Kaposi's sarcoma DNA encodes a growth factor that is a member of the FGF family. *Cell*, **50**, 729–37.

Dickson C. & Peters G. (1987) Potential oncogene product related to growth factors [letter]. *Nature*, **326**, 833.

Dionne C.A., Crumley G., Bellot F., Kaplow J.M., Searfoss G., Ruta M., Burgess W.H., Jaye M. & Schlessinger J. (1990) Cloning and expression of two distinct high-affinity receptors cross-reacting with acidic and basic fibroblast growth factors. *EMBO Journal*, **9**, 2685–92.

Edwards D.R., Murphy G., Reynolds J.J., Whitham S.E., Docherty A.J., Angel P. & Heath J.K. (1987) Transforming growth factor beta modulates the expression of collagenase and metalloproteinase inhibitor. *EMBO Journal*, **6**, 1899–1904.

Finch P.W., Rubin J.S., Miki T., Ron D. & Aaronson S.A. (1989) Human KGF is FGF-related with properties of a paracrine effector of epithelial cell growth. *Science*, **245**, 752–5.

Forough R., Xi Z., MacPhee M., Friedman S., Engleka K.A., Sayers T., Wiltrout R.H. & Maciag T. (1993) Differential transforming abilities of non-secreted and secreted forms of human fibroblast growth factor-1. *Journal of Biological Chemistry*, **268**, 2960–8.

Fujimoto J., Fujita H., Hosoda S., Okada H. & Tanaka N.G. (1989) Effect of medroxyprogesterone acetate on secondary spreading of endometrial cancer. *Invasion and Metastasis*, **9**, 209–15.

Fujimoto K., Ichimori Y., Kakizoe T., Okajima E., Sakamoto H., Sugimura T. & Terada M. (1991) Increased serum levels of basic fibroblast growth factor in patients with renal cell carcinoma. *Biochemical and Biophysical Research Communications*, **180**, 386–92.

Gallagher J.T. & Turnbull J.E. (1992) Heparan sulphate in the binding and activation of basic fibroblast growth factor. *Glycobiology*, **2**, 523–8.

Gimenez Gallego G., Rodkey J., Bennett C., Rios Candelore M., DiSalvo J. & Thomas K. (1985) Brain-derived acidic fibroblast growth factor: complete amino acid sequence and homologies. *Science*, **230**, 1385–8.

Glazer L. & Shilo B.Z. (1991) The *Drosophila* FGF-R homolog is expressed in the embryonic tracheal system and appears to be required for directed tracheal cell extension. *Genes and Development*, **5**, 697–705.

Goldfarb M., Deed R., MacAllan D., Walther W., Dickson C. & Peters G. (1991) Cell transformation by Int-2–a member of the fibroblast growth factor family. *Oncogene*, **6**, 65–71.

Goldfarb M. (1990) The fibroblast growth factor family. *Cell Growth and Differentiation*, **1**, 439–45.

Harper J.W. & Lobb R.R. (1988) Reductive methylation of lysine residues in acidic fibroblast growth factor: effect on mitogenic activity and heparin affinity. *Biochemistry*, **27**, 671–8.

Hattori Y., Odagiri H., Nakatani H., Miyagawa K., Naito K., Sakamoto H., Katoh O., Yoshida T., Sugimura T. & Terada M. (1990) K-*sam*, an amplified gene in stomach cancer, is a member of the heparin-binding growth factor receptor genes. *Proceedings of the National Academy of Sciences of the United States of America*, **87**, 5983–7.

Haub O. & Goldfarb M. (1991) Expression of the fibroblast growth factor-5 gene in the mouse embryo. *Development*, **112**, 397–406.

Hou J., Kan M., Wang F., Xu J.M., Nakahara M., McBride G., McKeehan K. & McKeehan W.L. (1992) Substitution of putative half-cystine residues in heparin-binding fibroblast growth factor receptors. Loss of binding activity in both two and three loop isoforms. *Journal of Biological Chemistry*, **267**, 17804–8.

Houssaint E., Blanquet P.R., Champion Arnaud P., Gesnel M.C., Torriglia A., Courtois Y. & Breathnach R. (1990) Related fibroblast growth factor receptor genes exist in the human genome. *Proceedings of National Academy of Science of the United States of America*, **87**, 8180–4.

Huang Y.Q., Li J.J., Moscatelli D., Basilico C., Nicolaides A., Zhang W.G., Poiesz B.J. & Friedman Kien A.E. (1993) Expression of *int*-2 oncogene in Kaposi's sarcoma lesions. *Journal of Clinical Investigations*, **91**, 1191–7.

Iida S., Yoshida T., Naito K., Sakamoto H., Katoh O., Hirohashi S., Sato T., Onda M., Sugimura T. & Terada M. (1992) Human *hst*-2 (FGF-6) oncogene: cDNA cloning and characterization. *Oncogene*, **7**, 303–9.

Imamura T., Engleka K., Zhan X., Tokita Y., Forough R., Roeder D., Jackson A., Maier J.A., Hla T. & Maciag T. (1990) Recovery of mitogenic activity of a growth factor mutant with a nuclear translocation sequence. *Science*, **249**, 1567–70.

Isaacs H.V., Tannahill D. & Slack J.M. (1992) Expression of a novel FGF in the *Xenopus* embryo. A new candidate inducing factor for mesoderm formation and anteroposterior specification. *Development*, **114**, 711–20.

Jackson A., Friedman S., Zhan X., Engleka K.A., Forough R. & Maciag T. (1992) Heat shock induces the release of fibroblast growth factor 1 from NIH 3T3 cells. *Proceedings of the National Academy of Sciences of the United States of America*, **89**, 10691–5.

Jaye M., Schlessinger J. & Dionne C.A. (1992) Fibroblast growth factor receptor tyrosine kinases: molecular analysis and signal transduction. *Biochimica et Biophysica Acta*, **1135**, 185–99.

Johnson D.E. & Williams L.T. (1993) Structural and functional diversity in the FGF receptor multigene family. *Advances in Cancer Research*, **60**, 1–41.

Johnson D.E., Lu J., Chen H., Werner S. & Williams L.T. (1991) The human fibroblast growth factor receptor genes: a common structural arrangement underlies the mechanisms for generating receptor forms that differ in their third immunoglobulin domain. *Molecular and Cellular Biology*, **11**, 4627–34.

Johnson D.E., Lee P.L., Lu J. & Williams L.T. (1990) Diverse forms of a receptor for acidic and basic fibroblast growth factors. *Molecular and Cellular Biology*, **10**, 4728–36.

Jouanneau J., Gavrilovic J., Caruelle D., Jaye M., Moens G., Caruelle J.P. & Thiery J.P. (1991) Secreted or nonsecreted forms of acidic fibroblast growth factor produced by transfected epithelial cells influence cell morphology, motility, and invasive potential. *Proceedings of the National Academy of Sciences of the United States of America*, **88**, 2893–7.

Kan M., Wang F., Xu J., Crabb J.W., Hou J. & McKeehan W.L. (1993) An essential heparin-binding domain in the fibroblast growth factor receptor kinase. *Science*, **259**, 1918–21.

Kan M., Shi E.G. & McKeehan W.L. (1991) Identification and assay of fibroblast growth factor receptors. *Methods in Enzymology*, **198**, 158–71.

Kasayama S., Saito H., Kouhara H., Sumitani S. & Sato B. (1993) Suramin interrupts androgen-inducible autocrine loop involving heparin binding growth factor in mouse mammary cancer (Shionogi carcinoma 115) cells. *Journal of Cellular Physiology*, **154**, 254–61.

Keegan K., Johnson D.E., Williams L.T. & Hayman M.J. (1991) Isolation of an additional member of the fibroblast growth factor receptor family, FGFR-3. *Proceedings of the National Academy of Sciences of the United States of America*, **88**, 1095–9.

Kerbel R.S. (1991) Inhibition of tumor angiogenesis as a strategy to circumvent acquired resistance to anti-cancer therapeutic agents. *Bioessays*, **13**, 31–6.

Kiefer P., Peters G. & Dickson C. (1993) Retention of fibroblast growth factor 3 in the Golgi complex may regulate its export from cells. *Molecular and Cellular Biology*, **13**(9), 5781–93.

Kiefer P., Peters G. & Dickson C. (1991) The Int-2/Fgf-3 oncogene product is secreted and associates with extracellular matrix: implications for cell transformation. *Molecular and Cellular Biology*, **11**, 5929–36.

Kim E.G., Kwon H.M., Burrow C.R. & Ballermann B.J. (1993) Expression of rat fibroblast growth factor receptor 1 as three splicing variants during kidney development. *American Journal of Physiology*, **264**, F66-73.

Kimelman D. & Kirschner M.W. (1989) An antisense mRNA directs the covalent modification of the transcript encoding fibroblast growth factor in *Xenopus* oocytes. *Cell*, **59**, 687–96.

Klagsbrun M. & Baird A. (1991) A dual receptor system is required for basic fibroblast growth factor activity. *Cell*, **67**, 229–31.

Klagsbrun M. (1990) The affinity of fibroblast growth factors (FGFs) for heparin; FGF-heparan sulfate interactions in cells and extracellular matrix. *Current Opinion in Cell Biology*, **2**, 857–63.

Kornbluth S., Paulson K.E. & Hanafusa H. (1988) Novel tyrosine kinase identified by phosphotyrosine antibody screening of cDNA libraries. *Molecular and Cellular Biology*, **8**, 5541–4.

Kramer R., Vogel K.G. & Nicolson G. (1982) Solubilization and degradation of subendothelial matrix glycoproteins and proteoglycans by metastatic tumor cells. *Journal of Biological Chemistry*, **257**, 2678–86.

Kurebayashi J., McLeskey S.W., Johnson M.D., Lippman M.E., Dickson R.B. & Kern F.G. (1993) Quantitative demonstration of spontaneous metastasis by MCF-7 human breast cancer cells cotransfected with fibroblast growth factor 4 and LacZ. *Cancer Research*, **53**, 2178–87.

Lappi D.A., Maher P.A., Martineau D. & Baird A. (1991) The basic fibroblast growth factor-saporin mitotoxin acts through the basic fibroblast growth factor receptor. *Journal of Cellular Physiology*, **147**, 17–26.

Lappi D.A. & Baird A. (1990) Mitotoxins: growth factor-targeted cytotoxic molecules. *Progress in Growth Factor Research*, **2**, 223–36.

Lee P.L., Johnson D.E., Cousens L.S., Fried V.A. & Williams L.T. (1989) Purification and complementary DNA cloning of a receptor for basic fibroblast growth factor. *Science*, **245**, 57–60.

Li L., Zhou J., James G., Heller Harrison R., Czech M.P. & Olson E.N. (1992) FGF inactivates myogenic helix-loop-helix proteins through phosphorylation of a conserved protein kinase C site in their DNA-binding domains. *Cell*, **71**, 1181–94.

Li Y., Koga M., Kasayama S., Matsumoto K., Arita N., Hayakawa T. & Sato B. (1992) Identification and characterization of high molecular weight forms of basic fibroblast growth factor in human pituitary adenomas. *Journal of Clinical Endocrinology and Metabolism*, **75**, 1436–41.

Lidereau R., Callahan R., Dickson C., Peters G., Escot C. & Ali I.U. (1988) Amplification of the int-2 gene in primary human breast tumors. *Oncogene Research*, **2**, 285–91.

Liscia D.S., Merlo G.R., Garrett C., French D., Mariani Costantini R. & Callahan R. (1989) Expression of int-2 mRNA in human tumors amplified at the int-2 locus. *Oncogene*, **4**, 1219–24.

Mach H., Volkin D.B., Burke C.J., Middaugh C.R., Linhardt R.J., Fromm J.R., Loganathan D. & Mattsson L. (1993) Nature of the interaction of heparin with acidic fibroblast growth factor. *Biochemistry*, **32**, 5480–9.

MacNicol A.M., Muslin A.J. & Williams L.T. (1993) *Raf*-1 kinase is essential for early *Xenopus* development and mediates the induction of mesoderm by FGF. *Cell*, **73**, 571–83.

Marics I., Adelaide J., Raybaud F., Mattei M.G., Coulier F., Planche J., De Lapeyriere O. & Birnbaum D. (1989) Characterization of the HST-related FGF.6 gene, a new member of the fibroblast growth factor gene family. *Oncogene*, **4**, 335–40.

Matuo Y., McKeehan W.L., Yan G.C., Nikolaropoulos S., Adams P.S., Fukabori Y., Yamanaka H. & Gaudreau J. (1992) Potential role of HBGF (FGF) and TGF-beta on prostate growth. *Advances in Experimental Medicine and Biology*, **324**, 107–14.

McDonald F. & Heath J., (1993) Developmentally regulated expression of fibroblast factor receptor genes and splice variants by murine embryogenic stem and embryonal carcinoma cells. *Developmental Genetics*, (in press).

McLeskey S.W., Kurebayashi J., Honig S.F., Zwiebel J., Lippman M.E., Dickson R.B. & Kern F.G. (1993) Fibroblast growth factor 4 transfection of MCF-7 cells produces cell lines that are tumorigenic and metastatic in ovariectomized or tamoxifen-treated athymic nude mice. *Cancer Research*, **53**, 2168–77.

Merwin J.R., Lynch M.J., Madri J.A., Pastan I. & Siegall C.B. (1992) Acidic fibroblast growth factor-*Pseudomonas* exotoxin chimeric protein elicits antiangiogenic effects on endothelial cells. *Cancer Research*, **52**, 4995–5001.

Meyers S.L. & Dudley J.P. (1992) Sequence analysis of the int-2/fgf-3 gene in aggressive human breast carcinomas. *Molecular Carcinogenesis*, **6**, 243–51.

Miki T., Bottaro D.P., Fleming T.P., Smith C.L., Burgess W.H., Chan A.M. & Aaronson S.A. (1992) Determination of ligand-binding specificity by alternative splicing: two distinct growth factor receptors encoded by a single gene. *Proceeding of the National Academy of Sciences of the United States of America*, **89**, 246–50.

Miki T., Fleming T.P., Bottaro D.P., Rubin J.S., Ron D. & Aaronson S.A. (1991) Expression cDNA cloning of the KGF receptor by creation of a transforming autocrine loop. *Science*, **251**, 72–5.

Miyamoto M., Narmo K., Seko C., Matsumoto S., Kondo T. & Kurokawa T. (1993) Molecular cloning of a novel cytokine cDNA encoding the ninth member of the fibroblast growth factor family, which has a unique secretion property. *Molecular and Cellular Biology*, **13**(7), 4251–9.

Mohammadi M., Dionne C.A., Li W., Li N., Spivak T., Honegger A.M., Jaye M. & Schlessinger J. (1992) Point mutation in FGF receptor eliminates phosphatidylinositol hydrolysis without affecting mitogenesis. *Nature*, **358**, 681–4.

Mohammadi M., Honegger A.M., Rotin D., Fischer R., Bellot F., Li W., Dionne C.A., Jaye M., Rubinstein M. & Schlessinger J. (1991) A tyrosine-phosphorylated carboxy-terminal peptide of the fibroblast growth factor receptor (Flg) is a binding site for the SH2 domain of phospholipase C-gamma 1. *Molecular and Cellular Biology*, **11**, 5068–78.

Morrison D.K., Kaplan D.R., Rapp U. & Roberts T.M. (1988) Signal transduction from membrane to cytoplasm: growth factors and membrane-bound oncogene products increase *Raf*-1 phosphorylation and associated protein kinase activity. *Proceedings of the National Academy of Sciences of the United States of America*, **85**, 8855–9.

Moscatelli D. (1987) High and low affinity binding sites for basic fibroblast growth factor on cultured cells: absence of a role for low affinity binding in the stimulation of plasminogen activator production by bovine capillary endothelial cells. *Journal of Cellular Physiology*, **131**, 123–30.

Murakami A., Tanaka H. & Matsuzawa A. (1990) Association of *hst* gene expression with metastatic phenotype in mouse mammary tumors. *Cell Growth and Differentiation,* **1**, 225–31.

Murphy M., Draggo J. & Bartlett P.F. (1990) Fibroblast growth factor stimulates the proliferation and differentiation of neural precursor cells *in vitro. Journal of Neuroscience Research,* **25**(4), 463–75.

Musci T.J., Amaya E. & Kirschner M.W. (1990) Regulation of the fibroblast growth factor receptor in early *Xenopus* embryos. *Proceedings of the National Academy of Sciences of the United States of America,* **87**, 8365–9.

Myers R.L., Payson R.A., Chotani M.A., Deaven L.L. & Chiu I. (1993) Gene structure and differential expression of acidic fibroblast growth factor mRNA: identification and distribution of four different transcripts. *Oncogene,* **8**, 341–9.

Nabel E.G., Yang Z.Y., Plautz G., Forough R., Zhan X., Haudenschild C.C., Maciag T. & Nabel GJ. (1993) Recombinant fibroblast growth factor-1 promotes intimal hyperplasia and angiogenesis in arteries in vivo. *Nature,* **362**, 844–6.

Nakamoto T., Chang C.S., Li A.K. & Chodak G.W. (1992) Basic fibroblast growth factor in human prostate cancer cells. *Cancer Research,* **52**, 571–7.

Nakanishi Y., Kihara K., Mizuno K., Masamune Y., Yoshitake Y. & Nishikawa K. (1992) Direct effect of basic fibroblast growth factor on gene transcription in a cell-free system. *Proceedings of the National Academy of Sciences of the United States of America,* **89**, 5216–20.

Nakatami. (1986) Detection of amplified sequences in gastric carcinomas by a renaturation method in gel. *Japanese Journal of Cancer Research,* **77**, 849–53.

New B.A. & Yeoman L.C. (1992) Identification of basic fibroblast growth factor sensitivity and receptor and ligand expression in human colon tumor cell lines. *Journal of Cellular Physiology,* **150**, 320–6.

Niswander L. & Martin G.R. (1992) Fgf-4 expression during gastrulation, myogenesis, limb and tooth development in the mouse. *Development,* **114**, 755–68.

Nurcombe V., Ford M.D., Wildschut J.A. & Bartlett P.F. (1993) Developmental regulation of neural response to FGF-1 and FGF-2 by heparan sulfate proteoglycan. *Science,* **260**, 103–6.

Ornitz D.M. & Leder P. (1992) Ligand specificity and heparin dependence of fibroblast growth factor receptors 1 and 3. *Journal of Biological Chemistry,* **267**, 16305–11.

Ornitz D.M., Yayon A., Flanagan J.G., Svahn C.M., Levi E. & Leder P. (1992) Heparin is required for cell-free binding of basic fibroblast growth factor to a soluble receptor and for mitogenesis in whole cells. *Molecular and Cellular Biology,* **12**, 240–7.

Partanen J., Makela T.P., Eerola E., Korhonen J., Hirvonen H., Claesson Welsh L. & Alitalo K. (1991) FGFR-4, a novel acidic fibroblast growth factor receptor with a distinct expression pattern. *EMBO Journal,* **10**, 1347–54.

Partanen J., Makela T.P., Alitalo R., Lehvaslaiho H. & Alitalo K. (1990) Putative tyrosine kinases expressed in K-562 human leukemia cells. *Proceedings of the National Academy of Sciences of the United States of America,* **87**, 8913–7.

Pastan I. & FitzGerald D. (1991) Recombinant toxins for cancer treatment. *Science,* **254**, 1173–7.

Paterno G.D., Gillespie L.L., Dixon M.S., Slack J.M. & Heath J.K. (1989) Mesoderm-inducing properties of INT-2 and kFGF: two oncogene-encoded growth factors related to FGF. *Development*, **106**, 79–83.

Peters K.G., Marie J., Wilson E., Ives H.E., Escobedo J., Del Rosario M., Mirda D. & Williams L.T. (1992) Point mutation of an FGF receptor abolishes phosphatidylinositol turnover and Ca2+ flux but not mitogenesis. *Nature*, **358**, 678–81.

Powell P.P. & Klagsbrun M. (1991) Three forms of rat basic fibroblast growth factor are made from a single mRNA and localize to the nucleus. *Journal of Cellular Physiology*, **148**, 202–10.

Prats H., Kaghad M., Prats A.C., Klagsbrun M., Lelias J.M., Liauzun P., Chalon P., Tauber J.P., Amalric F., Smith J.A. et al. (1989) High molecular mass forms of basic fibroblast growth factor are initiated by alternative CUG codons. *Proceedings of the National Academy of Sciences of the United States of America*, **86**, 1836–40.

Ravery V., Jouanneau J., Gil Diez S., Abbou C.C., Caruelle J.P., Barritault D. & Chopin D.K. (1992) Immunohistochemical detection of acidic fibroblast growth factor in bladder transitional cell carcinoma. *Urological Research*, **20**, 211–4.

Reiland J. & Rapraeger A. (1993) Heparan sulfate proteoglycan and FGF receptor target basic FGF to different intracellular destinations. *Journal of Cell Science*, **105**, 1085–93.

Rogelj S., Weinberg R.A., Fanning P. & Klagsbrun M. (1988) Basic fibroblast growth factor fused to a signal peptide transforms cells. *Nature*, **331**, 173–5.

Roghani M. & Moscatelli D. (1992) Basic fibroblast growth factor is internalized through both receptor-mediated and heparan sulfate-mediated mechanisms. *Journal of Biological Chemistry*, **267**, 22156–62.

Rosen A., Sevelda P., Klein M., Dobianer K., Hruza C., Czerwenka K., Hanak H., Vavra N., Salzer H., Leodolter S. et al. (1993) First experience with FGF-3 (INT-2) amplification in women with epithelial ovarian cancer. *British Journal of Cancer*, **67**, 1122–5.

Ruta M., Burgess W., Givol D., Epstein J., Neiger N., Kaplow J., Crumley G., Dionne C., Jaye M. & Schlessinger J. (1989) Receptor for acidic fibroblast growth factor is related to the tyrosine kinase encoded by the fms-like gene (FLG). *Proceedings of the National Academy of Sciences of the United States of America*, **86**, 8722–6.

Safran A., Avivi A., Orr Urtereger A., Neufeld G., Lonai P., Givol D. & Yarden Y. (1990) The murine flg gene encodes a receptor for fibroblast growth factor. *Oncogene*, **5**, 635–43.

Sano H., Forough R., Maier J.A., Case J.P., Jackson A., Engleka K., Maciag T. & Wilder R.L. (1990) Detection of high levels of heparin binding growth factor-1 (acidic fibroblast growth factor) in inflammatory arthritic joints. *Journal of Cell Biology*, **110**, 1417–26.

Saunders S., Jalkanen M., O'Farrell S. & Bernfield M. (1989) Molecular cloning of syndecan, an integral membrane proteoglycan. *Journal of Cell Biology*, **108**, 1547–56.

Shi E., Kan M., Xu J., Wang F., Hou J. & McKeehan W. (1993) Control of fibroblast growth factor receptor kinase signal transduction by heterodimerization of combinatorial splice variants. *Molecular and Cellular Biology*, **13**(7), 3907–18.

Shiurba R.A., Jing N., Sakakura T. & Godsave S.F. (1991) Nuclear translocation of fibroblast growth factor during *Xenopus* mesoderm induction. *Development,* **113**, 487–93.

Siegall C.B., Epstein S., Speir E., Hla T., Forough R., Maciag T., Fitzgerald D.J. & Pastan I. (1991) Cytotoxic activity of chimeric proteins composed of acidic fibroblast growth factor and *Pseudomonas* exotoxin on a variety of cell types. *FASEB Journal,* **5**, 2843–9.

Speir E., Sasse J., Shrivastav S. & Casscells W. (1991) Culture-induced increase in acidic and basic fibroblast growth factor activities and their association with the nuclei of vascular endothelial and smooth muscle cells. *Journal of Cellular Physiology,* **147**, 362–73.

Takahashi J.A., Fukumoto M., Igarashi K., Oda Y., Kikuchi H. & Hatanaka M. (1992) Correlation of basic fibroblast growth factor expression levels with the degree of malignancy and vascularity in human gliomas. *Journal of Neurosurgery,* **76**, 792–8.

Takahashi J.B., Hoshimaru M., Jaye M., Kikuchi H. & Hatanaka M. (1992) Possible activity of acidic fibroblast growth factor as a progression factor rather than a transforming factor. *Biochemical and Biophysical Research Communications,* **189**, 398–405.

Talarico D., Ittmann M.M., Bronson R. & Basilico C. (1993) A retrovirus carrying the K-*fgf* oncogene induces diffuse meningeal tumors and soft-tissue fibrosarcomas. *Molecular and Cellular Biology,* **13**, 1998–2010.

Talarico D. & Basilico C. (1991) The K-*fgf/hst* oncogene induces transformation through an autocrine mechanism that requires extracellular stimulation of the mitogenic pathway. *Molecular and Cellular Biology,* **11**, 1138–45.

Tanaka A., Miyamoto K., Minamino N., Takeda M., Sato B., Matsuo H. & Matsumoto K. (1992) Cloning and characterization of an androgen-induced growth factor essential for the androgen-dependent growth of mouse mammary carcinoma cells. *Proceedings of the National Academy of Sciences of the United States of America,* **89**, 8928–32.

Taylor W.R., Greenberg A.H., Turley E.A. & Wright J.A. (1993) Cell motility, invasion, and malignancy induced by overexpression of K-FGF or bFGF. *Experimental Cell Research,* **204**, 295–301.

Tessler S. & Neufeld G. (1990) Basic fibroblast growth factor accumulates in the nuclei of various bFGF-producing cell types. *Journal of Cellular Physiology,* **145**, 310–7.

Theillet C., Le Roy X., De Lapeyriere O., Grosgeorges J,. Adnane J., Raynaud S.D., Simony Lafontaine J., Goldfarb M., Escot C. & Birnbaum D. (1989) Amplification of FGF-related genes in human tumors: possible involvement of HST in breast carcinomas [published erratum appears in *Oncogene* 1989 Dec.;4(12):1537]. *Oncogene,* **4**, 915–22.

Thompson J. & Slack J.M. (1992) Over-expression of fibroblast growth factors in *Xenopus* embryos. *Mechanisms of Devopment,* **38**, 175–82.

Thompson J.A., Anderson K.D., DiPietro J.M., Zwiebel J.A., Zametta M., Anderson W.F. & Maciag T. (1988) Site-directed neovessel formation in vivo. *Science,* **241**, 1349–52.

Turnbull J.E., Fernig D.G., Ke Y., Wilkinson M.C. & Gallagher J.T. (1992) Identification of the basic fibroblast growth factor binding sequence in fibroblast heparan sulfate. *Journal of Biolical Chemistry,* **267**, 10337–41.

Tutrone R.F., Jr., Ball R.A., Ornitz D.M., Leder P. & Richie J.P. (1993) Benign prostatic hyperplasia in a transgenic mouse: a new hormonally sensitive investigatory model. *Journal of Urology,* **149**, 633–9.

Ueno H., Gunn M., Dell K., Tseng A., Jr. & Williams L. (1992) A truncated form of fibroblast growth factor receptor 1 inhibits signal transduction by multiple types of fibroblast growth factor receptor. *Journal of Biological Chemistry*, **267**, 1470–6.

Ullrich A. & Schlessinger J. (1990) Signal transduction by receptors with tyrosine kinase activity. *Cell*, **61**, 203–12.

Vainikka S., Partanen J., Bellosta P., Coulier F., Basilico C., Jaye M. & Alitalo K. (1992) Fibroblast growth factor receptor-4 shows novel features in genomic structure, ligand binding and signal transduction. *EMBO Journal*, **11**, 4273–80.

Volk R., Koster M., Poting A., Hartmann L. & Knochel W. (1989) An antisense transcript from the *Xenopus laevis* bFGF gene coding for an evolutionarily conserved 24 kd protein. *EMBO Journal*, **8**, 2983–8.

Wellstein A., Zugmaier G., Califano J.A., Kern F., Paik S. & Lippman M.E. (1991) Tumor growth dependent on Kaposi's sarcoma-derived fibroblast growth factor inhibited by pentosan polysulfate. *Journal of the National Cancer Institute*, **83**, 716–20.

Werner S., Weinberg W., Liao X., Peters K., Blessing M., Yuspa S.H., Weiner R. & Williams L. (1993) Targeted expression of a dominant-negative FGF receptor mutant in the epidermis of transgenic mice reveals a role of FGF in keratinocyte organization and differentiation. *EMBO Journal*, **12**(7), 2635–43.

Werner S., Duan D.S., de Vries C., Peters K.G., Johnson D.E. & Williams L.T. (1992) Differential splicing in the extracellular region of fibroblast growth factor receptor 1 generates receptor variants with different ligand-binding specificities. *Molecular and Cellular Biology*, **12**, 82–8.

Wilkinson D.G., Peters G., Dickson C. & McMahon A.P. (1988) Expression of the FGF-related proto-oncogene int-2 during gastrulation and neurulation in the mouse. *EMBO Journal*, **7**, 691–5.

Yan G., Fukabori Y., McBride G., Nikolaropolous S. & McKeehan W. (1993) Exon switching and activation of stromal and embryonic fibroblast growth factor (FGF)-FGF receptor genes in prostate epithelial cells accompany stromal independence and malignancy. *Molecular and Cellular Biology*, **13**(8), 4513–22.

Yayon A., Zimmer Y., Shen G.H., Avivi A., Yarden Y. & Givol D. (1992) A confined variable region confers ligand specificity on fibroblast growth factor receptors: implications for the origin of the immunoglobulin fold. *EMBO Journal*, **11**, 1885–90.

Yayon A., Klagsbrun M., Esko J.D., Leder P. & Ornitz D.M. (1991) Cell surface, heparin-like molecules are required for binding of basic fibroblast growth factor to its high affinity receptor. *Cell*, **64**, 841–8.

Yoshida M.C., Wada M., Satoh H., Yoshida T., Sakamoto H., Miyagawa K., Yokota J., Koda T., Kakinuma M., Sugimura T. et al. (1988) Human HST1 (HSTF1) gene maps to chromosome band 11q13 and coamplifies with the INT2 gene in human cancer. *Proceedings of the National Academy of Sciences of the United States of America*, **85**, 4861–4.

Yoshida T., Miyagawa K., Odagiri H., Sakamoto H., Little P.F., Terada M. & Sugimura T. (1987) Genomic sequence of *hst*, a transforming gene encoding a protein homologous to fibroblast growth factors and the int-2-encoded protein [published erratum appears in Proc. Natl. Acad. Sci. U.S.A., 1988, March;**85**(6):1967]. *Proceedings of the National Academy of Sciences of the United States of America*, **84**, 7305–9.

Zhan X., Hu X., Friedman S. & Maciag T. (1992) Analysis of endogenous and exogenous nuclear translocation of fibroblast growth factor-1 in NIH 3T3 cells. *Biochemical and Biophysical Research Communications,* **188**, 982–91.

Zhan X., Bates B., Hu X.G. & Goldfarb M. (1988) The human FGF-5 oncogene encodes a novel protein related to fibroblast growth factors. *Molecular and Cellular Biology,* **8**, 3487–95.

Zhan X., Culpepper A., Reddy M., Loveless J. & Goldfarb M. (1987) Human oncogenes detected by a defined medium culture assay. *Oncogene,* **1**, 369–76.

Zhu X., Komiya H., Chirino A., Faham S., Fox G.M., Arakawa T., Hsu B.T. & Rees D.C. (1991) Three-dimensional structures of acidic and basic fibroblast growth factors. *Science,* **251**, 90–3.

Zimmer Y., Givol D. & Yayon A. (1993) Multiple structural elements determine ligand binding of fibroblast growth factor receptors. Evidence that both Ig domain 2 and 3 define receptor specificity. *Journal of Biological Chemistry,* **268**, 7899–903.

Zuniga A., Borja M., Meijers C. & Zeller R. (1993) Expression of alternatively spliced bFGF first coding exons and antisense mRNAs during chicken embryogenesis. *Developmental Biology,* **157**, 110–18.

3

The Biological Role of Transforming Growth Factor Beta in Cancer Development

BRADLEY A. ARRICK AND RIK DERYNCK

INTRODUCTION

The examination of media conditioned by transformed cells for the presence of factors that regulate cell proliferation has led to the characterization of many distinct growth factors, including transforming growth factors-alpha and -beta (TGF-α and -β). The initial identification of TGF-β, now more than a decade ago, was based on its ability to induce phenotypic transformation of certain fibroblast cell lines. Often, depending on the particular cell line, the growth stimulatory effect of TGF-β was apparent only when TGF-α or epidermal growth factor (EGF) were added (Anzano et al., 1983). Despite the similarities in names, TGF-α and TGF-β bear no structural, functional or genetic commonality. TGF-β is a disulfide-linked homodimeric protein that exists as three distinct isoforms, each encoded by a separate gene (Derynck et al., 1988; ten Dijke et al., 1988). TGF-α and EGF, on the other hand, are structurally similar to each other and interact with a common receptor. This chapter will focus only on the role of TGF-β in cancer; we will not discuss the functions of TGF-α (reviewed in Derynck, 1992) except in so far as it relates to the action of TGF-β.

The rapid accumulation of knowledge on the biology of TGF-β and its involvement in a large variety of biological processes make it impossible to comprehensively review this cytokine in the space available. Thankfully, some excellent recent reviews make this unnecessary (Roberts & Sporn, 1993; Moses et al., 1990; Barnard et al., 1990; Rifkin et al., 1993; Derynck, 1994). Thus, we will not discuss the structure of TGF-β, nor will we consider its roles in nonmalignant processes, such as development, immunology and cellular physiology. Our consideration of the subject will have a distinctly cancerous focus.

This chapter is organized into five sections. Firstly, we will provide an overview of the range of biological activities of TGF-β as they relate to the processes of carcinogenesis and malignant progression. Secondly, we will review what is known regarding mechanisms by which production of TGF-β by tumour cells may be regulated, including hormonal regulation. Thirdly, we will review current data concerning the sensitivity of tumour cells to TGF-β and the rapidly expanding array of TGF-β receptors. In the penultimate section, we will consider the available data from in vivo experimental approaches that suggest important roles for TGF-β in various cancers. Finally, we will identify some possible future directions for research in this area.

BIOLOGICAL ACTIVITIES OF TGF-β

The three isoforms of TGF-β, TGF-β1, -β2 and -β3, are made by a large variety of cell types and often more than one isoform is expressed by a particular cell. TGF-β1 was the first isoform available in purified form. Because of its high abundance in platelets, a readily available source, this isoform is frequently the only one used to study the biological effects of TGF-β. The three TGF-β species exhibit similar biological activities; however, in part depending on the target cell used in the assay of TGF-β activity, differences among the isoforms in overall potency are often noted (Graycar et al., 1989; Jennings et al., 1988). In this chapter, unless we specify a specific isoform, we will use the term TGF-β to refer to the family as a whole. The similarity in biological activities is presumably based on the high degree (>70%) of amino acid homology between the mature polypeptide sequences of the TGF-β isoforms (Derynck et al., 1988; ten Dijke et al., 1988). Accordingly, competition experiments have revealed that the different TGF-β species interact with the same cell surface receptor population (Miyazono et al., 1993), although characterization of the cloned receptors has revealed a higher level of specificity and complexity than originally anticipated (for a review, see Derynck, 1994).

TGF-β exerts a wide range of biological activities, and TGF-β receptors are found on most cells in culture and a large variety of cell types in vivo. It is beyond the scope of this chapter to review comprehensively the physiological effects of TGF-β and its presumed role in normal physiology. We will focus on those aspects of the biology of TGF-β that directly relate to the processes of tumourigenesis and metastatic spread. The major activities of TGF-β that could influence or determine the behaviour of the tumour cells in vivo are the modulation of cell proliferation, extracellular matrix production and adhesion, localized immune response and cellular chemotaxis.

When considering the potential roles of TGF-β in tumours, its effects on cell proliferation become of primary interest. Whereas this factor was initially identified by its ability to stimulate the proliferation of a fibroblast cell line in vitro, TGF-β exhibits either a mitogenic or an antiproliferative effect depending on the specific cell line and experimental conditions. Most cells that are stimulated by TGF-β to proliferate are derived from mesenchyme. Examples of these cell types are fibroblasts, osteoblasts, smooth muscle cells and Schwann cells (Leof et al., 1986; Centrella et al., 1987; Battegay et al., 1990; Ridley et al., 1989). In contrast, TGF-β is a potent inhibitor of proliferation of many other cell types, especially epithelial cells of various origins, endothelial and hematopoietic cells. We and others have recently reviewed the effects of TGF-β on cell proliferation and the putative mechanistic bases of this growth regulation (Moses et al., 1990; Arrick & Derynck, 1993; Derynck, 1992, 1994).

The mitogenic effect of TGF-β on some cells has been determined to involve the secondary action of another growth factor, such as EGF or platelet-derived growth factor (PDGF) (Assoian et al., 1984; Leof et al., 1986; Soma & Grotendorst, 1989). Thus, the mitogenic effect of TGF-β could in some cases be attributed to increased PDGF production and autocrine responsiveness. As a result, the indirect growth stimulatory effect of TGF-β may be delayed in onset and dependent upon the presence of other factors (Chambard & Pouysségur, 1988).

As discussed below, there have been a few reports of "more malignant" cell clones of a tumour cell line, which are growth stimulated by TGF-β in contrast to the parental cells that respond to TGF-β with growth inhibition (Schwarz et al., 1988; Rodeck, 1993; Hsu et al., 1994). These differences in effects most likely represent a distinctly different mode of action of TGF-β and suggest that there has been a molecular switch that results in these two diametrically opposed effects. Such a change could obviously significantly impact the behaviour and tumourigenicity of the tumour cell in vivo.

The molecular basis of the antiproliferative effect of TGF-β has been the focus of many investigations. In most cell systems, the growth inhibitory effect of TGF-β seems to be direct (i.e., without altering the receptor availability or responsiveness for growth stimulatory factors). In some cases, however, TGF-β has been reported to act as a growth inhibitor by interfering with or attenuating the signal from another mitogen. For instance, TGF-β inhibited the fibroblast growth factor–stimulated proliferation of a fibroblast cell line without affecting other responses of this growth factor, including induction of c-*fos* and ornithine decarboxylase activity (Chambard & Pouysségur, 1988). Other examples of indirect growth inhibitory effects of

TGF-β include the down-regulation of PDGF receptors in smooth muscle cells and fibroblasts (Battegay et al., 1990; Paulsson et al., 1993), EGF and basic fibroblast growth factor receptors on endothelial and osteosarcoma cells (Takehara et al., 1987; Mioh & Chen, 1989) and interleukin-1 receptors on hematopoietic cells (Dubois et al., 1990).

The direct antiproliferative effect of TGF-β has been best evaluated in epithelial cells. Analysis of synchronized cells has revealed that the TGF-β induced inhibition of proliferation occurs rapidly and results in a cell cycle arrest late in the G_1 phase (Howe et al., 1991; Paulsson et al., 1993).

Analysis of the proliferative response of keratinocytes to TGF-β revealed a correlation between TGF-β–mediated growth inhibition and repression of endogenous c-*myc* expression in some cell lines. The subsequent determination that the effect of TGF-β on c-*myc* levels was transcriptional led to the functional identification of a 23-bp sequence in the c-*myc* promoter that was required for the TGF-β–mediated repression of transcription of c-*myc* and other genes (Pietenpol et al., 1990, 1991). Thus, it is possible that, at least in some cell lines, DNA-binding proteins that specifically recognize this TGF-β response element may be involved in TGF-β–mediated growth inhibition. Conceivably, loss or mutation of such DNA-binding proteins may underlie the diminished cellular responsiveness of some tumour cells to the growth inhibitory effect of TGF-β, which is occasionally observed with cells of enhanced malignancy. In some colon carcinoma cell lines, there is an association between growth inhibition by TGF-β and decreased expression of c-*myc* (Mulder et al., 1990a; Mulder et al., 1990b). However, alternative mechanisms of TGF-β–mediated inhibition of proliferation must operate, since growth inhibition of pancreatic and gastric carcinoma cells by TGF-β was not accompanied by decreased c-*myc* mRNA levels (Baldwin & Korc, 1993; Ito et al., 1992).

Expression of the transforming proteins from three DNA tumour viruses – E7 from HPV-16 virus, E1A from adenovirus and large T antigen from the SV40 virus – can effectively block the inhibition of c-*myc* transcription by TGF-β, thereby abrogating its growth inhibitory effect (Pietenpol et al., 1990). These proteins bind to critical growth regulatory cellular proteins that may themselves be involved in growth inhibition by TGF-β. A prominent example is the retinoblastoma gene product pRB. During the cell cycle, pRB undergoes phosphorylation and dephosphorylation, with the underphosphorylated form predominating in the G_1 phase (DeCaprio et al., 1989; Sherr, 1994). In these cells, the antiproliferative effect of TGF-β on epithelial cells was associated with decreased pRB phosphorylation, suggesting the possibility that TGF-β induces or stabilizes the hypophosphorylation of pRB, which in turn mediates inhibition of cell proliferation (Laiho et al., 1990). Thus, association of transforming proteins such as those listed above with pRB, resulting in inactivation or alteration of its function, might block the growth inhibitory activity of TGF-β in various tumour cell types.

In an analogous manner, nuclear factors other than pRB have been implicated in the growth regulatory response to TGF-β (Missero et al., 1991). This was anticipated with the reports of cell lines that lacked functional pRB yet retained sensitivity to the growth inhibitory effect of TGF-β (Ong et al., 1991). The p53 recessive oncogene is a candidate alternative mediator of growth inhibition by TGF-β for some cells. Recently, two groups have reported loss of cellular responsiveness to the growth inhibitory effect of TGF-β upon expression of mutant forms of p53 (Gerwin et al., 1992; Reiss et al., 1993). Similarly, the loss of function within colon cancer cells of another tumour suppressor gene product, DCC (for Deleted in Colorectal Cancer), may be involved in their acquired resistance to TGF-β (Goyette et al., 1992).

Recent characterization of multiple components of cell cycle regulatory machinery have facilitated the identification of important genes whose expression or function is affected by TGF-β. Thus, the effect of TGF-β on various cyclins and cyclin-dependent kinases has been evaluated. Analysis of human keratinocytes synchronized by serum deprivation identified cyclin E as one of the earliest and most completely repressed genes thus far reported (Geng & Weinberg, 1993). Furthermore, in these cells, serum-induced increases in mRNA levels for cyclin A, cyclin-dependent kinase 2 and cyclin-dependent kinase 4 were inhibited by TGF-β as well. Using a different epithelial cell line, other investigators confirmed that TGF-β down-regulated expression of cyclin-dependent kinase 4 (Ewen et al., 1993). Constitutive expression of this kinase conferred resistance to TGF-β in transfected cells, thus directly implicating cyclin-dependent kinase 4 in the TGF-β–induced growth inhibition (Ewen et al., 1993). In both studies, expression of cyclin D was unaffected by TGF-β (Geng & Weinberg, 1993; Ewen et al., 1993). Using differently synchronized cells, Koff et al. (1993) observed a diminished capacity of cyclin E and cyclin-dependent kinase 2 to assemble into functional complexes, even though the individual proteins were present in normal amounts (Koff et al., 1993). Finally, TGF-β has been reported to induce down-regulation of cyclin A expression as well (Geng & Weinberg, 1993; Landesman et al., 1992; Ralph et al., 1993). How TGF-β induces these changes in cyclins and cyclin-dependent kinases and whether these alterations are a direct consequence of the activity of TGF-β or a result of the stage-specific growth arrest at late G_1, is the subject of intense studies.

In addition to its effects on the cell cycle and consequent modulation of cell proliferation, TGF-β profoundly affects the cellular interactions with the surrounding extracellular matrix and/or basement membrane. Indeed, TGF-β is a potent inducer of expression of many components of the extracellular matrix, such as collagens, fibronectin, tenascin, thrombospondin, and proteoglycans (Ignotz et al. 1987; Laiho et al. 1991a). Thus, TGF-β treatment results in increased deposition of extracellular matrix components. Concomitantly, TGF-β also strongly alters the expression levels of proteases, gelatinases, and their respective protein inhibitors (Kawamata et al. 1993). Most frequently, the protease expression is decreased whereas the protease inhibitor expression is upregulated, resulting in a decreased extracellular matrix degradation. In addition, TGF-β treatment frequently increases the expression of some integrins, which is presumably at the basis of TGF-β-induced increase in cellular adhesion to the substrate. These alterations in interactions of the cell with the extracellular matrix, mediated through integrin-mediated signalling may affect gene expression and play a role in cellular differentiation (Damsky and Werb, 1992). The net effect of TGF-β on these parameters may vary, depending on the cells under study. For instance, Samuel et al. (1992) compared the effects of TGF-β in a *ras*-transformed fibrosarcoma cell line and its nontransformed parental fibroblast line. In the transformed cells, TGF-β treatment resulted in increased expression of collagenase IV and procathepsin L mRNA, whereas the expression of these genes was slightly downregulated by TGF-β in the nontransformed parental cells (Samuel et al. 1992). The modulation of the interactions of the cell with the extracellular matrix may be of particular relevance for the invasive and metastatic behaviour of the tumour cells. In this context, TGF-β treatment has been shown to result in increased invasion of extracellular matrix (Mukai et al., 1989; Welch et al., 1990; Mooradian et al., 1992).

Another aspect of the many biological activities of TGF-β that could be of major relevance for tumour development in vivo is the effect of TGF-β on the immune response. TGF-β is an extremely potent regulator of immune cell function of several effector cell types (for a review, see Ruscetti et al., 1993). Since many of the immunological response parameters affected by TGF-β depend upon cell proliferation, the inhibitory effect of TGF-β on cell cycle progression may form the basis for many of the immunosuppressive activities of TGF-β. In this category we include TGF-β–mediated inhibition of cytotoxic T cells, lymphokine-activated killer cells, and natural killer (NK) cells.

In addition, TGF-β inhibits the production and/or counteracts the actions of a wide range of cytokines, including interferon-γ, tumour necrosis factors-α and -β and various interleukins. It is thus conceivable that TGF-β inhibits immune surveillance and the immune response to established tumours, thus stimulating tumour development in vivo. Evidence that the immunosuppressive effect of TGF-β may provide an advantage to the development of the malignancy has been provided by several studies (Torre-Amione et al., 1990; Hirte & Clark, 1991; Horst et al., 1992; Inge et al., 1992; Ruffini et al., 1993; Chang et al., 1993; Arteaga et al., 1993).

Also of potential importance to tumour development in vivo is the potent chemotactic activity of TGF-β on several cell types, especially monocytes and fibroblasts. The influx of these cells into the site of tumour formation combined with subsequent macrophage activation that results in release of various growth factors, may result not only in a better environment for tumour cell proliferation but could also increase the fibrosis of many solid tumours. The chemotactic activity of TGF-β could also play a role in tumour-induced angiogenesis. Angiogenesis, the formation of new blood vessels, represents the net result of a complex sequence of interactions between cells and their surrounding environment and is a prerequisite for the development and viability of the tumour mass. The ability of some tumours to induce the formation of new blood vessels is a critical talent of metastatic variants. Indeed, quantitative assessment of the number of new capillary buds in tumours may be of significant prognostic value in breast and prostate cancer (Weidner et al., 1991; Van Hoef et al., 1993; Weidner et al., 1993). In some experimental models, TGF-β has demonstrated proangiogenic activity (Roberts et al., 1986; Yang & Moses, 1990; Pepper et al., 1993) and augmentation of TGF-β production by a tumour cell line can increase its angiogenic prowess (Ueki et al., 1992). It is as yet unclear exactly how TGF-β influences angiogenesis. In some settings, mitogenic stimulation of a subset of capillary endothelial cells appears to play a role (Iruela-Arispe & Sage, 1993) even though TGF-β inhibits the proliferation of endothelial cells in culture. In other settings, the chemotactic activity of TGF-β, which causes an influx of macrophages and stromal cells and formation of capillaries, lies at the heart of TGF-β–mediated angiogenesis. The presence of other growth factors that stimulate endothelial cell proliferation and capillary formation, such as fibroblast growth factor, can greatly augment the angiogenic effect of TGF-β (Pepper et al., 1990; Gajdusek et al., 1993).

Our survey of the potential role played by TGF-β in tumours would be incomplete without mention of observations linking TGF-β

expression to apoptosis, whether it be induced by hormone withdrawal, chemotherapy or TGF-β itself (Armstrong et al., 1992; Lin & Chou, 1992; Yanagihara & Tsumuraya, 1992; Taetle et al., 1993; Jurgensmeier et al., 1994). It remains to be determined whether TGF-β is directly involved in the molecular events that constitute apoptosis, or represents a cellular response to (or resistance mechanism against) cell death.

Based on the multiple activities of TGF-β on tumour cells and tumour development, it is understandable that the net effect of TGF-β on such complex phenomena as carcinogenesis and metastatic spread is difficult to predict. In some tumour systems, a selective loss of the growth inhibitory effect of TGF-β may underlie malignant progression. In such settings, the immunosuppressive and/or proangiogenic activities of TGF-β may play a determining role. Examples of increased tumourigenesis and/or metastasis correlating with diminished sensitivity to the growth inhibitory effects of TGF-β include bladder cancer (Kawamata et al., 1993), colon cancer (Manning et al., 1991), transformed rat tracheal epithelial cells (Hubbs et al., 1989; Steigerwalt et al., 1992), transformed fibroblasts (Schwarz et al., 1990) and melanoma cells (Rodeck, 1993; Mooradian et al., 1990; Blanckaert et al., 1993). However, loss of responsiveness to the antiproliferative effect of TGF-β does not necessarily result in loss of sensitivity to its other activities; thus, such tumour cells may retain responsiveness to some nonproliferation-related activities of TGF-β (Rundhaug et al., 1992; Zentella et al., 1991).

It is clear from the above considerations that the extent to which an established tumour elaborates and activates TGF-β may play a pivotal role in determining the outcome of the host–tumour interaction and the resulting cancer development. This would not negate the possibility that, during the early steps of cancer formation, TGF-β could act predominantly in an anticarcinogenic mode as an inhibitor of proliferation. Indeed, the targeted overexpression of TGF-β in the mammary glands of female transgenic mice not only yielded no increase in the rate of spontaneous tumour formation (Pierce et al., 1993) but also served to counteract the development of oncogene- and carcinogen-induced mammary cancers (H.L. Moses, personal communication). Another recently reported direct demonstration of the ability of endogenous TGF-β to suppress malignant progression comes from studies in which keratinocytes derived from transgenic mice homozygous for a targeted TGF-β1 gene deletion were transformed with the v-Ha-*ras* oncogene and found to produce squamous carcinomas, whereas similar *ras*-mediated transformation of keratinocytes from normal mice formed papillomas only (Glick et al., 1994).

REGULATION OF EXPRESSION OF TGF-β BY TUMOUR CELLS

The TGF-β homodimer is synthesized as a precursor protein in which the C-terminal mature polypeptide sequence is preceded by a much larger precursor segment. TGF-β is typically secreted from cells as a latent or biologically inactive complex that is unable to bind to TGF-β receptors. In this complex, the active TGF-β dimer is non-covalently associated with two copies of the precursor segment and frequently with a fifth protein component, the latent TGF-β binding protein. Thus, latent TGF-β secretion by tumour cells may be without biological consequence unless this complex is activated, either by the tumour cells themselves or the surrounding target cells. Only then will TGF-β be able to interact with the receptors and exert its biological activities in an autocrine or paracrine fashion. Thus, in addition to changes in protein expression as a consequence of transcriptional and translational regulation, the liberation of active TGF-β from its latent complex is a potential mode of regulation.

Many studies have quantitated the secretion of TGF-β by tumour cell lines and its activation state in vitro. Based on a survey of tumour tissues and cell lines, endogenous TGF-β1 expression appears to be up-regulated in tumours both in vitro and in vivo (Derynck et al., 1987; Gomella et al., 1989; Ito et al., 1991; Travers et al., 1988). The TGF-β released by tumour cells into the medium is often mostly in the latent form, but, in various cases, a significant fraction of secreted TGF-β is in the active state (Schwarz et al., 1990; Jennings et al., 1991; Constam et al., 1992; Lokeshwar & Block, 1992). Two groups studying hormonally responsive breast cancer cell lines have reported that the proportion of secreted TGF-β in the active state was altered significantly by hormonal treatments (Knabbe et al., 1987; Colletta et al., 1990; Colletta et al., 1991). The mechanism responsible for activation of the latent TGF-β complex is presumably based on the degradation of the precursor segments by specific proteases. Indeed, latent TGF-β1 can be converted into active TGF-β1 using plasmin or cathepsins which proteolyse the precursor segments and, in this way, release active TGF-β from its complex. In addition, co-culturing of endothelial cells and smooth muscle cells or pericytes results in a significant activation of the secreted TGF-β, which is due to plasmin activity, in turn induced by plasminogen activator. This process can also be blocked by antibodies against the cell surface mannose-6-phosphate receptors, indicative that the activation occurs at the cell surface. These observations and the synthesis and release of plasminogen activators and cathepsins by many tumour cells thus suggests the involvement of these proteases in the generation of active TGF-β by the tumour cells. Furthermore, the dissimilarity between the precursor sequences of the TGF-β isoforms suggests that different proteases or physiological conditions may be required for activation of the three TGF-β species. An intriguing suggestion that some cells are capable of isoform-specific activation of TGF-β has been provided by studies showing that the prostate carcinoma cell line PC3 could be induced to activate TGF-β2 but not TGF-β1 following exposure to cyclic adenosine monophosphate (AMP) analog (Bang et al., 1992). Clearly, much remains to be determined regarding the mechanisms used by tumour cells to activate TGF-β isoforms from their latent complexes.

The percentage of active TGF-β in conditioned media of tumour cells may not accurately reflect the full magnitude of the effect of TGF-β on cells. Indeed, activation of latent TGF-β by cells is associated with the cell surface (Antonelli-Orlidge et al., 1989; Sato et al., 1990), suggesting that release of significant levels of active TGF-β in the surrounding medium is not necessarily a consequence of the cell surface activation of TGF-β by the target cell. In support of this hypothesis, in two cell systems, cells overexpressing latent TGF-β1 as a result of transfection with a cDNA expression plasmid have been found to exhibit characteristics typical of cells exposed to active TGF-β (Arrick et al., 1992; Beauchamp et al., 1992).

Genes that encode the TGF-β isomers are located on separate chromosomes, and exhibit distinct patterns of transcriptional regulation. As yet, little is known about the complexity of the transcriptional regulation, but a comparison of the promoter regions for the three TGF-β species and their predicted regulatory sequences strongly suggests a complex transcriptional regulation distinct for each TGF-β isoform (Kim et al., 1989; O'Reilly et al., 1992; Lafyatis et al., 1990; Geiser et al., 1993). This has been illustrated by, for example, the marked induction of TGF-β2 but not TGF-β1 mRNA synthesis by retinoic acid (Glick et al., 1989). Also, oestrogen down-regulates TGF-β2 and TGF-β3 mRNA, but has no effect on TGF-β1 mRNA levels (Arrick et al., 1990). Finally, treatment of cells by TGF-β itself can differentially affect the expression of the three TGF-β isoforms, leading to an induction of TGF-β1 and a down-regulation of TGF-β2 and -β3 mRNA expression (Bascom et al., 1989). Examination of tissue expression patterns has confirmed the hypothesis that distinct regulatory controls determine the temporal and spatial production of the TGF-β isoforms, especially during development (Pelton et al., 1990; Flanders et al., 1991; Roberts & Sporn, 1992).

All three TGF-β genes encode mRNA transcripts with uncommonly long 5′ noncoding regions, ranging from 840 nucleotides in full-length TGF-β1 mRNA to 1.35 and 1.1 kb in the mRNAs for TGF-β2 and -β3, respectively (Kim et al., 1989; Noma et al., 1991; Lafyatis et al., 1990; Arrick et al., 1991). In addition, the 5′ noncoding region of the TGF-β3 mRNA contains 11 upstream AUG triplet sequences that may initiate short reading frames. These features stand in sharp contrast with most other mRNAs, which contain short 5′ untranslated regions lacking upstream AUGs (Kozak, 1987), and strongly suggest a regulation or attenuation of translation of these TGF-β proteins. In accordance with the scanning model for the initiation of mRNA translation (Kozak, 1989), the mRNAs for TGF-β1 and -β3 have been shown to be inefficiently translated (Kim et al., 1992; Arrick et al., 1991). It is possible that altered translational regulation may result in increased TGF-β secretion. This mechanism may in part be responsible for the increased TGF-β secretion in breast cancer cells following various hormonal treatments (Knabbe et al., 1987; Colletta et al., 1991).

One possible mechanism by which cells might increase production of TGF-β is to generate an mRNA transcript with a truncated 5′ noncoding region, which would have a much higher translation efficiency than the one with the long untranslated region. Indeed, the gene for TGF-β1 has two promoters. The 3′ most promoter can initiate transcription within the sequence which serves as 5′ noncoding sequence, when transcription is initiated from the upstream promoter, thereby generating a 5′ truncated transcript. The translational efficiency of the latter mRNA is expected to be considerably higher, since the 5′ untranslated region is not only much shorter but also lacks a very stable hairpin loop, which is present in the 5′ untranslated region of the longer mRNA and plays a major role in its translational repression (Kim et al., 1992; Romeo et al., 1993). An analogous situation may occur for TGF-β3 in many breast cancer cell lines, which produce a 5′ truncated TGF-β3 mRNA transcript that is more actively engaged in translation (Arrick et al., 1994). Interestingly, the downstream promoter that functions to produce the 5′ truncated TGF-β3 transcript in breast cancer cells has not been shown to be active in any other cell type. Thus, enhanced translational efficiency, which could be achieved by downstream transcription into an mRNA with a shorter 5′ noncoding region or by other regulatory mechanisms, may result in increased TGF-β production by tumour cells.

RESPONSIVENESS OF THE DEVELOPING TUMOUR TO TGF-β

The synthesis and secretion of endogenous TGF-β by tumour cells has autocrine action and paracrine effects. In this way, tumour-derived TGF-β can stimulate fibroblast proliferation, stroma formation, extracellular matrix deposition and angiogenesis, as well as inhibit the local immune response. To evaluate the autocrine responsiveness of the tumour cells to its TGF-β synthesis, numerous studies have measured the effect on proliferation of the tumour cells in vitro. Whereas many tumour cell lines are stimulated or inhibited in their proliferation by TGF-β, a lack of sensitivity to the growth modulatory effects of TGF-β is often seen. Thus, many carcinomas are resistant to the antiproliferative effect of TGF-β, in contrast to untransformed epithelial cells. This resistance to the growth modulatory effects of TGF-β is often considered as a general unresponsiveness of these cells to TGF-β, even though other responses to TGF-β such as the changes in cell-matrix interactions and extracellular matrix production are maintained (Laiho et al., 1991, Arrick et al., 1992). Indeed, inactivation of the growth inhibitory effect of TGF-β either spontaneously or by functional inactivation of pRB or the type II receptor-mediated signaling pathway does not decrease the cellular responses related to cell-matrix interactions and extracellular matrix production (Laiho et al., 1991, Arrick et al., 1992, Chen et al., 1993). As an example, the proliferation of 293 tumour cells in vitro is not affected by TGF-β, but TGF-β treatment induces increased fibronectin and extracellular matrix production and enhances adhesion to the culture substrate. Similarly, cells that are oncogenically transformed by Polyoma middle T, SV40 large T or adenovirus E1A proteins are still responsive to TGF-β by inducing the synthesis of c-*jun*, the protease inhibitor PAI-1 and fibronectin, yet are not affected in their proliferation rate in culture. The selective loss of the antiproliferative response to TGF-β may be considered as a contributory step in the progression of cells towards autonomous growth and a full malignant phenotype (Hubbs et al., 1989; Wakefield and Sporn, 1990; Haddow et al., 1991; Manning et al., 1991).

To further evaluate the responsiveness of tumour cells to TGF-β, the levels of cell surface TGF-β receptor expression has been evaluated using chemical crosslinking of radiolabelled TGF-β to cells, followed by gel electrophoretic analysis of the cross-linked products. Our current understanding of the biology of the TGF-β receptors is as yet minimal and it is only recently that cDNAs for the most common types of the TGF-β receptors have been cloned, thus allowing the prediction of their polypeptide structures. Using radioiodinated TGF-β1 as ligand, most normal and tumour cells have been shown to contain surface proteins that have been classified based on their size by gel electrophoresis after ligand crosslinking (reviewed by Lin & Lodish, 1993; Derynck, 1994). The three best characterized, and perhaps most widely expressed TGF-β receptors, are known as types I, II and III receptors, of which types I and II are thought to mediate most of the activities of TGF-β (Laiho, Weis et al., 1991; Geiser et al., 1992; Chen et al., 1993). The type III receptor, also referred to as betaglycan, is a large (280–330 kDa) transmembrane proteoglycan that exhibits no known signalling motif within its short cytoplasmic portion. Possible insight into the function of this protein, and its homologue endoglin, derives from the observation that expression of the type III receptor in cells that also expressed types I and II receptors enhances the binding of TGF-β to the type II receptor (López-Casillas et al., 1991; Wang et al., 1991; López-Casillas et al., 1993; Moustakas et al., 1993).

Both the type II and type I TGF-β receptors are transmembrane serine-threonine kinases (Lin et al., 1992). These receptors have a short extracellular domain, rich in cysteines, and a long cytoplasmic domain, which largely consists of the kinase domains. Mutation analysis has indicated that, at least in the case of the type II receptor, the kinase function is essential for signal transduction and biological activity (Wrana et al., 1992). Several type I receptors have been cloned and shown to bind TGF-β. Interestingly, these receptors do not have the ability to bind TGF-β by themselves but require co-expression of the type II receptor for efficient TGF-β binding (Ebner et al., 1993; Franzen et al., 1993; Bassing et al., 1994). The required co-expression of the type II receptor for cell surface transport and/or TGF-β binding to the type I receptor is consistent with observations in mutant cell lines that the type II receptor can rescue cell surface binding to the type I receptor (Wrana et al., 1992; Inagaki et al., 1993). Furthermore, when these type I receptors are co-expressed with the type II activin receptor, they can bind activin as well, suggesting that the type II receptor determines ligand specificity and binding properties of the type I receptor. Finally, co-immunoprecipitation analysis has indicated that the type I and type II receptors can physically associate.

The possible functional interdependence between type II and type I receptors for functional deployment at the cell surface has complicated the determination of their specific roles in TGF-β's many activities. Whereas both receptor types are required for the complete spectrum of biological activities of TGF-β, it is likely that two signalling pathways exist in association with these receptors. A functional type II receptor is required for the antiproliferative effect of TGF-β (Wrana et al., 1992; Chen et al., 1993; Ebner et al., 1993; Inagaki et al., 1993; Brand et al., 1993; Wieser et al., 1993). However, overexpression of a truncated type II receptor, which functions as a dominant negative mutant, abolishes the antiproliferative effect of TGF-β, but suggests that signalling through the type II receptor is not required for the induction of expression of several genes by TGF-β (Chen et al., 1993). The dissociation of the antiproliferative response from other effects of TGF-β in tumour cells suggests that this may be the case. Further work is required to define the respective roles of these two receptor types and the exact nature of the functional receptor complexes, as well as the physical and physiological interactions of the types I, II and III receptors at the cell surface. The ability of several type I receptors, which are structurally closely related, to bind TGF-β further complicates the analysis of the functional role of these receptors. However, only one of these type I receptors has been shown to restore biological responsiveness in receptor-deficient cells (Franzén et al., 1993). Unfortunately, the limited availability of model systems greatly hampers the demonstration of the ability of these type I receptors to mediate the diversity of biological activities of TGF-β in different cell contexts.

The recent cDNA characterization of the receptors has as yet precluded an analysis of the involvement of TGF-β receptor signalling in tumour cells. So far, the analysis of the receptors in tumour cells has been largely limited to a determination of the different receptor types at the cell surface. From these analyses, no correlation is apparent between the cell surface expression and availability of the receptors and the responsiveness of the tumour cells. Thus, the lack of the antiproliferative response to TGF-β in tumour cells does not consistently correlate with a decreased expression or loss of type II receptors or any alterations in the receptor profile. These findings suggest that malignant transformation may not necessarily affect receptor expression, but have downstream intracellular effects and this is consistent with our current understanding of the deregulation of tyrosine kinase receptor signalling and growth control in tumour cells. Without any doubt, much progress will be made in the elucidation of the TGF-β signalling both in normal and tumour cells during the next few years.

TGF-β AND CANCER: THE EVIDENCE

As illustrated above, the different biological activities of TGF-β on normal and tumour cells suggest a number of potential ways in which this factor might affect the biology and behaviour of tumours. Based on these considerations, various in vivo tumour studies have been developed to evaluate the effect of alterations in TGF-β expression on tumour development. This section will review the evidence that TGF-β can be an important factor in malignant progression.

Based on its antiproliferative effect on a variety of tumour cells, TGF-β could function as an autocrine negative growth regulator of tumour growth. Most of the evidence for this possible role is derived from in vitro experiments in which exogenous TGF-β inhibits the growth rate. Accordingly, the proliferation of tumour cells can be increased in the presence of neutralizing anti–TGF-β antibody. Three recent examples are lymphoma, sarcoma and ovarian cancer (Newcom et al., 1992; Berchuck et al., 1992; Chang et al., 1993). In addition, it is possible that the effect of tamoxifen on hormonally responsive breast cancer cell lines may in part reflect the autocrine growth inhibitory effects of increased TGF-β synthesis.

It is, however, the case for most locally acting factors that experimental data based solely on the exogenous administration of purified factor or neutralizing antibody can only approximate the in vivo situation. Even more caution with such extrapolations has to be applied for TGF-β, considering its wide diversity of autocrine and paracrine effects, the possible importance of cell-associated activation of the latent complex and its potential for functional interactions with other cytokines. For these reasons, various studies have addressed the role of TGF-β in tumour development using in vivo tumourigenicity assays in which mice are inoculated with tumour cells transfected with TGF-β expression plasmids.

Two of the first reports using this approach yielded different conclusions, although the differences may be ascribed to the use of two different model systems. Wu et al. (1992) transfected a colon carcinoma cell line, normally inhibited in its proliferation by TGF-β, with an expression vector for TGF-β1–specific antisense RNA. This transfection resulted in reduced expression of TGF-β and the stably transfected cells showed enhanced growth both in vitro in culture and as tumours in nude mice. These results thus suggested a growth inhibitory role for endogenous TGF-β in accordance with the in vitro results. In contrast, Steiner and Barrack transfected a rat prostate cancer cell line, itself growth inhibited in culture by TGF-β, with a TGF-β1 cDNA expression plasmid that directed the production of increased amounts of latent TGF-β. Transfected cells, despite demonstrating a somewhat decreased growth in vitro, formed larger tumours in rats and metastasized more frequently to the lung and lymph nodes. In both studies, it was hard to evaluate the respective contributions of the direct growth modulatory effects and the other autocrine and paracrine activities of TGF-β. We therefore studied the effects of increased endogenous TGF-β1 expression of tumourigenicity using 293 cells that are unresponsive to growth regulation by TGF-β. Their lack of growth inhibition by TGF-β is presumably due to the expression of the adenovirus E1A protein, which inactivates the retinoblastoma susceptibility gene. Transfection with a modified TGF-β1 expression plasmid, which led to secretion of active TGF-β1, resulted in increased tumourigenicity and tumour growth, even though there was no effect on tumour cell growth in vitro. No differences between the histology of the tumours from the parent and transfected cells were apparent (Arrick et al., 1992).

Based on our current knowledge, increased tumourigenesis as a consequence of increased endogenous TGF-β synthesis does not relate to the growth modulatory effects of TGF-β on these tumour cells. Instead, the increased adhesiveness and matrix formation of tumour cells may be important by creating an environment that is more permissive for tumour cell proliferation. Thus, increased extracellular matrix formation and stroma formation may provide an advantage to the tumour cells. In this context, Ueki et al. (1993) have reported that transfected Chinese hamster ovary cells overexpressing TGF-β1 exhibited a notable increase in angiogenesis and were more metastatic. Furthermore, the local immunosuppressive effect of TGF-β released by tumour cells may also support tumour development (Torre-Amione et al., 1990). This would be consistent with the decrease in NK cell activity in the presence of TGF-β (Arteaga et al., 1993) and may help explain why even tumour cells that are growth inhibited by TGF-β in culture are much more tumourigenic when their TGF-β expression is increased following transfection (Chang et al., 1993). Finally, an interconnection between endogenous TGF-β expression and hormonal dependence of breast cancer has been suggested by the finding that overexpression of TGF-β1 in the otherwise estrogen-dependent MCF7 cell line led to hormone-independent tumour formation in ovariectomized nude mice (Arteaga et al., 1993). In summary, the current evidence suggests that increased TGF-β expression may provide an advantage to tumour development, even though in vitro data may be indicative of an antiproliferative effect of TGF-β.

Based on the findings summarized above, it is conceivable that there may be a correlation between the level of TGF-β1 expression and the development and prognosis of the cancer in patients. However, the analysis of clinical specimens has provided only some suggestive information; these studies are limited by intratissue heterogeneity as well as interpatient variability. A number of investigators have examined expression of TGF-β by breast cancers to determine if any association with clinical outcome was evident. Some reports have suggested that increased expression of TGF-β correlated with more aggressive disease (Walker & Dearing, 1992; Gorsch et al., 1992; Dalal et al., 1993), whereas others observed the opposite association (Mizukami et al., 1990; Murray et al., 1993). Using a similar type of analysis, increased expression of TGF-β isoforms by pancreatic cancer has been reported to correlate with poor clinical outcome (Friess et al., 1993).

CONCLUSION

The TGF-β system of ligands and receptors represents a highly complex and versatile cytokine network. Many of the multiple activities of TGF-β bear directly on critical stages of tumour formation, local invasion and distant spread. The impact of TGF-β on tumour development in any given circumstance depends on multiple factors, including the nature of the cell types involved, the complexity of the cell surface TGF-β receptor population and the intracellular regulation of the signal transduction pathways involved in the sensitivity of the tumour cells to TGF-β, and the presence of other cytokines. Thus, generalizations concerning the endogenous role of TGF-β in cancer development and metastasis should only be made with caution. Accordingly, the desirability of specific pharmacological manipulations of TGF-β either to prevent cancer development or to treat an established tumour, cannot be assessed with certainty without further study. As an example, the net effect of localized production of TGF-β in mammary tissue may be an inhibition of carcinogenesis or a decreased preinvasive growth of malignant cells. Once breast cancer cells cease to be responsive to the growth inhibitory effect of TGF-β, however, the other activities of TGF-β may come to the fore, serving to promote angiogenesis, tissue invasion and immunosuppression. Considering the autocrine and paracrine nature of TGF-β action, in vivo models are best suited to address these important issues.

In recent years, observations from many laboratories have provided examples in which no one TGF-β–related effect, but rather a composite of multiple activities is important. Given that potentially distinct signal transduction pathways mediate different TGF-β responses, it is understandable, perhaps likely, that some mutations within those pathways – for example, mutations affecting the TGF-β receptors or distinct downstream signalling events – might tip the balance in favor of tumour growth and malignant progression. A loss of function mutation of this sort might thereby identify a candidate tumour suppressor gene. Such a mutation might best be sought by studying highly malignant tumours that produce high levels of TGF-β, are not growth inhibited by this factor and contain normal p53 and pRB activity.

Clinical studies that further evaluate the prognostic value of the expression level of TGF-β in a tumour should be pursued, ideally within the context of a clinical therapeutic trial so that the effect of therapy on the clinical outcome can be monitored. In addition, if we can determine the molecular mechanisms that underlie these clinical correlations, we might be able to construct rational therapeutic strategies. For instance, if TGF-β–induced angiogenesis is a major contributor to a particular tumour's malignant behaviour, then the clinical use of inhibitors of angiogenesis may limit tumour growth.

Finally, the effects of TGF-β on cells of the immune system suggest potential implications for immunotherapy. In certain circumstances, the production of TGF-β by the tumour, or in the case of adoptive immunotherapy the autocrine TGF-β activity level within the effector cells, may be a critical and potentially manipulatable determinant of clinical outcome.

REFERENCES

Antonelli-Orlidge A., Saunders K.B., Smith S.R. & D'Amore P.A. (1989) An activated form of transforming growth factor β is produced by cocultures of endothelial cells and pericytes. *Proceedings of the National Academy of Sciences of the United States of America*, **86**, 4544–8.

Anzano M.A., Roberts A.B., Smith J.M., Sporn M.B. & DeLarco J.E. (1983) Sarcoma growth factor from conditioned medium is composed of both type alpha and type beta transforming growth factors. *Proceedings of the National Academy of Sciences of the United States of America*, **80**, 6264–8.

Armstrong D.K., Isaacs J.T., Ottaviano Y.L. & Davidson N.E. (1992) Programmed cell death in an estrogen-independent human breast cancer cell line, MDA-MB-468. *Cancer Research*, **52**, 3418–24.

Arrick B.A. & Derynck R. (1993) Growth-regulation by transforming growth factor-β. In Benz C. & Liu E.T., (Eds.) *Oncogenes and Tumor Suppressor Genes in Human Malignancies*, pp. 255–64. Kluwer Academic Publishers, Boston.

Arrick B.A., Grendell R.L. & Griffin L.A. (1994) Enhanced translational efficiency of a novel transforming growth factor-β3 mRNA in human breast cancer cells. *Molecular and Cellular Biology*, **14**, 619–28.

Arrick B.A., Korc M. & Derynck R. (1990) Differential regulation of expression of three transforming growth factor β species in human breast cancer cell lines by estradiol. *Cancer Research*, **50**, 299–303.

Arrick B.A., Lee A.L., Grendell R.L. & Derynck R. (1991) Inhibition of translation of transforming growth factor-β3 mRNA by its 5′ untranslated region. *Molecular and Cellular Biology*, **11**, 4306–13.

Arrick B.A., Lopez A.R., Elfman F., Ebner R., Damsky C.H. & Derynck R. (1992) Altered metabolic and adhesive properties and increased tumorigenesis associated with increased expression of transforming growth factor β1. *Journal of Cell Biology*, **118**, 715–26.

Arteaga C.L., Carty-Dugger T., Moses H.L., Hurd S.D. & Pietenpol J.A. (1993) Transforming growth factor β1 can induce estrogen-independent tumorigenicity of human breast cancer cells in athymic mice. *Cell Growth and Differentiation*, **4**, 193–201.

Arteaga C.L., Hurd S.D., Winnier A.R., Johnson M.D., Fendly B.M. & Forbes J.T. (1993) Antitransforming growth factor (TGF)-β1 antibodies inhibit breast cancer cell tumorigenicity and increase mouse spleen natural killer cell activity. *Journal of Clinical Investigation,* **92**, 2569–76.

Assoian R.K., Frolik C.A., Roberts A.B., Miller D.M. & Sporn M.B. (1984) Transforming growth factor beta controls receptor levels for epidermal growth factor in NRK fibroblasts. *Cell,* **36**, 35–41.

Baldwin R.L. & Korc M. (1993) Growth inhibition of human pancreatic carcinoma cells by transforming growth factor beta-1. *Growth Factors* **8**, 22–34.

Bang Y.-J., Kim S.-J., Danielpour D. et al. (1992) Cyclic AMP induces transforming growth factor β2 gene expression and growth arrest in the human androgen-independent prostate carcinoma cell line PC-3. *Proceedings of the National Academy of Sciences of the United States of America,* **89**, 3556–60.

Barnard J.A., Lyons R.M. & Moses H.L. (1990) The cell biology of transforming growth factor β. *Biochimica et Biophysica Acta Reviews of Cancer,* **1032**, 79–87.

Bascom C.C., Wolfshohl J.R., Coffey R.J., Jr. et al. (1989) Complex regulation of transforming growth factor β1, β2, and β3 mRNA expression in mouse fibroblasts and keratinocytes by transforming growth factors β1 and *b*2. *Molecular and Cellular Biology,* **9**, 5508–15.

Bassing C.H., Yingling J.M., Howe D.J., Wang T., He W.W., Gustafson M.L., Shah P., Donahoe P.K. & Wang X.-F. (1994) A transforming growth factor β type I receptor that signals to activate gene expression. *Science,* **263**, 87–9.

Battegay E.J., Raines E.W., Seifert R.A., Bowen-Pope D.F. & Ross R. (1990) TGF-β induces bimodal proliferation of connective tissue cells via complex control of an autocrine PDGF loop. *Cell,* **63**, 515–24.

Beauchamp R.D., Sheng H.-M., Bascom C.C. et al. (1992) Phenotypic alterations in fibroblasts and fibrosarcoma cells that overexpress latent transforming growth factor-β1. *Endocrinology,* **130**, 2476–86.

Berchuck A., Rodriguez G., Olt G. et al. (1992) Regulation of growth of normal ovarian epithelial cells and ovarian cancer cell lines by transforming growth factor-β. *American Journal of Obstetrics and Gynecology,* **166**, 676–84.

Blanckaert V.D., Schelling M.E., Elstad C.A. & Meadows G.G. (1993) Differential growth factor production, secretion, and response by high and low metastatic variants of B16BL6 melanoma. *Cancer Research,* **53**, 4075–81.

Brand T., MacLellan W.R. & Schneider M.D. (1993) A dominant-negative receptor for type β transforming growth factors created by deletion of the kinase domain. *Journal of Biological Chemistry,* **268**, 11500–3.

Centrella M., McCarthy T.L. & Canalis E. (1987) Transforming growth factor β is a bifunctional regulator of replication and collagen synthesis in osteoblast-enriched cell cultures from fetal rat bone. *Journal of Biological Chemistry,* **262**, 2869–74.

Chambard J.-C. & Pouysségur J. (1988) TGF-β inhibits growth factor-induced DNA synthesis in hamster fibroblasts without affecting the early mitogenic events. *Journal of Cellular Physiology,* **135**, 101–7.

Chang H.-L., Gillett N., Figari I., Lopez A.R., Palladino M.A. & Derynck R. (1993) Increased transforming growth factor β inhibits cell proliferation *in vitro,* yet increases tumorigenicity and tumor growth of Meth A sarcoma cells. *Cancer Research,* **53**, 4391–8, 1993.

Chen R.-H., Ebner R. & Derynck R. (1993) Inactivation of the type II receptor reveals two receptor pathways for the diverse TGF-β activities. *Science*, **260**, 1335–8.

Colletta A.A., Wakefield L.M., Howell F.V., Danielpour D., Baum M. & Sporn M.B. (1991) The growth inhibition of human breast cancer cells by a novel synthetic progestin involves the induction of transforming growth factor beta. *Journal of Clinical Investigation*, **87**, 277–83.

Colletta A.A., Wakefield L.M., Howell F.V. et al. (1990) Anti-oestrogens induce the secretion of active transforming growth factor beta from human fetal fibroblasts. *British Journal of Cancer*, **62**, 405–9.

Constam D.B., Philipp J., Malipiero U.V., Ten Dijke P., Schachner M. & Fontana A. (1992) Differential expression of transforming growth factor-β1, -β2, and -β3 by glioblastoma cells, astrocytes, and microglia. *Journal of Immunology*, **148**, 1404–10.

Dalal B.I., Keown P.A. & Greenberg A.H. (1993) Immunocytochemical localization of secreted transforming growth factor-β_1 to the advancing edges of primary tumors and to lymph node metastases of human mammary carcinoma. *American Journal of Pathology*, **143**, 381–9.

Damsky C.H. & Werb Z. (1992) Signal transduction by integrin receptors for extracellular matrix: cooperative processing of extracellular information. *Current Opinion in Cell Biology*, **4**, 772–81.

DeCaprio J.A., Ludlow J.W., Lynch D. et al. (1989) The product of the retinoblastoma susceptibility gene has properties of a cell cycle regulatory element. *Cell*, **58**, 1085.

Derynck, R. (1992) The physiology of transforming growth factor-α. *Advances in Cancer Research*, **58**, 27–52.

Derynck, R. (1994) TGF-β receptor-mediated signaling. *Trends in Biochemical Sciences*, **19**, 548–553.

Derynck R, Lindquist P.B., Lee A. et al. (1988) A new type of transforming growth factor-β, TGF-β3. *EMBO Journal*, **7**, 3737–43.

Dubois C.M., Ruscetti F.W., Palaszynski E.W., Falk L.A., Oppenheim J.J. & Keller J.R. (1990) Transforming growth factor β is a potent inhibitor of interleukin 1 (IL-1) receptor expression: proposed mechanism of inhibition of IL-1 action. *Journal of Experimental Medicine*, **172**, 737–44.

Ebner R., Chen R.-H., Shum L. et al. (1993) Cloning of a type I TGF-β receptor and its effect on TGF-β binding to the type II receptor. *Science*, **260**, 1344–8.

Ewen M.E., Sluss H.K., Whitehouse L.L. & Livingston D.M. (1993) TGFβ inhibition of Cdk4 synthesis is linked to cell cycle arrest. *Cell*, **74**, 1009–20.

Flanders K.C., Ludecke G., Engels S. et al. (1991) Localization and actions of transforming growth factor-βs in the embryonic nervous system. *Development*, **113**, 183–91.

Franzén P., Ichijo H. & Miyazono K. (1993) Different signals mediate transforming growth factor-β1-induced growth inhibition and extracellular matrix production in prostatic carcinoma cells. *Experimental Cell Research*, **207**, 1–7.

Franzén P., ten Dijke P., Ichijo H. et al. (1993) Cloning of a TGFβ type I receptor that forms a heteromeric complex with the TGFβ type II receptor. *Cell*, **75**, 681–92.

Friess H., Yamanaka Y., Buchler M. et al. (1993) Enhanced expression of transforming growth factor-β isoforms in pancreatic cancer correlates with decreased survival. *Gastroenterology*, **105**, 1846–56.

Gajdusek C.M., Luo Z. & Mayberg M.R. (1993) Basic fibroblast growth factor and transforming growth factor beta-1: synergistic mediators of angiogenesis in vitro. *Journal of Cellular Physiology*, **157**, 133–44.

Geiser A.G., Burmester J.K., Webbink R., Roberts A.B. & Sporn M.B. (1992) Inhibition of growth by transforming growth factor-β following fusion of two nonresponsive human carcinoma cell lines. Implication of the type II receptor in growth inhibitory responses. *Journal of Biological Chemistry*, **267**, 2588–93.

Geiser A.G., Busam K.J., Kim S.-J. et al. (1993) Regulation of the transforming growth factor-β1 and -β3 promoters by transcription factor Sp1. *Gene*, **129**, 223–8.

Geng Y. & Weinberg R.A. (1993) Transforming growth factor β effects on expression of G_1 cyclins and cyclin-dependent protein kinases. *Proceedings of the National Academy of Sciences of the United States of America*, **90**, 10315–19.

Gerwin B.I., Spillare E., Forrester K. et al. (1992) Mutant p53 can induce tumorigenic conversion of human bronchial epithelial cells and reduce their responsiveness to a negative growth factor, transforming growth factor β_1. *Proceedings of the National Academy of Sciences of the United States of America*, **89**, 2759–63.

Glick A.B., Flanders K.C., Danielpour D., Yuspa S.H. & Sporn M.B. (1989) Retinoic acid induces transforming growth factor-β2 in cultured keratinocytes and mouse epidermis. *Cell Regulation*, **1**, 87–97.

Glick A.B., Lee M.M., Kulkarni A.B., Karlsson S. & Yuspa S.A. (1994) Rapid malignant progression of epidermal tumors derived from TGF-β1 null keratinocytes. *Proceedings of the American Association for Cancer Research*, **35**, 611.

Gorsch S.M., Memoli V.A., Stukel T.A., Gold L.I. & Arrick B.A. (1992) Immunohistochemical staining for transforming growth factor β_1 associates with disease progression in human breast cancer. *Cancer Research*, **52**, 6949–52.

Goyette M.C., Cho K., Fasching C.L. et al. (1992) Progression of colorectal cancer is associated with multiple tumor suppressor gene defects but inhibition of tumorigenicity is accomplished by correction of a single defect via chromosome transfer. *Molecular and Cellular Biology*, **12**, 1387–95.

Graycar J.L., Miller D.A., Arrick B.A., Lyons R.M., Moses H.L. & Derynck R. (1989) Human transforming growth factor-β3: Recombinant expression, purification, and biological activities in comparison with transforming growth factors-β1 and β2. *Molecular Endocrinology*, **3**, 1977–86.

Haddow S., Fowlis D.J., Parkinson K., Akhurst R.J. & Balmain A. (1991) Loss of growth control by TGF-β occurs at a late stage of mouse skin carcinogenesis and is independent of *ras* gene activation. *Oncogene*, **6**, 1465–70.

He W.W., Gustafson M.L., Hirobe S. & Donahoe P.K. (1993) Developmental expression of four novel serine/threonine kinase receptors homologous to the activin/transforming growth factor-β type II receptor family. *Developmental Dynamics*, **196**, 133–42.

Hirte H. & Clark D.A. (1991) Generation of lymphokine-activated killer cells in human ovarian carcinoma ascitic fluid: identification of transforming growth factor-β as a suppressive factor. *Cancer Immunology, Immunotherapy*, **32**, 296–302.

Horst H.-A., Scheithauer B.W., Kelly P.J. & Kovach J.S. (1992) Distribution of transforming growth factor-β1 in human astrocytomas. *Human Pathology*, **23**, 1284–8.

Howe P.H., Dobrowolski S.F., Reddy K.B. & Stacey D.W. (1993) Release from G_1 growth arrest by transforming growth factor β1 requires cellular *ras* activity. *Journal of Biological Chemistry*, **268**, 21448–52.

Howe P.H., Draetta G. & Leof E.B. (1991) Transforming growth factor β1 inhibition of $p34^{cdc2}$ phosphorylation and histone H1 kinase activity is associated with G1/S phase growth arrest. *Molecular and Cellular Biology*, **11**, 1185–94.

Hsu S., Huang F., Hafez M., Winawer S. & Friedman E. (1994) Colon carcinoma cells switch their response to transforming growth factor β_1 with tumor progression. *Cell Growth & Differentiation*, **5**, 267–75.

Hubbs A.F., Hahn F.F. & Thomassen D.G. (1989) Increased resistance to transforming growth factor beta accompanies neoplastic progression of rat tracheal epithelial cells. *Carcinogenesis*, **10**, 1599–605.

Ignotz R.A., Endo T. & Massague J. (1987) Regulation of fibronectin and type I collagen mRNA levels by transforming growth factor-β. *Journal of Biological Chemistry*, **262**, 6443–6.

Inagaki M., Moustakas A., Lin H.Y., Lodish H.F. & Carr B.I. (1993) Growth inhibition by transforming growth factor β (TGF-β) type I is restored in TGF-β-resistant hepatoma cells after expression of TGF-β receptor type II cDNA. *Proceedings of the National Academy of Sciences of the United States of America*, **90**, 5359–63.

Inge T.H., Hoover S.K., Susskind B.M., Barrett S.K. & Bear H.D. (1992) Inhibition of tumor-specific cytotoxic T-lymphocyte responses by transforming growth factor β_1. *Cancer Research*, **52**, 1386–92.

Iruela-Arispe M.L. & Sage E.H. (1993) Endothelial cells exhibiting angiogenesis in vitro proliferate in response to TGF-β1. *Journal of Biological Chemistry*, **52**, 414–30.

Ito M., Yasui W., Kyo E. et al. (1992) Growth inhibition of transforming growth factor β on human gastric carcinoma cells: receptor and postreceptor signaling. *Cancer Research*, **52**, 295–300.

Jennings J.C., Mohan S., Linkhart T.A., Widstrom R. & Baylink D.J. (1988) Comparison of the biological actions of TGF-beta 1 and TGF-beta 2: differential activity in endothelial cells. *Journal of Cellular Physiology*, **137**, 167–72.

Jennings M.T., Maciunas R.J., Carver R. et al. (1991) TGFβ1 and TGFβ2 are potent growth regulators for low-grade and malignant gliomas in vitro: evidence in support of an autocrine hypothesis. *International Journal of Cancer*, **49**, 129–39.

Jurgensmeier J.M., Schmitt C.P., Viesel E., Hofler P. & Bauer G. (1994) Transforming growth factor β-treated fibroblasts eliminate transformed fibroblasts by induction of apoptosis. *Cancer Research*, **54**, 393–8.

Kawamata H., Kameyama S., Kawai K. & Oyasu R. (1993) Effect of epidermal growth factor and transforming growth factor β1 on growth and invasive potentials of newly established rat bladder carcinoma cell lines. *International Journal of Cancer*, **55**, 968–73.

Kim S.-J., Glick A., Sporn M.B. & Roberts A.B. (1989) Characterization of the promoter region of the human transforming growth factor-β1 gene. *Journal of Biological Chemistry*, **264**, 402–8.

Kim S.-J., Park K., Koeller D. et al. (1992) Post-transcriptional regulation of the human transforming growth factor-β1 gene. *Journal of Biological Chemistry*, **267**, 13702–7.

Knabbe C., Lippman M.E., Wakefield L.M. et al. (1987) Evidence that transforming growth factor-β is a hormonally regulated negative growth factor in human breast cancer cells. *Cell,* **48**, 417–28.

Koff A., Ohtsuki M., Polyak K., Roberts J.M. & Massagué J. (1993) Negative regulation of G1 in mammalian cells: inhibition of cyclin E-dependent kinase by TGF-β. *Science,* **260**, 536–9.

Kozak M. (1987) An analysis of 5′-noncoding sequences from 699 vertebrate messenger RNAs. *Nucleic Acids Research,* **15**, 8125–47.

Kozak M. (1989) The scanning model for translation: an update. *Journal of Cell Biology,* **108**, 229–41.

Kozak M. (1991) An analysis of vertebrate mRNA sequences: intimations of translational control. *Journal of Cell Biology,* **115**, 887–03.

Lafyatis R., Lechleider R., Kim S.-J., Jakowlew S., Roberts A.B. & Sporn M.B. (1990) Structural and functional characterization of the transforming growth factor β3 promoter. A cAMP-responsive element regulates basal and induced transcription. *Journal of Biological Chemistry,* **265**, 19128–36.

Laiho M., DeCaprio J.A., Ludlow J.W., Livingston D.M. & Massagué J. (1990) Growth inhibition by TGF-β linked to suppression of retinoblastoma protein phosphorylation. *Cell,* **62**, 175–85.

Laiho M., Ronnstrand L., Heino J. et al. (1991) Control of JunB and extracellular matrix protein expression by transforming growth factor-β1 is independent of simian virus 40 T antigen-sensitive growth-inhibitory events. *Molecular and Cellular Biology,* **11**, 972–8.

Laiho M., Weis F.M.B., Boyd F.T., Ignotz R.A. & Massagué J. (1991) Responsiveness to transforming growth factor-beta (TGF-beta) restored by genetic complementation between cells defective in TGF-beta receptors I and II. *Journal of Biological Chemistry,* **266**, 9108–12.

Landesman Y., Pagano M., Draetta G., Rotter V., Fusenig N.E. & Kimchi A. (1992) Modifications of cell cycle controlling nuclear proteins by transforming growth factor β in the HaCaT keratinocyte cell line. *Oncogene,* **7**, 1661–5.

Lawler S., Candia A.F., Ebner R., Shum L., Lopez A.R., Moses H.L., Wright C.V. & Derynck R. (1994) The murine type II TGF-β receptor has a coincident embryonic expression and binding preference for TGF-β1. *Development,* **120**, 165–75.

Leof E.B., Proper J.A., Goustin A.S., Shipley G.D., DiCorleto P.E. & Moses H.L. (1986) Induction of c-*sis* mRNA and activity similar to platelet-derived growth factor by transforming growth factor β: a proposed model for indirect mitogenesis involving autocrine activity. *Proceedings of the National Academy of Sciences of the United States of America,* **83**, 2453–7.

Lin H.Y. & Lodish H.F. (1993) Receptors for the TGF-β superfamily: multiple polypeptides and serine/threonie kinases. *Trends in Cell Biology,* **3**, 14–19.

Lin H.Y., Wang X.-F., Ng-Eaton E., Weinberg R.A. & Lodish H.F. (1992) Expression cloning of the TGF-β type II receptor, a functional transmembrane serine/threonine kinase. *Cell,* **68**, 775–85.

Lin J.-K. & Chou C.-K. (1992) *In vitro* apoptosis in the human hepatoma cell line induced by transforming growth factor β_1. *Cancer Research,* **52**, 385–8.

Lokeshwar B.L. & Block N.L. (1992) Isolation of a prostate carcinoma cell proliferation-inhibiting factor from human seminal plasma and its similarity to transforming growth factor β. *Cancer Research,* **52**, 5821–5.

Longstreet M., Miller B. & Howe P.H. (1992) Loss of transforming growth factor β1 (TGF-β1)-induced growth arrest and p34^{cdc2} regulation in *ras*-transfected epithelial cells. *Oncogene*, **7**, 1549–56.

López-Casillas F., Cheifetz S., Doody J., Andres J.L., Lane W.S. & Massagué J. (1991) Structure and expression of the membrane proteoglycan betaglycan, a component of the TGF-β receptor system. *Cell*, **67**, 785–95.

López-Casillas F., Wrana J.L. & Massagué J. (1993) Betaglycan presents ligand to the TGFβ signaling receptor. *Cell*, **73**, 1435–44.

Manning A.M., Williams A.C., Game S.M. & Paraskeva C. (1991) Differential sensitivity of human colonic adenoma and carcinoma cells to transforming growth factor β (TGF-β): Conversion of an adenoma cell line to a tumorigenic phenotype is accompanied by a reduced response to the inhibitory effects of TGF-β. *Oncogene*, **6**, 1471–6.

Mioh H. & Chen J.K. (1989) Differential inhibitory effects of TGF-β on EGF-, PDGF-, and HBGF-1-stimulated MG63 human osteosarcoma cell growth: possible involvement of growth facter interactions at the receptor and postreceptor levels. *Journal of Cellular Physiology*, **139**, 509–16.

Missero C., Filvaroff E. & Dotto G.P. (1991) Induction of transforming growth factor β_1 resistance by the E1A oncogene requires binding to a specific set of cellular proteins. *Proceedings of the National Academy of Sciences of the United States of America*, **88**, 3489–93.

Miyazono K., Ichijo H. & Heldin C.-H. (1993) Transforming growth factor-β: Latent forms, binding proteins and receptors. *Growth Factors*, **8**, 11–22.

Mizukami Y., Nonomura A., Yamada T. et al. (1990) Immunohistochemical demonstration of growth factors, TGF-α, TGF-β, IGF-I and *neu* oncogene product in benign and malignant breast tissues. *Anticancer Research*, **10**, 1115–26.

Mooradian D.L., McCarthy J.B., Komanduri K.V. & Furcht L.T. (1992) Effects of transforming growth factor-β1 on human pulmonary adenocarcinoma cell adhesion, motility, and invasion in vitro. *Journal of the National Cancer Institute*, **84**, 523–7.

Mooradian D.L., Purchio A.F. & Furcht L.T. (1990) Differential effects of transforming growth factor β1 on the growth of poorly and highly metastatic murine melanoma cells. *Cancer Research*, **50**, 273–7.

Moses H.L., Yang E.Y. & Pietenpol J.A. (1990) TGF-β stimulation and inhibition of cell proliferation: new mechanistic insights. *Cell*, **63**, 245–7.

Moustakas A., Lin H.Y., Henis Y.I., Plamondon J., O'Connor-McCourt M.D. & Lodish H.F. (1993) The transforming growth factor β receptors types I, II, and III form hetero-oligomeric complexes in the presence of ligand. *Journal of Biological Chemistry*, **268**, 22215–18.

Mukai M., Shinkai K., Komatsu K. & Akedo H. (1989) Potentiation of invasive capacity of rat ascites hepatoma cells by transforming growth factor-beta. *Japanese Journal of Cancer Research*, **80**, 107–10.

Mulder K.M., Humphrey L.E., Gene Choi H., Childress-Fields K.E. & Brattain M.G. (1990a) Evidence for c-*myc* in the signaling pathway for TGF-β in well-differentiated human colon carcinoma cells. *Journal of Cellular Physiology*, **145**, 501–7.

Mulder K.M., Zhong Q., Choi H.G., Humphrey L.E. & Brattain M.G. (1990b) Inhibitory effects of transforming growth factor β_1 on mitogenic response, transforming growth factor α, and c-*myc* in quiescent, well-differentiated colon carcinoma cells. *Cancer Research*, **50**, 7581–6.

Murray P.A., Barrett-Lee P., Travers M., Luqmani Y., Powles T. & Coombes R.C. (1993) The prognostic significance of transforming growth factors in human breast cancer. *British Journal of Cancer*, **67**, 1408–12.

Newcom S.R., Tagra K.K. & Kadin M.E. (1992) Neutralizing antibodies against transforming growth factor β potentiate the proliferation of Ki-1 positive lymphoma cells: Further evidence for negative autocrine regulation by transforming growth factor β. *American Journal of Pathology*, **140**, 709–18.

Noma T., Glick A.B., Geiser A.G. et al. (1991) Molecular cloning and structure of the human transforming growth factor-β2 gene promoter. *Growth Factors*, **4**, 247–55.

O'Reilly M.A., Geiser A.G., Kim S.-J. et al. (1992) Identification of an activating transcription factor (ATF) binding site in the human transforming growth factor-β2 promoter. *Journal of Biological Chemistry*, **267**, 19938–43.

Ong G., Sikora K. & Gullick W.J. (1991) Inactivation of the retinoblastoma gene does not lead to loss of TGF-β receptors or response to TGF-β in breast cancer cell lines. *Oncogene*, **6**, 761–3.

Paulsson Y., Karlsson C., Heldin C.-H. & Westermark B. (1993) Density-dependent inhibitory effect of transforming growth factor-β1 on human fibroblasts involves the down-regulation of platelet-derived growth factor α-receptors. *Journal of Cellular Physiology*, **157**, 97–103.

Pelton R.W., Hogan B.L.M., Miller D.A. & Moses H.L. (1990) Differential expression of genes encoding TGFs β1, β2, and β3 during murine palate formation. *Developmental Biology*, **141**, 456–60.

Pepper M.S., Berlin D., Montesano R., Orci L. & Vassalli J.D. (1990) Transforming growth factor-beta 1 modulates basic fibroblast growth factor-induced proteolytic and angiogenic properties of endothelial cells in vitro. *Journal of Cell Biology*, **111**, 743–55.

Pepper M.S., Vassalli J.-D., Orci L. & Montesano R. (1993) Biphasic effect of transforming growth factor-β_1 on *in vitro* angiogenesis. *Experimental Cell Research*, **204**, 356–63.

Pierce D.R., Jr., Johnson M.D., Matsui Y., Robinson S.D., Gold L.I., Purchio A.F., Daniel C.W., Hogan B.L.M. & Moses H.L. (1993) Inhibition of mammary duct development but not alveolar outgrowth during pregnancy in transgenic mice expressing active TGF-β1. *Genes & Development*, **7**, 2308–17.

Pietenpol J.A., Holt J.T., Stein R.W. & Moses H.L. (1990) Transforming growth factor β1 suppression of c-*myc* gene transcription: role in inhibition of keratinocyte proliferation. *Proceedings of the National Academy of Sciences of the United States of America*, **87**, 3758–62.

Pietenpol J.A., Munger K., Howley P.M., Stein R.W. & Moses H.L. (1991) Factor-binding element in the human c-*myc* promoter involved in transcriptional regulation by transforming growth factor β1 and the retinoblastoma gene product. *Proceedings of the National Academy of Sciences of the United States of America*, **88**, 10227–31.

Pietenpol J.A., Stein R.W., Moran E. et al. (1990) TGF-β1 inhibition of c-*myc* transcription and growth in keratinocytes is abrogated by viral transforming proteins with pRB binding domains. *Cell*, **61**, 777–85.

Ralph D., McClelland M. & Welsh J. (1993) RNA fingerprinting using arbitrarily primed PCR identifies differentially regulated RNAs in mink lung (Mv1Lu) cells growth arrested by transforming growth factor β1. *Proceed-*

ings of the National Academy of Sciences of the United States of America, **90**, 10710–14.

Reiss M., Vellucci V.F. & Zhou Z. (1993) Mutant p53 tumor suppressor gene causes resistance to transforming growth factor β_1 in murine keratinocytes. *Cancer Research,* **53**, 899–904.

Ridley A.J., Davis J.B., Stroobant P. & Land H. (1989) Transforming growth factors-β1 and β2 are mitogens for rat Schwann cells. *Journal of Cell Biology,* **109**, 3419–24.

Rifkin D.B., Kojima S., Abe M. & Harpel J.G. (1993) TGF-β: structure, function, and formation. *Thrombosis and Haemostasis,* **70**, 177–9.

Roberts A.B. & Sporn M.B. (1992) Differential expression of the TGF-β isoforms in embryogenesis suggests specific roles in developing and adult tissues. *Molecular Reproduction and Development,* **32**, 91–8.

Roberts A.B. & Sporn M.B. (1993) Physiological actions and clinical applications of transforming growth factor-β (TGF-β). *Growth Factors,* **8**, 1–9.

Roberts A.B., Sporn M.B., Assoian R.K. et al. (1986) Transforming growth factor beta: rapid induction of fibrosis and angiogenesis in vivo and stimulation of collagen formation in vitro. *Proceedings of the National Academy of Sciences of the United States of America,* **83**, 4167–71.

Rodeck U. (1993) Growth factor independence and growth regulatory pathways in human melanoma development. *Cancer and Metastasis Reviews,* **12**, 219–26.

Romeo D.S., Park K., Roberts A.B., Sporn M.B. & Kim S.-J. (1993) An element of the transforming growth factor-β1 5′-untranslated region represses translation and specifically binds a cytosolic factor. *Molecular Endocrinology,* **7**, 759–66.

Ruffini P.A., Rivoltini L., Silvani A., Boiardi A. & Parmiani G. (1993) Factors, including transforming growth factor β, released in the glioblastoma residual cavity, impair activity of adherent lymphokine-activated killer cells. *Cancer Immunology, Immunotherapy,* **36**, 409–16.

Rundhaug J.E., Gray T., Steigerwalt R.W. & Nettesheim P. (1992) Changes in responsiveness of rat tracheal epithelial cells to transforming growth factor-beta 1 with time in culture. *Journal of Cellular Physiology,* **152**, 281–91.

Ruscetti F., Varesio L., Ochoa A. & Ortaldo J. (1993) Pleiotropic effects of transforming growth factor-β on cells of the immune system. *Annals of the New York Academy of Sciences,* **685**, 488–500.

Samuel S.K., Hurta R.A.R., Kondaiah P. et al. (1992) Autocrine induction of tumor protease production and invasion by a metallothionein-regulated TGF-β_1 (Ser223, 225). *EMBO Journal,* **11**, 1599–1605.

Sato Y., Tsuboi R., Lyons R., Moses H. & Rifkin D.B. (1990) Characterization of the activation of latent TGF-β by co-cultures of endothelial cells and pericytes or smooth muscle cells: a self-regulating system. *Journal of Cell Biology,* **111**, 757–63.

Schwarz L.C., Gingras M.-C., Goldberg G., Greenberg A.H. & Wright J.A. (1988) Loss of growth factor dependence and conversion of transforming growth factor-β_1 inhibition to stimulation in metastatic H-*ras*-transformed murine fibroblasts. *Cancer Research,* **48**, 6999–7003.

Schwarz L.C., Wright J.A., Hall A. et al. (1990) Enhanced secretion of activated TGF-β1 and post-receptor blockade to TGF-β1 signaling in highly malignant fibrosarcomas. *Annals of the New York Academy of Sciences,* **593**, 315–17.

Sherr, C.J. (1994) The ins and outs of RB: coupling gene expression to the cell cycle clock. *Trends in Cell Biology*, **00**, 15–18.

Soma Y. & Grotendorst G.R. (1989) TGF-β stimulates primary human skin fibroblast DNA synthesis via an autocrine production of PDGF-related peptides. *Journal of Cellular Physiology*, **140**, 246–53.

Steigerwalt R.W., Rundhaug J.E. & Nettesheim P. (1992) Transformed rat tracheal epithelial cells exhibit alterations in transforming growth factor-β secretion and responsiveness. *Molecular Carcinogenesis*, **5**, 32–40.

Steiner M.S. & Barrack E.R. (1992) Transforming growth factor-β1 overproduction in prostate cancer: effects on growth *in vivo* and *in vitro*. *Molecular Endocrinology*, **6**, 15–25.

Taetle R., Payne C., Dos Santos B., Russell M. & Segarini P. (1993) Effects of transforming growth factor β1 on growth and apoptosis of human acute myelogenous leukemia cells. *Cancer Research*, **53**, 3386–93.

Takehara K., LeRoy E.C. & Grotendorst G.R. (1987) TGF-β inhibition of endothelial cell proliferation: alteration of EGF binding and EGF-induced growth-regulatory (competence) gene expression. *Cell*, **49**, 415–22.

ten Dijke P., Hansen P., Iwata K.K., Pieler C. & Foulkes J.G. (1988) Identification of another member of the transforming growth factor type β gene family. *Proceedings of the National Academy of Sciences of the United States of America*, **85**, 4715–19.

Torre-Amione G., Beauchamp R.D., Koeppen H. et al. (1990) A highly immunogenic tumor transfected with a murine transforming growth factor type β_1 cDNA escapes immune surveillance. *Proceedings of the National Academy of Sciences of the United States of America*, **87**, 1486–90.

Ueki N., Nakazato M., Ohkawa T. et al. (1992) Excessive production of transforming growth-factor β1 can play an important role in the development of tumorigenesis by its action for angiogenesis: validity of neutralizing antibodies to block tumor growth. *Biochimica et Biophysica Acta Molecular Cell Research*, **1137**, 189–96.

Ueki N., Ohkawa T., Yokoyama Y. et al. (1993) Potentiation of metastatic capacity by transforming growth factor-β1 gene transfection. *Japanese Journal of Cancer Research*, **84**, 589–93.

Van Hoef M.E.H.M., Knox W.F., Dhesi S.S., Howell A. & Schor A.M. (1993) Assessment of tumour vascularity as a prognostic factor in lymph node negative invasive breast cancer. *European Journal of Cancer*, **29A**:1141–5.

Walker R.A. & Dearing S.J. (1992) Transforming growth factor beta$_1$ in ductal carcinoma in situ and invasive carcinomas of the breast. *European Journal of Cancer*, **28**, 641–4.

Wang X.-F., Lin H.Y., Ng-Eaton E., Downward J., Lodish H.F. & Weinberg R.A. (1991) Expression cloning and characterization of the TGF-β type III receptor. *Cell*, **67**, 797–805.

Weidner N., Carrol P.R., Flax J., Blumenfeld W. & Folkman J. (1993) Tumor angiogenesis correlates with metastasis in invasive prostate carcinoma. *American Journal of Pathology*, **143**, 401–9.

Weidner N., Semple J.P., Welch W.R. & Folkman J. (1991) Tumor angiogenesis and metastasis—correlation in invasive breast carcinoma. *New England Journal of Medicine*, **324**, 1–8.

Welch D.R., Fabra A. & Nakajima M. (1990) Transforming growth factor β stimulates mammary adenocarcinoma cell invasion and metastatic potential. *Proceedings of the National Academy of Sciences of the United States of America*, **87**, 7678–82.

Wieser R., Attisano L., Wrana J.L. & Massagué J. (1993) Signaling activity of transforming growth factor β type II receptors lacking specific domains in the cytoplasmic region. *Molecular and Cellular Biology*, **13**, 7239–47.

Wrana J.L., Attisano L., Cárcamo J. et al. (1992) TGFβ signals through a heteromeric protein kinase receptor complex. *Cell*, **71**, 1003–14.

Wu S., Theodorescu D., Kerbel R.S. et al. (1992) TGF-β1 is an autocrine-negative growth regulator of human colon carcinoma FET cells in vivo as revealed by transfection of an antisense expression vector. *Journal of Cell Biology*, **116**, 187–96.

Yanagihara K. & Tsumuraya M. (1992) Transforming growth factor β_1 induces apoptotic cell death in cultured human gastric carcinoma cells. *Cancer Research*, **52**, 4042–45.

Yang E.Y. & Moses H.L. (1990) Transforming growth factor β1-induced changes in cell migration, proliferation, and angiogenesis in the chicken chorioallantoic membrane. *Journal of Cell Biology*, **111**, 731–41.

Zentella A., Weis F.M.B., Ralph D.A., Laiho M. & Massagué J. (1991) Early gene responses to transforming growth factor-β in cells lacking growth-suppressive RB function. *Molecular and Cellular Biology*, **11**, 4952–8.

4

Bombesin and Its Receptor

MICHAEL J. SECKL AND ENRIQUE ROZENGURT

INTRODUCTION

Multicellular organisms have developed highly efficient regulatory networks to control cell proliferation. These involve cellular interactions with positive and negative diffusible modulators as well as with the extracellular matrix proteins. In fully mature organisms, the cells of many tissues and organs are maintained in a nonproliferating state, but can be stimulated to resume DNA synthesis and cell division in response to external stimuli such as hormones, antigens or growth factors. In this manner the growth of individual cells is regulated according to the requirements of the whole organism. The regulation of normal cell proliferation is therefore central to many physiological processes, including embryogenesis, growth and development, selective cell survival, tissue repair and immune responses.

It has become evident that cultured cancer cells, which are characterized by unrestrained proliferation, acquire complete or partial independence of mitogenic signals in the extracellular environment through different mechanisms (Cross & Dexter, 1991; Westermark & Heldin, 1991). These include production of growth factors that act on the same cells that produced them or on adjacent cells, alterations in the number or structure of cellular receptors and changes in the activity of postreceptor signalling pathways that either stimulate or suppress cell growth (Bishop, 1991; Sager, 1989). For these reasons the identification of the extracellular factors that modulate cell proliferation and the elucidation of the molecular mechanisms involved have emerged as fundamental problems in cancer biology.

In recent years an increasing number of small regulatory peptides or neuropeptides including bombesin/gastrin releasing peptide (GRP) have been discovered in the neural and neuroendocrine cells of the gastrointestinal tract and central nervous system (Walsh, 1987). Defining the physiological functions of these peptides is complicated by the different modes of action of these molecules. Some are localized in neurons and act as neurotransmitters in the central or peripheral nervous system, while others are released by endocrine cells and have effects both as systemic hormones circulating through the bloodstream and by acting in a paracrine or autocrine fashion. Moreover, a number of peptides are found in both neuronal and endocrine cells, and a major effect of some regulatory peptides in vivo (e.g., bombesin/GRP) is to stimulate the release of other biologically active peptides. The role of these peptides as fast-acting neurohumoural signallers has recently been expanded by the discovery that they also stimulate cell proliferation (Zachary, Woll & Rozengurt, 1987; Rozengurt 1991). Furthermore, indirect evidence is accumulating that the mitogenic effects of neuropeptides such as bombesin may be relevant for a number of normal and abnormal biological processes, and in particular tumourigenesis. Consequently, it is very important to understand in detail the receptors and signal transduction pathways that mediate the mitogenic action of bombesin and other neuropeptides because they may provide potential targets for therapeutic intervention.

Many studies to identify the molecular pathways by which neuropeptide mitogens elicit cellular growth have exploited cultured murine 3T3 cells as a model system (Rozengurt, 1985, 1986). The list of neuropeptides that can act as mitogens in these cells has now grown considerably and includes bombesin, bradykinin, endothelin, vasopressin and vasoactive intestinal peptide (Rozengurt, Legg & Pettican, 1979; Rozengurt & Sinnett-Smith, 1983; Woll & Rozengurt, 1988a; Zurier et al., 1988; Takuwa et al., 1989; Sethi & Rozengurt, 1991a, 1991b, 1992). Evidence for direct growth-promoting activities of several other peptides including cholecystokinin, galanin, gastrin and neurotensin has recently come from work in another cultured cell model system, namely, cell lines established from small-cell lung carcinoma (SCLC). This work will be reviewed in a later section. Some fundamental features of the mechanism of action of bombesin as a growth factor in 3T3 cells will be discussed in the following review.

EARLY SIGNALLING EVENTS INDUCED BY BOMBESIN

The early cellular and molecular responses elicited by bombesin and structurally related peptides in 3T3 cells (Figure 4.1) have been

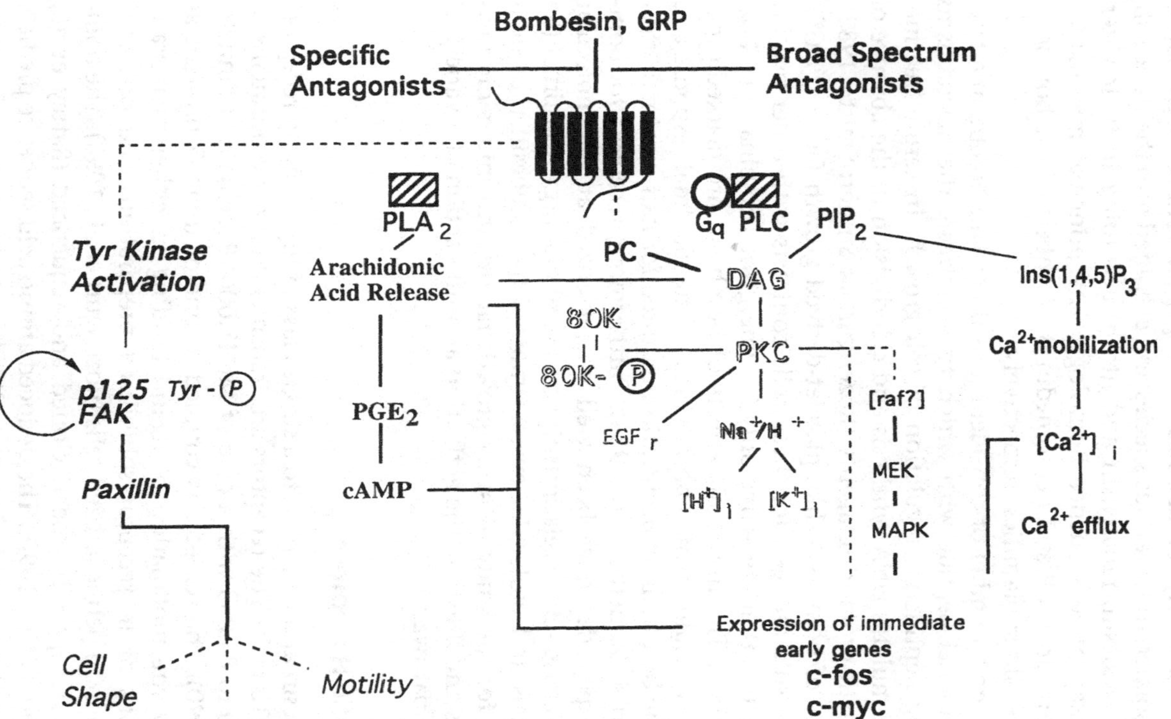

Figure 4.1 Signal transduction pathways activated by bombesin. Detailed explanation can be found in the text.

elucidated in detail. Bombesin is a 14 amino acid peptide first isolated from the skin of the frog *Bombina bombina* (Anastasi, Erspamer & Bucci, 1971). Many bombesin-related peptides have been subsequently isolated from various species and classified into the three subfamilies bombesin, ranatensin and litorin according to their C-terminal hexapeptide sequence homology. The principal mammalian counterparts are GRP and neuromedin B, members of the bombesin and ranatensin subfamilies, respectively.

There are a number of considerations that make bombesin attractive as a model peptide with which to investigate the mechanisms underlying peptidergic regulation of cell growth. In serum-free medium it stimulates DNA synthesis and cell division in the absence of other growth-promoting agents (Rozengurt & Sinnett-Smith, 1983). The ability of bombesin, like platelet-derived growth factor (PDGF), to act as a sole mitogen for these cells contrasts with other peptide growth factors that are active only in synergistic combinations (Rozengurt, 1986). The mitogenic effects of bombesin are markedly potentiated by insulin, which both increases the maximal response and reduces the bombesin concentration required for half-maximal effect (Rozengurt & Sinnett-Smith, 1983). Furthermore, receptors for bombesin-like peptides have been well characterized at the molecular level. The cause–effect relationships and temporal organization of the early signals and molecular events induced by bombesin provide a paradigm for the study of other growth factors and mitogenic neuropeptides and illustrate the activation and interaction of a variety of signalling pathways.

Specific Receptors

Bombesin and GRP bind to a single class of high-affinity receptors in Swiss 3T3 cells. The receptors are transmembrane glycoproteins of Mr 75,000 to 85,000 with a core of Mr 43,000 (Rozengurt & Sinnett-Smith, 1990). The receptor is coupled to one or more G proteins as judged by the modulation of ligand binding in either membrane preparations or in receptor solubilized preparations and of signal transduction in permeabilized cells (Rozengurt et al., 1990). The bombesin/GRP receptor has been cloned and sequenced (Battey et al., 1990; Spindel et al., 1990). The deduced amino acid sequence predicts a polypeptide core of Mr 43,000 and demonstrates that it belongs to the superfamily of heterotrimeric G-protein coupled receptors. These receptors are characterized by seven hydrophobic domains thought to traverse the cytoplasmic membrane and cluster to form a ligand-binding packet (Battey et al., 1990; Spindel et al., 1990).

The neuromedin-B receptor has also been cloned and shown to be another member of the heterotrimeric G-protein receptor superfamily (Wada et al., 1991). The predicted amino acid sequence has 56% homology with the GRP receptor and in stably transfected cells, the neuromedin-B receptor binds GRP with low affinity and neuromedin-B with high affinity (Wada et al., 1991).

Mutational analysis of these receptors is beginning to reveal which parts of the receptors are important for ligand binding, G-protein interaction and receptor internalization. Thus, the fifth transmembrane domain of the neuromedin-B receptor has been shown to reduce or abolish neuromedin-B binding, suggesting that this part of the receptor is critical for ligand binding (Fathi et al., 1993). The carboxyl cytoplasmic tail of the GRP receptor has been truncated, resulting in diminished rates of receptor internalization following ligand binding, without affecting the affinity of the receptor for ligand or activation of the heterotrimeric G protein (Benya et al., 1993). In a number of other members of the seven transmembrane domain receptor superfamily, the third cytoplasmic loop appears to be particularly critical in determining G-protein coupling to the activated receptor–ligand complex (Probst et al., 1992). Other neuropeptide mitogens with seven transmembrane domain receptors include endothelin, vasopressin, bradykinin, substance K and substance P (reviewed in Strosberg, 1991).

Inositol Phosphatidyl Turnover, Ca^{2+} Mobilization and Activation of Protein Kinase C

Binding of bombesin/GRP to its receptor initiates a cascade of intracellular signals culminating in DNA synthesis 10 to 15 hours later (Figure 4.1). One of the earliest events to occur after the binding of bombesin to its specific receptor is the activation of the heterotrimeric G protein, which in turn stimulates phospholipase C (PLC) catalyzed hydrolysis of phosphatidyl inositol 4,5-bisphosphate (PIP_2) in the plasma membrane. This reaction produces inositol 1,4,5-trisphosphate ($Ins[1,4,5]P_3$), which, as a second messenger binds to an intracellular receptor and induces the release of Ca^{2+} from internal stores (Berridge, 1993). Bombesin causes a rapid increase in $Ins(1,4,5)P_3$, which coincides with a transient increase in the intracellular concentration of Ca^{2+} ($[Ca^{2+}]_i$) and with Ca^{2+} efflux from the cells (Mendosa et al., 1986; Lopez-Rivas et al., 1987; Nanberg & Rozengurt, 1988).

Our understanding of the molecular identity of the G proteins and phospholipases involved has been greatly enhanced by the cloning, expression and in vitro reconstitution of activity of these proteins. The binding of bombesin to its receptor causes activation of pertussis toxin-insensitive G proteins (Zachary et al., 1987; Erusalimsky, Freidberg & Rozengurt, 1988; Erusalimsky & Rozengurt, 1989; Coffer et al., 1990, Murphy & Rozengurt, 1992) probably of the G_q subfamily (Strathmann & Simon, 1990; Wilkie et al., 1991). Recently, neuropeptide activated $G_{\alpha q}$ has been shown to stimulate the PLC-β isoform of PLC (Blank, Ross & Exton, 1991; Gutowski et al., 1991; Shenker et al., 1991; Smrcka et al., 1991; Taylor et al., 1991; Berstein et al., 1992). This, however, has not been specifically shown for bombesin-activated receptors. Furthermore, while there is direct evidence indicating that the $\gamma 1$ isoform of PLC is a target for growth factor receptors with intrinsic tyrosine kinase activity, it is less clear which of the three PLC-β isoforms play the most important role in G-protein linked bombesin-stimulated signal transduction. Likewise, the role of the $\beta\gamma$ subunits of the heterotrimeric G protein remains poorly defined (reviewed in Sternweis & Smrcka, 1992). In summary, a role of PLC-β and G_q in the mechanism of action of bombesin and other growth-promoting peptides is plausible, but definitive evidence is not yet available.

PLC-mediated hydrolysis of PIP_2 also generates 1,2-diacylglycerol (DAG). DAG can also be generated from other sources, such as phosphatidylcholine (PC) hydrolysis, and acts as a second messenger in the activation of protein kinase C (PKC) by multiple extracellular stimuli (Nishizuka, 1988) including bombesin (Erusalimsky et al., 1988). In accord with this, bombesin strikingly increases the phosphorylation of a major protein kinase C substrate that migrates with an apparent molecular mass of 80 kDa termed '80K' (Rozengurt, Rodriguez-Pena & Smith, 1983; Erusalimsky et al., 1991). Recently, the cDNA encoding this substrate from Swiss 3T3 cells has been cloned (Brooks et al., 1991). 80K has been shown to have 66 to 74% homology with a myristoylated alanine rich C-kinase substrate (MARCKS) cloned from human and bovine brain, but only one 80K/MARCKS gene exists in each species (Herget et al., 1992). This implies that rodent 80K and bovine and human MARCKS are not distinct members of a gene family (Herget et al., 1992). Interestingly, PKC activation induced by bombesin causes a dramatic down-regulation of the expression of mRNA and protein of the 80K/MARCKS substrate in Swiss 3T3 cells through a post-transcriptional mechanism (Brooks et al., 1991; Brooks et al., 1992). This novel result suggests that this PKC substrate, which appears to be a calmodulin- and actin-binding protein (Blackshear, 1993), may play a suppressor role in the control of cell proliferation.

As depicted in Figure 4.1, bombesin/GRP also stimulates a rapid exchange of Na^+, H^+ and K^+ ions across the cell membrane, leading to cytoplasmic alkalinization and increased intracellular [K^+] and induces a striking PKC-dependent transmodulation of the epidermal growth factor (EGF) receptor (Rozengurt & Sinnett-Smith, 1990).

Role of Mitogen-Activated Protein Kinase

Mitogen-activated protein (MAP) kinase is an important intermediate in the signal transduction pathways initiated by both heterotrimeric G-protein–linked receptors and receptors that possess intrinsic tyrosine kinase activity (Crews & Erikson, 1993; Davis, 1993). The signalling pathways that lead from the activated receptor to MAP kinase are different for these two classes of receptors. Thus PDGF or EGF induce tyrosine phosphorylation of their respective receptors, which permits the association of the two linking molecules Grb2/SEM 5 and Sos. This complex facilitates the activation of the oncoprotein, *ras*, by exchanging GDP for GTP on the *ras* protein. The active GTP-bound *ras* then directly associates with the serine/threonine kinase, *Raf*, which in turn stimulates MAP kinase kinase (MEK). Subsequently, MEK activates MAP kinase by tyrosine and serine phosphorylation (Egan & Weinberg, 1993).

The pathways leading from the activated heterotrimeric G-protein–linked receptors to MAP kinase activation is less clear. Bombesin has recently been shown to stimulate MAP kinase via PKC activation, while EGF uses an alternative pathway that involves *ras* activation in Swiss 3T3 cells (Pang, Decker & Saltiel, 1993). However, in Rat-1 fibroblasts, EGF and 1-oleoyl-lyso-phosphatidic acid (LPA; like bombesin signals via heterotrimeric G proteins), have both been shown to activate MAP kinase via a *ras*-dependent pathway (Cook et al., 1993). In addition, LPA has been shown in Swiss 3T3 cells to activate MAP kinase in two phases the second of which appears to be dependent on tyrosine phosphorylation mediated by the small GTP-binding *ras*-related protein, *rho* p21 (Kumagai et al., 1993). These data indicate that different G-protein linked receptors may activate MAP kinase via separate pathways in different cells.

Furthermore, there is very little evidence to suggest that *ras* is involved in signalling induced by bombesin in Swiss 3T3 cells (Satoh et al., 1990; Zachary, 1991). However, the recent finding that bombesin and bradykinin increase the relative amount of *ras*-GAP in phosphotyrosine and *ras*-GAP immunoprecipitates in Swiss 3T3 cells has reopened the issue (Leeb-Lundberg & Song, 1993).

In summary, it is probable that bombesin stimulates MAP kinase via PKC in Swiss 3T3 cells (see Figure 4.1). The events that take place between PKC and MAP kinase activation following bombesin stimulation are under investigation. MAP kinase is itself activated by MEK. This in turn has a number of activators termed "MAP kinase kinase kinases" which include MEK kinase and *Raf*. The latter is not only involved in PDGF or EGF signalling as discussed above, but may play a role in bombesin signalling as it is phosphorylated and activated by PKC (Crews & Erikson, 1993; Davis, 1993). Interestingly, PKC translocates to the plasma membrane for activation by DAG, while activated MAP kinase subsequently translocates to the nucleus to phosphorylate a number of substrates that directly cause induction of early response genes such as c-*fos* (Davis, 1993).

Arachidonic Acid Release and Prostaglandin Synthesis: Differential Effects of Bombesin and Vasopressin

While bombesin and structurally related mammalian peptides stimulate DNA synthesis in the absence of other factors, vasopressin is mitogenic for Swiss 3T3 cells only in synergistic combination with other factors (Rozengurt et al., 1979; Rozengurt & Sinnett-Smith, 1983). Binding of vasopressin to its distinct receptor on quiescent cultures of Swiss 3T3 cells causes a rapid production of Ins(1,4,5)P_3, mobilization of Ca^{2+} from intracellular stores and sustained activation of PKC via a G-protein linked transduction pathway (reviewed in Rozengurt, 1991). Since the initiation of DNA synthesis is triggered by independent signal-transduction pathways that act synergistically in mitogenic stimulation, the ability of bombesin to act as a sole mitogen could be due to activation of a signalling pathway not stimulated by vasopressin.

Recently, bombesin, but not vasopressin, has been shown to induce a marked, biphasic release of arachidonic acid into the extracellular medium (Millar & Rozengurt, 1990a; Domin & Rozengurt, 1993). A first phase involves rapid activation of phospholipase A_2 (PLA_2). These results showed a clear difference in the pattern of early signals induced by the neuropeptides bombesin and vasopressin in Swiss 3T3 cells. The stimulation of arachidonic acid release by bombesin is likely to contribute to bombesin-induced mitogenesis because externally applied arachidonic acid potentiates mitogenesis induced by agents that stimulate polyphosphoinositide breakdown but not arachidonic acid release (e.g., vasopressin) (Millar & Rozengurt, 1990a).

Arachidonic acid released by bombesin is converted into E-type prostaglandins which, acting in an autocrine and paracrine manner, enhance cyclic adenosine monophosphate (cAMP) accumulation in the cell (Figure 4.1). Since elevated cAMP levels constitute a mitogenic signal for Swiss 3T3 cells (Rozengurt, 1991), at least one consequence of arachidonic acid release may be the modulation of intracellular cAMP levels. However, other arachidonic acid metabolites may also play a role in mitogenic signal transduction by bombesin.

Bombesin Induction of the Proto-Oncogenes c-*fos* and c-*myc*

In addition to the events in the membrane and cytosol described above, bombesin rapidly and transiently induces the expression of the cellular oncogenes c-*fos* and c-*myc* in quiescent fibroblasts (Rozengurt & Sinnett-Smith, 1988). Since these cellular oncogenes encode nuclear proteins, it is plausible that their transient expression may play a role in the transduction of the mitogenic signal in the nucleus (Lewin, 1991). The demonstration that the product of the proto-oncogene c-*jun*, identified as a major component of the transacting factor AP-1, forms a tight complex with *fos* protein is consistent with a role for c-*fos* in the regulation of gene transcription (Lewin, 1991).

There has been considerable interest in elucidating the signal transduction pathways involved in c-*fos* induction. There is increasing evidence implicating PKC activation in the sequence of events linking receptor occupancy and proto-oncogene induction (Rozengurt & Sinnett-Smith, 1988; Rozengurt & Sinnett-Smith, 1990). Accordingly, bombesin-induced oncogene expression is markedly reduced by down-regulation of PKC. As mentioned above, PKC activation leads to the activation of MAP kinase, which directly phosphorylates transcription factor regulators resulting in the increased expression of c-*fos* (Treisman, 1992; Davis, 1993). However, neither direct activation of PKC by phorbol esters nor addition of vasopressin evoke a maximal increase in c-*fos* mRNA levels. It is likely that the induction of c-*fos* by bombesin is mediated by the coordinated effects of PKC activation, Ca^{2+} mobilization and an additional pathway dependent on arachidonic acid release (Rozengurt, 1991).

Bombesin Stimulation of Tyrosine Phosphorylation: Focal Adhesion Kinase ($p125^{FAK}$) and Paxillin; Cytoskeletal Link

It has been unequivocally established that the receptor for peptides of the bombesin family is coupled to G proteins and does not possess intrinsic tyrosine kinase activity. Recently, however, bombesin has been shown to increase rapidly tyrosine phosphorylation of multiple substrates in intact quiescent Swiss 3T3 cells (Zachary et al., 1991). Vasopressin and endothelin elicit a similar response. The substrates for neuropeptide tyrosine phosphorylation in these cells appear to be unrelated to known targets for the PDGF receptor including the GTPase-activating protein (GAP), the PLC-γ and the phosphatidylinositol 3′ kinase (Westermark & Heldin, 1991). Thus, bombesin and other neuropeptides that act through receptors linked to G proteins can increase tyrosine phosphorylation of protein substrates in intact cells (Figure 4.1). Furthermore, the stimulation of tyrosine phosphorylation by neuropeptides is due to activation of cellular tyrosine kinases (Zachary, Sinnett-Smith & Rozengurt, 1991).

A novel cytosolic protein tyrosine kinase was recently identified in the search for substrates of the oncogene pp60^{v-src} tyrosine kinase (Schaller et al., 1992). This new kinase co-localized with several components of cellular focal adhesions, such as tensin, vinculin and talin, which are important in regulating cytoskeletal structure and probably signal transduction (Schaller et al., 1992). It was therefore named focal adhesion kinase (p125^{FAK}) and was subsequently shown to be regulated by activation of the adhesive receptors of the integrin family. It is now recognized that p125^{FAK} is a major substrate for bombesin-stimulated tyrosine phosphorylation in Swiss 3T3 cells (Zachary, Sinnett-Smith & Rozengurt, 1992). Thus, p125^{FAK} appears to be a point of convergence in the action of neuropeptides, integrins and oncogenes and could be involved in the regulation of cell shape, adhesion and motility (Zachary & Rozengurt, 1992).

At present, it is not known how the bombesin receptor is linked to p125^{FAK} phosphorylation. Stimulation of p125^{FAK} tyrosine phosphorylation by bombesin is not dependent on either PKC activation or Ca^{2+} mobilization (Sinnett-Smith et al., 1993). There is evidence from studies of cytoskeletal changes induced by bombesin in Swiss 3T3 cells, that the small GTP-binding *ras*-related protein, *rho* p21, may be associated with p125^{FAK} phosphorylation (Ridley & Hall, 1992). Thus, bombesin promotes a rapid increase in actin stress fibers and focal adhesions that can be blocked by inhibitors of *rho* (Ridley & Hall, 1992). Cytochalasin D, an agent that selectively disrupts the network of actin microfilaments, completely inhibits bombesin-induced p125^{FAK} tyrosine phosphorylation (Sinnett-Smith et al., 1993). Furthermore, LPA, which induces similar cytoskeletal changes to bombesin, is unable to stimulate tyrosine phosphorylation of p125^{FAK} when *rho* is inactivated by ADP-ribosylation with botulinum C3 exoenzyme (Kumagai et al., 1993). Thus it is attractive to speculate that

$p125^{FAK}$ tyrosine phosphorylation induced by bombesin is triggered by a change in microfilament organization that in turn is mediated by *rho* p21 activation. However, other possibilities exist including *rho* p21 activation of both $p125^{FAK}$ and, for example, a parallel pathway that mediates cytoskeletal changes. Another intriguing problem that remains to be solved is the precise nature by which the bombesin receptor activates *rho* p21 and whether this in turn directly activates $p125^{FAK}$. However, the exact function of $p125^{FAK}$ is far from clear.

Paxillin is a 68-kDa tyrosine phosphorylated protein that also localizes to focal adhesions and binds to vinculin (Turner, Glenney & Burridge, 1990). Like $p125^{FAK}$, paxillin is tyrosine phosphorylated by integrin activation and by bombesin stimulation (Burridge, Turner & Romer, 1992; Zachary et al., 1993). Similarly, the pathway leading from the bombesin receptor to tyrosine phosphorylation of paxillin does not involve PKC activation or Ca^{2+} mobilization, but it is critically dependent on the integrity of the actin filament network (Zachary et al., 1993). The coordinated regulation of tyrosine phosphorylation of $p125^{FAK}$ and paxillin may reflect the fact that paxillin could be a direct substrate of $p125^{FAK}$ (Turner, Schaller & Parsons, 1993).

Interestingly, high concentrations of PDGF inhibit tyrosine phosphorylation of $p125^{FAK}$ and paxillin and cytoskeletal changes, which are normally seen when Swiss 3T3 cells are stimulated with low concentrations of PDGF (Rankin & Rozengurt, 1994). Furthermore, high concentrations of PDGF abolish the ability of bombesin to stimulate both cytoskeletal changes and tyrosine phosphorylation of $p125^{FAK}$ and paxillin (Rankin & Rozengurt, 1994). This suggests at least two conclusions. Firstly, that the cytoskeletal changes induced by PDGF are associated with $p125^{FAK}$. Secondly, there is a novel cross talk between PDGF and bombesin on the tyrosine phosphorylation of $p125^{FAK}$ and paxillin that occurs as a result of their opposing effects on the integrity of focal adhesions and the actin cytoskeleton (Rankin & Rozengurt, 1994).

Given the importance of tyrosine phosphorylation in the action of growth factors and nonreceptor oncogenes, it is plausible that this novel event plays a role in neuropeptide mitogenic signalling. The tyrphostins are a series of cell-permeable molecules that inhibit the tyrosine kinase activity of various receptors and block cell proliferation (Levitzki, 1992). They provide potential antiproliferative agents that could inhibit cell proliferation through a novel mechanism. Recent studies have shown that tyrphostin selectively inhibits bombesin stimulation of tyrosine phosphorylation including $p125^{FAK}$ in Swiss 3T3 cells (Seckl & Rozengurt, 1993). Since tyrphostin also inhibited bombesin-induced DNA synthesis over a similar concentration range and to a similar degree, it is tempting to speculate that tyrosine phosphorylation plays an important role in bombesin-mediated mitogenesis (Seckl & Rozengurt, 1993).

Regulation of Cellular Responsiveness to Bombesin-Stimulated Mitogenesis

Exposure of cells to many peptide hormones or neurotransmitters decreases the subsequent response of target cells to further challenge with the same ligand (homologous desensitization) or with a structurally unrelated ligand that elicits responses through a separate receptor (heterologous desensitization). Desensitization has been well documented for hormones that elicit short-term metabolic responses and is increasingly recognized as an important part of the regulation of cell growth.

The mitogenic response induced by bombesin in Swiss 3T3 cells is sensitive to at least two distinct desensitization mechanisms. Prolonged treatment of the cells with bombesin or structurally related peptides causes homologous desensitization of both mitogenic stimulation and generation of early signals by progressive down-regulation of cell surface receptors (Millar & Rozengurt, 1990b). In contrast, prolonged pretreatment with vasopressin induces a selective and reversible heterologous desensitization of the mitogenic activity of bombesin and GRP (Millar & Rozengurt, 1989). The block to bombesin-stimulated mitogenesis occurs at a postreceptor locus, namely, the liberation of arachidonic acid, which represents a novel target for heterologous desensitization (Millar & Rozengurt, 1990a).

Interestingly, acute bombesin stimulation, which does not alter the number or affinity of bombesin receptors, also results in homologous desensitization of the calcium response (Millar & Rozengurt, 1990b). Since the bombesin/GRP receptor has three potential PKC phosphorylation sites, one possible explanation of acute homologous desensitization could involve receptor down-regulation by PKC. This hypothesis was supported by the fact that two of the PKC phosphorylation sites occurred in areas known to be involved in G-protein coupling by the receptor. Furthermore, the β_2- and α_1-adrenergic receptors are known to be phosphorylated by activated PKC, leading to decreased G-protein coupling and desensitization (Leeb-Lundberg et al., 1987; Bouvier, Guilbault & Bonin, 1991). However, inhibition of PKC activity either by chronic phorbol ester exposure or by a specific inhibitor did not block acute homologous desensitization induced by bombesin in Swiss 3T3 cells (Walsh, Bouzyk & Rozengurt, 1993).

The existence of homologous and heterologous mitogenic desensitization suggests that the control of cell proliferation by neuropeptides may result from a delicate interplay between growth-stimulatory and growth-inhibitory signals.

BOMBESIN AND SCLC

The growth-promoting activity of bombesin and the elucidation of the signalling pathways that mediates its activity assume an added importance in view of the increasing recognition that bombesin and other neuropeptides may play a role in sustaining the proliferation of cancer cells. Bombesin has been implicated in carcinomas from lung, colon and breast. Recent evidence implicating bombesin and other neuropeptides in mediating proliferation in lung cancer and the use of antibombesin antibodies and antagonists as potential anticancer agents will be discussed below.

Lung cancer is the commonest fatal malignancy in the developed world. SCLC constitutes 25% of the total and follows an aggressive clinical course, despite initial sensitivity to chemotherapy and radiotherapy. SCLC is characterized by its ability to secrete many hormones and neuropeptides including bombesin, neurotensin, cholecystokinin and vasopressin (Sethi et al., 1991). Among these, only bombesin-like peptides, which include GRP, have been shown to act as autocrine growth factors for certain SCLC cell lines (Cuttitta et al., 1985; Mahmoud et al., 1991). These lines express the bombesin receptor, secrete bombesin and show increased DNA synthesis and clonal growth in response to bombesin. Furthermore, in the presence of either antibombesin antibodies or a bombesin-specific antagonist, the growth of certain SCLC lines in semisolid media or as xenografts in nude mice is markedly inhibited (Cuttitta et al., 1985; Mahmoud et al., 1991). These observations led to the belief that antibombesin antibodies or bombesin-specific antagonists could be utilized as new therapies in the treatment of SCLC. Unfortunately, in a phase I clinical study with monoclonal antibombesin antibodies, no inhibition of tumour growth in patients with SCLC was seen (Mulshine et al., 1988). In a subsequent phase II study of twelve SCLC patients previously treated with at least one cisplatinum-containing compound, one patient had a complete response to antibombesin monoclonal antibody therapy lasting 5 months (Kelly et al., 1993). This responding patient had measurable GRP in the serum but no evidence of GRP receptors on tumour biopsy, and thus the mechanism of the response is unclear. Although this result warrants further investigation, it is unlikely that a strategy based on eliminating the effects of a single growth factor will be sufficient to inhibit the growth of SCLC, which is now known to be a tumour driven by multiple neuropeptide growth factors.

Multiple Neuropeptides Stimulate Early Signal Transduction and Clonal Growth in SCLC Cell Lines

GRP stimulates mobilization of intracellular Ca^{2+} and inositol phosphate production in SCLC cells as previously elucidated in murine 3T3 cells (Figure 4.1) (Heikkila et al., 1987). In a subsequent study, multiple neuropeptides were screened for their ability to induce a rapid increase in $[Ca^{2+}]_i$ in different SCLC cell lines (Woll & Rozengurt, 1989). This assay should be regarded as an indicator of a productive ligand–receptor interaction. Ca^{2+} mobilization is one of the components of a complex array of signalling events rather than the signal that promotes cell growth (Figure 4.1). Woll and Rozengurt (1989) demonstrated that multiple neuropeptides induce a rapid and transient increase in $[Ca^{2+}]_i$ in SCLC cell lines. The Ca^{2+}-mobilizing effects are mediated by distinct receptors as shown by the use of specific antagonists and by the induction of homologous desensitization (Sethi & Rozengurt, 1991a, 1991b). The expression of these receptors is heterogeneous among these lines. Studies carried out in other laboratories are in agreement with these findings (Bunn et al., 1990).

In view of these findings, it has been hypothesized that SCLC growth is regulated by multiple autocrine or paracrine circuits involving Ca^{2+}-mobilizing neuropeptides. In line with this hypothesis, growth in culture of SCLC cells has been shown to be stimulated by many neuropeptides, including bombesin, bradykinin, cholecystokinin, neurotensin and vasopressin (Sethi & Rozengurt, 1991b). Further studies showed that galanin and gastrin also act as cellular growth factors for SCLC cells (Sethi & Rozengurt, 1991a, 1992). These novel findings are important because they suggest that the previously identified autocrine growth loop of bombesin-like peptides is only one of an extensive network of paracrine and autocrine circuits that sustain the proliferation of SCLC. Approaches designed to block SCLC growth must take into account this mitogenic complexity.

Blocking the Action of Multiple Neuropeptides: Broad-Spectrum Antagonists

As our understanding of the effects of growth factors in cancer increases, it has become possible to plan rational therapeutic interventions. Disrupting autocrine and paracrine growth loops and blocking mitogenesis. In this context it is thought that SCLC constitutes a special case in which unrestrained proliferation appears driven, at least in part, by multiple autocrine and paracrine circuits involving Ca^{2+}-mobilizing neuropeptides. Consequently, broad-spectrum growth factor antagonists capable of blocking the biological effects of multiple neuropeptides could provide an effective approach in the treatment of SCLC.

This role could be filled by a number of substance P analogues (Woll & Rozengurt, 1988b; Woll & Rozengurt, 1990). These compounds inhibit the biological effects of many Ca^{2+}-mobilizing neuropeptides including bombesin, its homologues and vasopressin in both Swiss 3T3 and SCLC cells (Zachary & Rozengurt, 1985; Zachary, Sinnett-Smith & Rozengurt, 1986; Woll & Rozengurt, 1988b, 1990). Moreover, these peptides block the growth of SCLC in liquid culture, semisolid media and as xenografts in nude mice (Langdon et al., 1992; Sethi et al., 1991; Woll & Rozengurt, 1990). The antagonists inhibit ligand binding at 37°C (Zachary & Rozengurt, 1985; Woll & Rozengurt, 1988a; Sinnett-Smith, Lehmann & Rozengurt, 1990), Ca^{2+} mobilization (Mendosa et al., 1986; Woll & Rozengurt, 1990; Langdon et al., 1992), PKC activation (Erusalimsky et al., 1988), tyrosine phosphorylation (Zachary et al., 1991), c-*fos* and c-*myc* induction (Rozengurt & Sinnett-Smith, 1988) and stimulation of DNA synthesis (Zachary & Rozengurt, 1985; Zachary et al., 1986; Woll & Rozengurt, 1988b, 1990) in Swiss 3T3 cells. In contrast, they do not affect mitogenesis stimulated by noncalcium mobilizing neuropeptides such as vasoactive intestinal peptide (VIP) (Woll & Rozengurt, 1988b), which induces cAMP accumulation via the heterotrimeric G-protein subclass G_s. The antagonists also do not inhibit the action of polypeptide growth factors such as PDGF (Woll & Rozengurt, 1990), which signal through receptors with intrinsic tyrosine kinase activity and mobilize calcium via activation of PI-PLC-γ. Thus substance P analogue antagonists show specificity against Ca^{2+}-mobilizing neuropeptides.

The conclusion that the substance P analogues compete with neuropeptide binding to their corresponding receptors is surprising in view of the lack of structural similarity between these agonists and antagonists. Classic antagonists compete at the same site as ligand for receptor binding and are thus specific to one ligand. These antagonists have been employed to analyze hormone function, ligand receptor interaction and receptor diversity and are under investigation as therapeutic agents. The substance P analogues constitute a different family of antagonists which may also function as novel antiproliferative agents in SCLC.

BOMBESIN IN BREAST AND COLON CANCER

The addition of bombesin to cultures of several breast cancer cell lines stimulates cell proliferation, but the magnitude of the stimulation is small as compared to the effects obtained in 3T3 cells or in

SCLC cell lines (Yano et al., 1992). The growth-promoting effects of bombesin on breast cancer cells were elicited when the cells were cultured in steroid stripped media. Interestingly, a bombesin-receptor antagonist inhibits the growth of MCF-7 human breast cancer xenografts in nude mice (Yano et al., 1992). These results suggest that bombesin/GRP may play a role as growth factors in some human breast cancer cells.

Several reports have demonstrated the expression of neuropeptide receptors in human colon cancer cell lines (Sethi & Rozengurt, 1993). In particular, gastrin has been shown to exert a growth-promoting effect on colon cancer cell lines and although it has been suggested that this hormone could act as an autocrine growth factor in this malignancy, there is no experimental evidence that this is the case (Sethi & Rozengurt, 1993).

The role of bombesin as a growth factor in colon cancer is less clear. However, a recent study using newly characterized human colon cancer cell lines demonstrated receptors for bombesin/GRP, gastrin, vasoactive intestinal peptide and substance P (Frucht et al., 1992). In addition, there has been one report showing significant inhibition of human colon cancer xenograft growth by the bombesin/GRP antagonist RC-3095 (Radulovic, Miller & Schally, 1991). Since these neuropeptides have been shown to act as cellular growth factors in other cellular systems, it is likely that the growth of colon carcinoma cells is also regulated by multiple autocrine/paracrine loops. Further, experimental work will be needed to test this hypothesis.

CONCLUSIONS

Bombesin and other neuropeptides are implicated in the control of cell proliferation and their mechanisms of action are attracting interest. Peptides of the bombesin family bind to specific surface receptors and initiate a complex cascade of signalling events that culminate in the stimulation of DNA synthesis and cell division in Swiss 3T3 cells. These peptides may also act as autocrine growth factors for certain SCLC cell lines. The autocrine growth loop of bombesin-like peptides may be only a part of an extensive network of autocrine and paracrine interactions involving a variety of Ca^{2+}-mobilizing neuropeptides in SCLC. In the context of the multistage evolution of cancer, neuropeptide mitogenesis may play a role at an early stage as tumour promoters in initiated cells or later as growth factors that sustain the unrestrained growth of the fully developed SCLC tumour. Bombesin and other neuropeptides are also implicated as growth factors for breast and colon cancer cells.

It is most likely that a detailed understanding of the receptors and signal transduction pathways that mediate the mitogenic action of regulatory peptides will identify novel targets for therapeutic intervention.

REFERENCES

Anastasi, A., Erspamer V. & Bucci M. (1971) Isolation and structure of bombesin and alytesin, two analogous active peptides from the skin of the European amphibians *Bombina* and *Alytes. Experimentia*, **27**, 166–7.

Battey, J.F., Way, J.M., Corjay, M.H., Shapira, H., Kusano, K., Harkins, R., Wu, J.M., Slattery, T., Mann, E. & Feldman, R.I. (1990) Molecular cloning of the bombesin/GRP receptor from Swiss 3T3 cells. *Proceedings of the National Academy of Sciences of the United States of America*, **88**, 395–9.

Benya, R., Faithi, Z., Battey, J.F. & Jenson, R.T. (1993) Serines and threonines in the gastrin-releasing peptide receptor carboxyl terminus mediate internalization. *Journal of Biological Chemistry*, **268**, 20285–90.

Berridge M.J. (1993) Inositol trisphosphate and calcium signalling. *Nature*, **361**, 315–25.

Berstein, G., Blank, J.L., Smrka, A.V., Higashijima, T., Sternweis, P.C., Exton J.H. & Ross E.M. (1992) Reconstitution of agonist-stimulated phosphatidylinositol 4,5-bisphosphate hydrolysis using purified m1 muscarinic receptor, Gq/11, and phospholipase C-β1. *Journal of Biological Chemistry*, **267**, 8081–8.

Bishop J.M. (1991) Molecular themes in oncogenesis. *Cell*, **64**, 235–48.

Blackshear P.J. (1993) The MARCKS family of cellular protein kinase C substrates. *Journal of Biological Chemistry*, **268**, 1501–4.

Blank J.L., Ross A.H. & Exton J.H. (1991) Purification and characterization of two G-proteins that activate the β1 isozyme of phosphoinositide-specific phospholipase C. *Journal of Biological Chemistry*, **266**, 18206–16.

Bouvier M., Guilbault N. & Bonin H. (1991) Phorbol-eter-induced phosphorylation of the B2-adrenergic receptor decreases its coupling to Gs. *European Journal of Biochemistry*, **279**, 243–8.

Brooks S.F., Herget T., Erusalimsky J.D. & Rozengurt E. (1991) Protein kinase C activation potently down-regulates the expression of its major substrate, 80K, in Swiss 3T3 cells. *EMBO Journal*, **10**(9), 2497–505.

Brooks S., Herget T., Broad S. & Rozengurt E. (1992) The expression of 80K/MARCKS, a major substrate of PKC, is down-regulated through both PKC-dependent and -independent pathways. *Journal of Biological Chemistry*, **267**, 14212–18.

Bunn P.A., Dienhart D.G., Chan D., Puck T.T., Tagawa M., Jewett P.B. & Braunschweiger E. (1990) Neuropeptide stimulation of calcium flux in human lung cancer cells: delineation of alternative pathways. *Proceedings of the National Academy of Sciences of the United States of America*, **87**, 2162–6.

Burridge K., Turner C.E. & Romer L.H. (1992) Tyrosine phosphorylation of paxillin and $p125^{FAK}$ accompanies cell adhesion to extracellular matrix: a role in cytoskeletal assembly. *Journal of Cell Biology*, **119**, 893–903.

Coffer A., Fabregat I., Sinnett-Smith J. & Rozengurt E. (1990) Solubilisation of the bombesin receptor from Swiss 3T3 cell membranes: functional association to a guanine nucleotide regulatory protein. *FEBS Letters*, **263**, 80–4.

Cook S., Rubinfeld B., Albert I. & McCormick F. (1993) RapV12 antagonizes Ras-dependent activation of ERK1 and ERK2 by LPA and EGF in Rat-1 fibroblasts. *EMBO Journal*, **12**, 3475–85.

Crews C.M. & Erikson R.L. (1993) Extracellular signals and reversible protein phosphorylation: what to Mek of it all. *Cell*, **74**, 215–17.

Cross M. & Dexter T.M. (1991) Growth factors in development, transformation and tumorigenesis. *Cell*, **64**, 271–80.

Cuttitta F., Carney D.N., Mulshine J., Moody T.W., Fedorko J., Fischler A. & Minna J.D. (1985) Bombesin like peptides can function as autocrine growth factors in human small cell lung cancer. *Nature*, **316**, 823–6.

Davis R. (1993) The mitogen-activated protein kinase signal transduction pathway. *Journal of Biological Chemistry*, **268**, 14553–6.

Domin J. & Rozengurt E. (1993) Platelet-derived growth factor stimulates a biphasic mobilization of arachidonic acid in Swiss 3T3 cells. The role of phospholipase A_2. *Journal of Biological Chemistry*, **268**, 8927–8934.

Egan S.E. & Weinberg R.A. (1993) The pathway to signal achievement. *Nature*, **365**, 781–3.

Erusalimsky J., Freidberg I. & Rozengurt E. (1988) Bombesin, diacylglycerol, and phorbol esters rapidly stimulate the phosphorylation of an Mr=80,000 protein kinase C substrate in permiablized 3T3 cells. *Journal of Biological Chemistry*, **263**, 19188–94.

Erusalimsky J. & Rozengurt E. (1989) Vasopressin rapidly stimulates protein kinase C in digitonin-permeabilized Swiss 3T3 cells: involvement of a pertussis toxin-insensitive guanine nucleotide binding protein. *Journal of Cellular Physiology*, **141**, 253–61.

Erusalimsky J.D., Brooks S.F., Herget T., Morris C. & Rozengurt E. (1991) Molecular cloning and characterization of the acidic 80-kda protein kinase c substrate from rat brain. Identification as a glycoprotein. *Journal of Biological Chemistry*, **266**(1), 7073–80.

Fathi Z., Benyas R.V., Shapira H., Jenson R.T. & Battey J.F. (1993) The fifth transmembrane segment of the neuromedin B receptor is critical for high affinity neuromedin B binding. *Journal of Biological Chemistry*, **268**, 14622–6.

Frucht H., Gazdar A.F., Park J.-A., Oie H. & Jenson R.T. (1992) Characterization of functional receptors for gastrointestinal hormones on human colon cancer cells. *Cancer Research*, **52**, 1114–22.

Gutowski S., Smrcka A.V., Nowak L., Wu D., Simon M. & Sternweis P.C. (1991) Antibodies to the α_q subfamily of guanine nucleotide-binding regulatory protein α subunits attenuate activation of phosphatidylinositol 4,5-bisphosphate hydrolysis. *Journal of Biological Chemistry*, **266**, 20519–24.

Heikkila R., Trepel J.B., Cuttitta F., Neckers L.M. & Sausville E.A. (1987) Bombesin-related peptides induce calcium mobilization in a subset of human small cell lung cancer cell lines. *Journal of Biological Chemistry*, **262**, 16456–60.

Herget T., Brooks S.F., Broad S. & Rozengurt E. (1992) Relationship between the major protein kinase C substrates acidic 80-kDa protein-kinase-C substrate (80K) and myristoylated alanine-rich C-kinase substrate (MARCKS). *European Journal of Biochemistry*, **209**, 7–14.

Kelly M.J., Avis I., Linnoila R.I., Richardson G., Snider R., Phares J., Ashburn R., Laskin W.B., Becker K., Boland C., Cuttitta F., Mulshine J. & Johnson

B.E. (1993) Complete response in a patient with small cell lung cancer (SCLC) treated on a phase II trial using a murine monoclonal antibody (2A11) directed against gastrin-releasing peptide (GRP). *Proceedings of the American Society of Clinical Oncology*, **12**, 339.

Kumagai N., Morii N., Fujisawa K., Nemoto Y. & Narumiya S. (1993) ADP-ribosylation of rho p21 inhibits lysophosphatidic acid-induced protein tyrosine phosphorylation and phosphatidylinositol 3-kinase activation in cultured Swiss 3T3 cells. *Journal of Biological Chemistry*, **238**, 24535–24538.

Langdon S.P., Sethi T., Ritchie A., Muir M., Smyth J. & Rozengurt E. (1992) Broad spectrum neuropeptide antagonists inhibit the growth of small cell lung cancer *in vivo*. *Cancer Research*, **52**, 4554–7.

Leeb-Lundberg L.M.F., Cotecchia S., DeBlasi A., Caron M.G. & Lefkowitz R.J. (1987) Regulation of adrenergic receptor function by phosphorylation: I antagonist promoted desensitization and phosphorylation of α1-adrenergic receptors coupled to inositol phospholipid metabolism in DDT1-MF-2 smooth muscle cells. *Journal of Biological Chemistry*, **262**, 3098–105.

Leeb-Lundberg L.M.F. & Song X.H. (1993) Identification of p125, a component of a group of 120-kDa proteins that are phosphorylated on tyrosine residues in response to bradykinin and bombesin stimulation, in anti-Ras-GTPase-activating proteins immunoprecipitates of Swiss 3T3 cells. *Journal of Biological Chemistry*, **268**(11), 8151–7.

Levitzki A. (1992) Tyrphostins: tyrosine kinase blockers as novel antiproliferative agents and dissectors of signal transduction. *FASEB Journal*, **6**, 3275–82.

Lewin B. (1991) Oncogenic conversion by regulatory changes in transcription factors. *Cell*, **64**, 303–12.

Lopez-Rivas A., Mendoza S.A., Nanberg E., Sinnett-Smith J. & Rozengurt E. (1987) Ca2+-mobilizing actions of platelet derived growth factor differ from those of bombesin and vasopressin in Swiss 3T3 mouse cells. *Proceedings of the National Academy of Sciences of the United States of America*, **84**, 5768–72.

Mahmoud S., Staley J., Taylor J., Bogden A., Moreau J.-P., Coy D., Avis I., Cuttitta F., Mulshine J.L. and Moody T.W. (1991) [Psi13,14] bombesin analogues inhibit growth of small cell lung cancer *in vitro* and *in vivo*. *Cancer Research*, **51**, 1798–802.

Mendosa S.A., Schneider J.A., Lopez-Rivas A., Sinnett-Smith J.W. & Rozengurt E. (1986) Early events elicited by bombesin and structurally related peptides in quiescent Swiss 3T3 cells. II. Changes in Na^+ and Ca^{2+} fluxes, Na^+/K^+ pump activity and intracellular pH. *Journal of Cell Biology*, **102**, 2223–33.

Millar J.B.A. & Rozengurt E. (1989) Heterologous desensitization of bombesin induced mitogenesis by prolonged exposure to vasopressin: a post-receptor signal transduction block. *Proceedings of the National Academy of Sciences of the United States of America*, **86**, 3204–8.

Millar J.B. & Rozengurt E. (1990a) Arachidonic acid release by bombesin: a novel post-receptor target for heterologous mitogenic desensitization. *Journal of Biological Chemistry*, **265**, 19973–9.

Millar J.B. & Rozengurt E. (1990b) Chronic desensitization to bombesin by progressive down-regulation of bombesin receptors in swiss 3t3 cells. Distinction from acute desensitization. *Journal of Biological Chemistry*, **265**(20), 12052–8.

Mulshine J.L., Avis I., Treston A.M., Mobley C., Kaspryzyk P., Carasquillo J.A., Larson S.M., Nakanishs Y., Merchant B., Minna J.D. & Cuttitta F. (1988) Clinical use of a monoclonal antibody to bombesin-like peptide in patients with lung cancer. *Annals of the New York Academy of Sciences*, **547**, 360–72.

Murphy A.C. & Rozengurt E. (1992) *Pasteurella multocida* toxin selectivity facilitates phosphatidylinositol 4,5-bisphosphate hydrolysis by bombesin, vasopressin, and endothelin. *Journal of Biological Chemistry*, **267**, 25296–303.

Nanberg E. & Rozengurt E. (1988) Temporal relationship between inositol polyphosphate formation and increases in cytosolic Ca2+ in quiescent 3T3 cells stimulated by platelet-derived growth factor, bombesin and vasopressin. *EMBO Journal*, **7**(9), 2741–7.

Nishizuka Y. (1988) The molecular heterogeneity of protein kinase C and its implications for cellular regulation. *Nature*, **334**, 661–5.

Pang L., Decker S.J. & Saltiel A.R. (1993) Bombesin and epidermal growth factor stimulate the mitogen-activated protein kinase through different pathways in Swiss 3T3 cells. *Biochemical Journal*, **289**, 283–7.

Probst W.C., Snyder L.A., Schuster D.I., Brosius J. & Sealfon S.C. (1992) Sequence alignment of the G-protein coupled receptor superfamily. *DNA and Cell Biology*, **11**(1), 1–20.

Radulovic S., Miller G. & Schally A.V. (1991) Inhibition of growth of HT-29 human colon cancer xenografts in nude mice by treatment with bombesin/gastrin releasing peptide antagonist (RC-3095). *Cancer Research*, **51**, 6006–9.

Rankin S. & Rozengurt E. (1994) Platelet-derived growth factor modulation of focal adhesion kinase ($p125^{FAK}$) and paxillin tyrosine phosphorylation in Swiss 3T3 cells. *Journal of Biological Chemistry*, **269**, 704–710.

Ridley A.J. & Hall A. (1992) The small GTP-binding protein rho regulates the assembly of focal adhesions and actin stress fibers in response to growth factors. *Cell*, **70**, 389–99.

Rozengurt E., Legg A. & Pettican P. (1979) Vasopressin stimulation of mouse 3T3 cell growth. *Proceedings of the National Academy of Sciences of the United States of America*, **76**, 1284–7.

Rozengurt E., Rodriguez-Pena A. & Smith K.A. (1983) Phorbol esters, phospholipase C, and growth factors rapidly stimulate the phosphorylation of a Mr 80,000 protein in intact quiescent 3T3 cells. *Proceedings of the National Academy of Sciences of the United States of America*, **80**, 7224–48.

Rozengurt E. & Sinnett-Smith J. (1983) Bombesin stimulation of DNA synthesis and cell division in cultures of Swiss 3T3 cells. *Proceedings of the National Academy of Sciences of the United States of America*, **80**, 2936–40.

Rozengurt E. (1985) The mitogenic response of cultures 3T3 cells: integration of early signals and synergistic effects in a unified framework. In P. Cohen & M. Houslay (Eds.) *Molecular mechanisms of transmembrane signalling*, pp. 429–52. Elsevier Science Publishers B.V., Amsterdam.

Rozengurt E. (1986) Early signals in the mitogenic response. *Science*, **234**, 161–6.

Rozengurt E. & Sinnett-Smith J. (1988) Early signals underlying the induction of the proto-oncogenes c-fos and c-myc in quiescent fibroblasts: studies with peptides of the bomobesin family and other growth factors. *Progress in Nucleic Acid Research and Molecular Biology*, **35**, 261–95.

Rozengurt E. & Sinnett-Smith J. (1990) Bombesin stimulation of fibroblast mitogenesis: specific receptors, signal transduction and early events. *Philosophical Transactions of the Royal Society of London. Series B: Biological Sciences*, **327**, 209–21.

Rozengurt E., Fabregat I., Coffer A., Gil J. & Sinnett-Smith J. (1990) Mitogenic signalling through the bombesin receptor: role of a guanine nuleotide regulatory protein. *Journal of Cell Science*, **13**(Suppl.), 13–56.

Rozengurt E. (1991) Neuropeptides as cellular growth factors. *European Journal of Clinical Investigation*, **21**, 123–34.

Sager R. (1989) Tumour suppressor genes: the puzzle and the promise. *Science*, **246**, 406–12.

Satoh T., Endo M., Nakafuku M., Nakamura S. & Kaziro Y. (1990) Platelet-derived growth factor stimulates formation of active $p21^{ras}$ GTP complex in Swiss mouse 3T3 cells. *Proceedings of the National Academy of Sciences of the United States of America*, **87**, 5993–7.

Schaller M.D., Borgman C.A., Cobb B.S., Vines R.R., Reynolds A.B. & Parsons J.T. (1992) $pp125^{FAK}$, a structurally unique protein tyrosine kinase associated with focal adhesions. *Proceedings of the National Academy of Sciences of the United States of America*, **89**, 5192–6.

Seckl M.J. & Rozengurt E. (1993) Tyrphostin inhibits bombesin stimulation of tyrosine phosphorylation, c-fos expression and DNA synthesis in Swiss 3T3 cells. *Journal of Biological Chemistry*, **268**, 9548–54.

Sethi T., Langdon S., Smyth J. & Rozengurt E. (1991) Growth of small cell lung cancer cells: stimulation by multiple neuropeptides and inhibition by broad spectrum antagonists in vitro and in vivo. *Cancer Research*, **52**, 2737s–42s.

Sethi T. & Rozengurt E. (1991a) Galanin stimulates ca2+ mobilization, inositol phosphate accumulation, and clonal growth in small cell lung cancer cells. *Cancer Research*, **51**(6), 1674–9.

Sethi T. & Rozengurt E. (1991b) Multiple neuropeptides stimulate clonal growth of small cell lung cancer: effects of bradykinin, vasopressin, cholecystokinin, galanin, and neurotensin. *Cancer Research*, **51**(13), 3621–3.

Sethi T. & Rozengurt E. (1992) Gastrin stimulates Ca^{2+} mobilization and clonal growth in small cell lung cancer cells. *Cancer Research*, **52**, 6031–5.

Sethi T. & Rozengurt E. (1993) Gastrin as a growth factor for small cell lung cancer cells in vitro. In J. Walsh (Ed.) *Gastrin*, pp. 395–406. Raven Press, New York.

Shenker A., Goldsmith P., Unson C.G. & Spiegel A.M. (1991) The G protein coupled to the thromboxane A2 receptor in human platelet is a member of the novel Gq family. *Science*, **266**, 9309–13.

Sinnett-Smith J., Lehmann W. & Rozengurt E. (1990) Bombesin receptor in membranes from Swiss 3T3 cells. *Biochemistry Journal*, **265**, 80–4.

Sinnett-Smith J., Zachary I., Valverde A.M. & Rozengurt E. (1993) Bombesin stimulation of p125 focal adhesion kinase tyrosine phosphorylation: role of protein kinase C, Ca^{2+} mobilization and the actin cytoskeleton. *Journal of Biological Chemistry*, **268**, 14261–8.

Smrcka A.V., Hepler J.R., Brown K.O. & Sternweis P.C. (1991) Regulation of polyphosphoinositide-specific phospholipase C activity by purified Gq. *Science*, **251**, 804–7.

Spindel E.R., Giladi E., Brehm P., Goodman R.J. & Segerson T.P. (1990) Cloning and functional characterisation of complementary DNA encoding the murine fibroblast bombesin/gastrin-releasing peptide receptor. *Molecular Endocrinology*, **4**, 1956–63.

Sternweis P.C. & Smrcka A.V. (1992) Regulation of phospholipase C by G proteins. *Trends in Biochemical Science*, **17**, 502–6.

Strathmann M. & Simon M.I. (1990) G protein diversity: a distinct class of α subunits is present in vertebrates and invertebrates. *Proceedings of the National Academy of Sciences of the United States of America*, **87**, 9113–17.

Strosberg A.D. (1991) Structure/function relationship of proteins belonging to the family of receptors coupled to GTP-binding proteins. *European Journal of Biochemistry*, **196**, 1–10.

Takuwa N., Takuwa Y., Yanagisawa M., Yamashita K. & Masaki T. (1989) A novel vasoactive peptide endothelin stimulates mitogenesis through inositol lipid turnover in Swiss 3T3 fibroblasts. *Journal of Biological Chemistry*, **264**, 7856–61.

Taylor S.J., Chae H.Z., Rhee S.G. & Exton J.H. (1991) Activation of the β1 isozyme of phospholipase C by α subunits of the Gq class of G proteins. *Nature*, **350**, 516–8.

Treisman R. (1992) The serum response element. *Trends in Biochemical Sciences*, **17**, 423–6.

Turner C.E., Glenney J.R. & Burridge K. (1990) Paxillin; a new vinculin binding protein present in focal adhesions. *Journal of Cell Biology*, **111**, 1059–68.

Turner C.E., Schaller M.D. & Parsons J.T. (1993) Tyrosine phosphorylation of the focal adhesion kinase $pp125^{FAK}$ during development: relation to paxillin. *Journal of Cell Science*, **105**, 637–45.

Wada E., Way J., Shapira H., Kusano K., Lebacq-Verheyden A.M., Coy D., Jenson R. & Battey J. (1991) cDNA cloning, characterization, and brain region-specific expression of a neuromedin-B-preferring bombesin receptor. *Neuron*, **6**, 421–30.

Walsh J.H. (1987) Gastrointestinal hormones. In L.R. Johnson (Ed.) *Physiology of the gastrointestinal tract*, 2nd ed., p. 181. Raven Press, New York.

Walsh J.H., Bouzyk M. & Rozengurt E. (1993) Homologous desensitization of bombesin-induced increases in intracellular Ca^{2+} in quiescent Swiss 3T3 cells involves a protein kinase C-independent mechanism. *Journal of Cellular Physiology*, **156**, 333–40.

Westermark B. & Heldin C.-H. (1991) Platelet-derived growth factor in autocrine transformation. *Cancer Research*, **51**, 5087–92.

Wilkie T.M., Scherle P.A., Strathmann M.P. & Slepak V.Z. (1991) Characterization of G-protein α subunits in the Gq class: expression in murine tissues and in stromal and hematopoietic cell lines. *Proceedings of the National Academy of Sciences of the United States of America*, **88**, 10049–53.

Woll P.J. & Rozengurt E. (1988a) Two classes of antagonist interact with receptors for the mitogenic neuropeptides bombesin, bradykinin and vasopressin. *Growth Factors*, **1**, 75–83.

Woll P.J. & Rozengurt E. (1988b) [D-Arg^1, D-Phe^5, D-$Trp^{7,9}$, Leu^{11}] Substance P, a potent bombesin antagonist in murine Swiss 3T3 cells, inhibits the growth of small cell lung cancer cells *in vitro*. *Proceedings of the National Academy of Sciences of the United States of America*, **85**, 1859–63.

Woll P.J. & Rozengurt E. (1989) Multiple neuropeptides mobilise calcium in small cell lung cancer: effects of vasopressin, bradykinin, cholecystokinin, galanin and neurotensin. *Biochemical and Biophysical Research Communications*, **164**, 66–73.

Anderson L., Hoyland J., Mason W.T. & Eidne K.A. (1992) Characterization of the gonadotrophin-releasing hormone calcium response in single αT3-1 pituitary gonadotroph cells. *Molecular and Cellular Endocrinology,* **86**, 167–75.

Anderson L., Milligan G. & Eidne K.A. (1993) Characterization of the gonadotrophin-releasing hormone receptor in αT3-1 pituitary gonadotroph cells. *Journal of Endocrinology,* **136**, 51–8.

Aten R.F., Williams A.T. & Behrman H.R. (1986) Ovarian gonatropin-releasing hormone-like protein(s): demonstration and characterization. *Endocrinology,* **118**, 961–7.

Baldwin J.M. (1993) The probable arrangement of the helices in G protein-coupled receptors. *EMBO Journal,* **12**, 1693–1703.

Bardon S., Vignon F., Montcourrier P. & Rochefort H. (1987) Steroid receptor-mediated cytotoxicity of an antiestrogen and an antiprogestin in breast cancer cells. *Cancer Research,* **47**, 1441–8.

Bauer-Dantoin A.C., Hollenberg A.N. & Jameson J.L. (1993) Dynamic regulation of gonadotropin-releasing hormone receptor mRNA levels in the anterior pituitary gland during the rat estrous cycle. *Endocrinology,* **133**, 1911–14.

Baumann K.H., Kiesel L., Kaufmann M., Bastert G. & Runnebaum B. (1993) Characterization of binding sites for a GnRH-agonist (Buserelin) in human breast cancer biopsies and their distribution in relation to tumor parameters. *Breast Cancer Research Treatment,* **25**, 37–46.

Benovic J.L., Strasser R.H., Daniel K. & Lefkowitz R.J. (1986) Beta-adrenergic receptor kinase: identification of a noval protein kinase that phosphorylates the agonist-occupied form of the receptor. *Proceedings of the National Academy of Sciences of the United States of America,* **83**, 2797–2801.

Billig H., Furuta I. & Hsueh A.J.W. (1994) Gonadotropin-releasing hormone directly induces apoptotic cell death in the rat ovary: biochemical and *in situ* detection of deoxyribonucleic acid fragmentation in granulosa cells. *Endocrinology,* **134**, 245–52.

Birnbaumer L., Shahabi N., Rivier J. & Vale W. (1985) Evidence for a physiological role of gonadotropin-releasing hormone (GnRH) or GnRH-like material in the ovary. *Endocrinology,* **116**, 1367–70.

Bond C.T., Hayflick J.S., Seeburg P.H. & Adelman J.P. (1989) The rat gonadotropin-releasing hormone: SH locus: structure and hypothalamic expression. *Molecular Endocrinology,* **3**, 1257–62.

Borgeat P., Chavancy G., Dupont A., Labrie F., Arimura A. & Schally A.V. (1972) Stimulation of adenosine 3′:5′-cyclic monophosphate accumulation in anterior pituitary gland *in vitro* by synthetic luteinizing hormone-releasing hormone. *Proceedings of the National Academy of Sciences of the United State of America,* **69**, 2677–81.

Bouvier M., Guilbault N. & Bonin H. (1991) Phorbol-ester-induced phosphorylation of the β_2-adrenergic receptor decreases its coupling to G_2. *FEBS Letters,* **279**, 243–48.

Bouvier M., Hausdorff W.P., de Blasio A., O'Dowd B.F., Kobilka B.K., Caroa M.G. & Lefkowitz R.J. (1988) Removal of phosphorylation sites from the β_2-adrenergic receptor delays onset of agonist-promoted desensitization. *Nature,* **333**, 370–3.

Braden T.D. & Conn P.M. (1992) Gonadotropin-releasing hormone and its actions. In P.M. Conn & W.F. Crowley (Eds.) *Modes of action of GnRH and GnRH analogs,* pp. 26–54. Springer-Verlag, New York.

Brooks J., Taylor P.L., Saunders P.T.K., Eidne K.A., Struthers W.J. & McNeilly A.S. (1993) Cloning and sequencing of the sheep pituitary gonadotropin-releasing hormone receptor and changes in expression of its mRNA during the estrous cycle. *Molecular and Cellular Endocrinology*, **94**, R23–7.

Chang J.P., McCoy E.E., Graeter J., Tasaka K. & Catt K.J. (1986) Participation of voltage-dependent calcium channels in the action of gonadotropin-releasing hormone. *Journal of Biological Chemistry*, **261**, 9105–8.

Compton M.M. & Cidlowski J.A. (1992) Thymocyte apoptosis. A model of programmed cell death. *Trends in Endocrinology and Metabolism*, **3**, 17–23.

Conn P.M. & Crowley W.F. (1991) Gonadotropin-releasing hormone and its analogues. *New England Journal of Medicine*, **324**, 93–103.

Conn P.M., Rodgers D.C. & Seay S.G. (1984) Biphasic regulation of the gonadotropin-releasing hormone receptor by receptor microaggregation and intracellular Ca^{2+} levels. *Molecular Pharmacology*, **25**, 51–5.

Cook J.V., Faccenda E., Anderson L., Couper G.G., Eidne K.A. & Taylor P.L. (1993) Effects of Asn^{87} and Asp^{318} mutations on ligand binding and signal transduction in the rat GnRH receptor. *Journal of Endocrinology*, **139**, R1–4.

Cronin M.J., Evans W.S., Hewlett E.L. & Thorner M.O. (1984) LH release is facilitated by agents that alter cyclic AMP-generating system. *American Journal of Physiology*, **246**, E44–51.

Croxton T.L., Ben-Jonathan N. & Armstrong W.M. (1988) Gonadotropin-releasing hormone induces oscillatory membrane currents in rat gonadotropes. *Endocrinology*, **123**, 1783–91.

Davidson J., van der Merwe P.A., Wakefield I. & Millar R.P. (1991) Mechanisms of luteinizing-hormone secretion – new insights from studies with permeabilized cells. *Molecular and Cellular Endocrinology*, **76**, 1–3.

Decensi A., Torrisi R., Fontana V., Marroni P., Padovani P., Guarneri D., Minuto F. & Boccardo F. (1993) Long-term endocrine effects of administration of either a non-steroidal antiandrogen or a luteinizing hormone-releasing hormone agonist in men with prostate cancer. *Acta Endocrinologica*, **129**, 315–21.

Dong K., Yu K. & Roberts J.L. (1993) Identification of a major upstream transcription start site for the human progonadotropin-releasing hormone gene used in reproductive tissues and cell lines. *Molecular Endocrinology*, **7**, 1654–66.

Eidne K.A., Flanagan C.A. & Millar R.P. (1985) Gonadotropin-releasing hormone binding sites in human breast carcinoma. *Science*, **229**, 989–91.

Eidne K.A., Flanagan C.A., Harris N.S. & Millar R.P. (1987) Gonadotropin-releasing hormone (GnRH)-binding sites in human breast cancer cell lines and inhibitory effects of GnRH antagonists. *Journal of Clinical Endocrinology and Metabolism*, **64**, 425–32.

Eidne K.A., McNiven A.I., Taylor P.L., Plant S., House C.R., Lincoln D.W. & Yoshida S. (1988) Functional expression of rat pituitary gonadotrophin-releasing hormone receptors in *Xenopus* oocytes. *Journal of Molecular Endocrinology*, **1**, R9–12.

Eidne K.A. (1991) The polymerase chain reaction and its uses in endocrinology. *Trends in Endocrinology and Metabolism*, **2**, 169–75.

Eidne K.A., Sellar R.E., Couper G., Anderson L. & Taylor P.L. (1992) Molecular cloning and characterisation of the rat pituitary gonadotropin-releasing hormone (GnRH) receptor. *Molecular and Cellular Endocrinology*, **90**, R5–9.

Eidne K.A. (1994) Expression of receptors in *Xenopus* oocytes. In G.W. Gould (Ed.) *Membrane protein expression systems*, pp. 275–300. Portland Press, London.

Emons G., Ortmann O., Becker M., Irmer G., Springer B., Laun R., Holzel F., Schulz K.D. & Schally A.V. (1993) High affinity binding and direct antiproliferative effects of LHRH analogues in human ovarian cancer cell lines. *Cancer Research*, **53**, 5439–46.

Fekete M., Bajusz S., Groot K., Csernus V.J. & Schally A.V. (1989) Comparison of different agonist and antagonists and of luteinizing hormone-releasing hormone for receptor-binding ability to rat pituitary and human breast cancer membranes. *Endocrinology*, **124**, 946–55.

Fraser H.M. & Eidne K.A. (1989) Extrapituitary actions of LHRH analogues and LHRH-like peptides. In R.W. Shaw & J.C. Marshall (Eds.) *LHRH and its analogues: their use in gynaecological practice*, pp. 64–9. Wright, London.

Gordon K. & Hodgen G.D. (1992) Evolving role of gonadotropin-releasing-hormone antagonists. *Trends in Endocrinology and Metabolism*, **3**, 259–63.

Harris N.S., Wilcox J.N., Dutlow C.M., Flanagan C.A., Prescott R.A., Roberts J.L., Eidne K.A. & Millar R.P. (1988) A putative autocrine role for GnRH in mammary. In F. Bresciani, R.J.B. King, M.E. Lippman & J.P. Raynaud (Eds.) *Hormones and cancer*, pp. 174–8. Raven Press, New York.

Harris N., Dutlow C., Eidne E., Dong K.-W., Roberts J. & Millar R. (1991) Gonadotropin-releasing hormone gene expression in MDA-MB-231 and ZR-75-1 breast carcinoma cell lines. *Cancer Research*, **51**, 2577–81.

Harvey H.A., Lipton A., Santen R.J., Escher G.C., Hardy M.A., Glode L.M., Segaloff A., Landau R.L., Schneir H., Max D.T. (1981) Phase II study of a gonadotropin-releasing hormone analogue (Leuprolide) in postmenopausal advanced breast cancer patients. *Proceedings of the American Association of Cancer Research*, **22**, 436.

Harwood J.P., Clayton R.N. & Catt K.J. (1980a) Ovarian gonadotropin releasing hormone receptors. I. Properties and inhibition of luteal cell function. *Endocrinology*, **107**, 407.

Harwood J.P., Clayton R.N., Chen G., Knox G. & Catt K.J. (1980b) Ovarian gonadotropin-releasing hormone receptors. II. Regulation and effects of ovarian development. *Endocrinology*, **107**, 414.

Hausdorff W.P., Bouvier M., O'Dowd B.F., Irons G.P., Caron M.G. & Lefkowitz R.J. (1989) Phosphorylation sites on two domains of the β_2-adrenergic receptor are involved in distinct pathways of receptor desensitization. *Journal of Biological Chemistry*, **264**, 12657–65.

Hawes B.E. & Conn P.M. (1992) Development of gonadotrope desensitization to gonadotropin-releasing hormone (GnRH) and recovery are not coupled to inositol phosphate production or GnRH receptor number. *Endocrinology*, **131**, 2681–90.

Hawes B.E., Marzen J.E., Waters S.B. & Conn P.M. (1992) Sodium fluoride provokes gonadotrope desensitization to GnRH and gonadotrope sensitization to A23187: evidence for multiple sites of G protein actions. *Endocrinology*, **130**, 2465–75.

Hawes B.E., Water S.B., Janovick J.A., Bleasdale J.E. & Conn P.M. (1992) Gonadotropin-releasing hormone-stimulated intracellular Ca^{2+} fluctuations and LH release can be uncoupled from inositol phosphate production. *Endocrinology*, 1**30**, 3475–83.

Hazum E. (1981) Some characteristics of GnRH receptors in rat-pituitary membranes: differences between an agonist and an antagonist. *Molecular and Cellular Endocrinology*, **23**, 275.

Henderson R., Baldwin J.M., Ceska T.A., Semlin F., Beckmann E. & Downing K.H. (1990) Model for the structure of bacteriorhodopsin based on high-resolution electron cryo-microscopy. *Journal of Molecular Biology*, **213**, 899–929.

Higashijima T., Burnier J. & Ross E.M. (1990) Regulation of G_i and G_o by mastoparan, related amphipathic peptides and hydrophobic amines. *Journal of Biological Chemistry*, **265**, 14176–86.

Horn F., Bilezikjian L.M., Perrin M.H., Bosma M.M., Windle J.J., Huber K.S., Blount A.L., Hille B., Vale W. & Mellon P.L. (1991) Intracellular responses to gonadotropin-releasing hormone in a clonal cell line of the gonadotrope lineage. *Molecular Endocrinology*, **5**, 347–55.

Hsieh K.-P. & Martin T.F.J. (1992) Thyrotropin-releasing hormone and gonadotropin-releasing hormone receptors activate phospholipase C by coupling to the guanosine triphosphate-binding proteins G_q and G_{11}. *Molecular Endocrinology*, **6**, 1673–81.

Hsueh A.J.W. & Erickson G.F. (1979) Extrapituitary action of gonadotropin-releasing hormone: direct inhibition of ovarian steroidogenesis. *Science*, **204**, 854.

Hsueh A.J.W. & Ling N.C. (1979) Effect of an antagonist analog of gonadotropin-releasing hormone upon ovarian granulosa cell function. *Life Sciences*, **25**, 1223.

Izumi S.I., Stojilkovic S.S., Iida T., Krsmanovic T., Omeljaniuk R.J. & Catt K.J. (1990) Role of voltage-sensitive calcium channels in (Ca^{2+}) (i) and secretory responses to activators of protein kinase C in pituitary gonadotrophs. *Biochemical and Biophysical Research Communications*, **170**, 359–67.

Jager W., Wildt L. & Lang N. (1989) Some observations on the effects of a GnRH analog in ovarian-cancer. *European Journal of Obstetrics, Gynecology, and Reproductive Biology*, **32**, 137–48.

Janovick J.A. & Conn P.M. (1993) A cholera toxin-sensitive guanyl nucleotide binding protein mediates the movement of pituitary luteinizing hormone into a releasable pool: loss of this event is associated with the onset of homologous desensitization to gonadotropin-releasing hormone. *Endocrinology*, **132**, 2131–5.

Janovick J.A., Haviv F., Fitzpatrick T.D. & Conn P.M. (1993) Differential orientation of a GnRH agonist and antagonist in the pituitary GnRH receptor. *Endocrinology*, **133**, 942–5.

Jones P.B.C., Conn P.M., Marian J. & Hsueh A.J.W. (1980) Binding of gonadotropin releasing hormone agonist to rat ovarian granulosa cells. *Life Sciences*, **27**, 2125–32.

Kakar S.S., Musgrove L.C., Devor D.C., Sellers J.C. & Neill J.D. (1992) Cloning, sequencing and expression of human gonadotrophin releasing hormone (GnRH) receptor. *Biochemical and Biophysical Research Communications*, **189**, 289–95.

Karten M.J. & Rivier J.E. (1986) Gonadotropin-releasing hormone analog design. Structure-function studies toward the development of agonists and antagonists: rationale and perspective. *Endocrine Reviews*, **7**, 44–66.

Kavanagh J.J., Roberts W., Townsend P. & Hewitt S. (1989) Leuprolide acetate in the treatment of refractory or persistent epithelial ovarian cancer. *Journal of Clinical Oncology*, **7**, 115–18.

Kennelly P.J. & Krebs E.G. (1991) Consensus sequences as substrate specificity determinants for protein kinases and protein phosphatases. *Journal of Biological Chemistry*, **266**, 1555–8.

Kepa J.K., Wang C., Neeley C.I., Raynolds M.V., Gordon D.F., Wood W.M. & Wierman M.E. (1992) Structure of the rat gonadotropin releasing hormone (rGnRH) gene promotor and functional analysis in hypothalamic cells. *Nucleic Acids Research*, **20**, 1393–9.

Klyn J.Y. & De Jong F.M. (1982) Treatment with a luteinizing hormone-releasing hormone analogue (Buserelin) in premenopausal patients with metastatic breast cancer. *Lancet*, **1**, 1213–16.

Kyprianou N. & Isaacs J.T. (1988) Activation of programmed cell death in the rat ventral prostate after castration. *Endocrinology*, **122**, 552–62.

Layman L.C. (1991) The genetics of gonadotropin genes and the GnRH/GAP gene. *Seminars in Reproductive Endocrinology*, **9**, 22–33.

Leong D.A. & Thorner M.O. (1991) A potential code of luteinizing hormone-releasing hormone-induced calcium ion responses in the regulation of luteinizing hormone secretion among individual gonadotropes. *Journal of Biological Chemistry*, **266**, 9016–22.

Limor R., Schvartz I., Hazum E., Ayalon D. & Naor S. (1989) Effect of guanine nucleotides on stimulus secretion coupling mechanism in permeabilized pituitary cells: relationship to gonadotropin releasing hormone action. *Biochemical and Biophysical Research Communications*, **159**, 51–8.

Lincoln D.W. (1995) Gonadotropin releasing hormone (GnRH). In *De Groot's Endocrinology*, 3rd ed. W.B. Saunders Company, Philadelphia, 218–229 .

Manni A., Santen R., Harvey H., Lipton A. & Max D. (1986) Treatment of breast cancer with gonadotropin-releasing hormone. *Endocrine Reviews*, **7**, 89–94.

Mason A.J., Hayflick J.S., Zoeller R.T., Young W.S. III, Phillips H.S., Nikolics K. & Seeburg P.H. (1986a) A deletion truncating the gonadotropin-releasing hormone gene is responsible for hypogonadism in the hpg mouse. *Science*, **234**, 1366–71.

Mason A.J., Pitts S.L., Nikolics K., Szonyi E., Wilcox J.N., Seerburg P.H. & Stewart T.A. (1986b) The hypogonadal mouse: reproductive functions restored by gene therapy. *Science*, **234**, 1372–8.

Mason W.T. & Sikdar S.K. (1988) Characterization of voltage-gated sodium channels in bovine gonadotrophs: relationship to hormone secretion. *Journal of Physiology*, **399**, 493–517.

McArdle C.A. & Poch A. (1992) Dependence of gonadotrophin-releasing hormone-stimulated luteinizing hormone release upon intracellular Ca^{2+} pools is revealed by desensitization and thapsigargin blockade. *Endocrinology*, **130**, 3567–74.

Meyerhof W., Morley S., Schwartz J. & Richer D. (1988) Receptors for neuropeptides are induced by exogenous poly(A)$^+$ RNA in oocytes from *Xenopus laevis*. *Proceedings of the National Academy of Sciences of the United States of America*, **85**, 714–17.

Millar R.P., Wormald P.J. & de L. Milton R.C. (1986) Stimulation of gonadotropin release by a non-GnRH peptide sequence of the GnRH precursor. *Science*, **232**, 68–70.

Miller W.R., Scott W.N., Morris R., Fraser H.M. & Sharpe R.M. (1985) LHRH agonists and human breast cancer cells. *Nature*, **329**, 770.

Milligan G. (1993) Mechanisms of multifunctional signalling by G protein-linked receptors. *Trends in Pharmacological Sciences*, **14**, 239–44.

Milovanovic S.R., Radulovic S. & Schally A.V. (1992) Evaluation of binding of cytotoxic analogs of luteinizing hormone-releasing hormone to human breast cancer and mouse MXT mammary tumor. *Breast Cancer Research and Treatment*, **24**, 147–58.

Momany F.A. (1976) Conformational energy analysis of the molecule, luteinizing hormone-releasing hormone. *Journal of the American Chemical Society*, **98**, 2990–6.

Morgan J.E., O'Neil C.E., Coy D.H., Hocart S.J. & Nekola M.V. (1986) Antagonistic analogs of luteinizing hormone-releasing hormone are mast cell secretagogues. *International Archives of Allergy and Immunology*, **80**, 70–5.

Morgan R.O., Chang J.P. & Catt K.J. (1987) Novel aspects of gonadotropin releasing hormone action on inositol phosphate metabolism in cultured pituitary gonadotrophs. *Journal of Biological Chemistry*, **262**, 1166–71.

Morrison N., Sellar R.E., Boyd E., Eidne K.A. & Connor J.M. (1994) Assignment of the gene encoding the human gonadotropin-releasing hormone receptor to 4q13.2-13.3 by fluorescence in situ hybridisation. *Human Genetics*, **93**, 714–715.

Mullen P., Bramley T., Menzies G. & Miller B. (1992) Failure to detect gonadotrophin-releasing hormone receptors in human benign and malignant breast tissue and in MCF-7 and MDA-MB-231 cancer cells. *European Journal of Cancer*, **29A**, 248–52.

Naor S., Zer J., Zakut H. & Hermon J. (1985) Characterization of pituitary calcium-activated, phospholipid-dependent protein-kinase redistribution by gonadotropin-releasing hormone. *Proceedings of the National Academy of Sciences of the United States of America*, **82**, 8203–7.

Naor Z., Fawcett C.P. & McCann S.M. (1979) Differential effects of castration and testosterone replacement on basal and LHRH-stimulated cAMP and cGMP accumulation and on gonadotropin release from the pituitary of the male rat. *Molecular and Cellular Endocrinology*, **14**, 191–8.

Nicholson R.I., Walker K.J., Turkes A., Turkes A.O., Dyas J., Blamey R.W., Campbell F.C., Robinson M.R.G. & Griffiths K. (1984) Therapeutic significance and the mechanism of action of the LH-RH agonist ICI 118630 in breast and prostate cancer. *Journal of Steroid Biochemistry*, **20**, 129.

Nikolics K., Mason A.J., Szonyi E., Ramachandran J. & Seeburg H. (1985) A prolactin-inhibiting factor within the precursor for human gonadotropin-releasing hormone. *Nature*, **316**, 511–17.

Nussenzveig D.R., Heinflink M. & Gershengorn M.C. (1993a) Agonist-stimulated internalization of the thyrotropin-releasing hormone receptor is dependent on two domains in the receptor carboxyl terminus. *Journal of Biological Chemistry*, **268**, 2389–92.

Nussenzveig D.R., Heinflink M. & Gershengorn M.C. (1993b) Decreased levels of internalized thyrotropin-releasing hormone receptors after uncoupling from guanine nucleotide-binding proteins and phospholipase-C. *Journal of Molecular Endocrinology*, **7**, 1105–11.

Oron Y., Straub R.E., Traktman P. & Gershengorn M.C. (1987) Decreased TRH receptor mRNA activity precedes homologues down-regulation: assay in oocytes. *Science*, **85**, 1406–8.

Parmar H., Nicoll J., Stockdale A., Cassoni A., Phillips R.H., Lightman S.L. & Schally A.V. (1985) Advanced ovarian carcinoma: response to the agonist D-Trp-6-LHRH. *Cancer Treatment Reports*, **69**, 1341–2.

Perrin M.H., Haas Y., Porter J., Rivier J. & Vale W. (1989) The gonadotropin-releasing hormone pituitary receptor interacts with a guanosine triphosphate-binding protein: differential effects of guanyl nucleotides on agonist and antagonist binding. *Endocrinology*, **124**, 798–803.

Petit C. (1993) Molecular basis of the X-chromosome-linked Kallman's syndrome. *TEMS*, **4**, 8–13.

Pieper D.R., Richards J.S. & Marshall J.C. (1981) Ovarian gonadotropin-releasing hormone (GnRH) receptors: characterization, distribution and induction by GnRH. *Endocrinology*, **108**, 1148–55.

Pinski J., Schally A.V., Yano T., Szepeshazi K., Halmos G., Groot K., Comaru Schally A.M., Radulovic S. & Nagy A. (1993) Inhibition of growth of experimental prostate cancer in rats by LH-RH analogs linked to cytotoxic radicals. *Prostate*, **23**, 165–78.

Plowman P.N., Nicholson R.I. & Walker K.J. (1986) Remission of postmenopausal breast cancer during treatment with the luteinising hormone-releasing hormone agonist. *British Journal of Cancer*, **54**, 903–9.

Prevost G., Mormont C., Gunning M. & Thomas F. (1993) Therapeutic use and perspectives of synthetic peptides in oncology. *Acta Oncologica*, **32**, 209–15.

Probst W.C., Snyder L.A., Schuster D.I., Brosius J. & Sealfon S.C. (1992) Sequence alignment of the G-protein coupled receptor superfamily. *Molecular and Cellular Biology*, **11**, 1–20.

Qayum A., Gullick W., Clayton R.C., Sikora K. & Waxman J. (1990a) The effects of gonadotropin releasing hormone analogues in prostate cancer are mediated through specific tumour receptors. *British Journal of Cancer*, **62**, 96–9.

Qayum A., Gullick W.J., Mellon K., Krausz T., Neal D., Sikora K. & Waxman J. (1990b) The partial purification and characterization of GnRH-like activity from prostatic biopsy specimens and prostatic cancer cell lines. *Journal of Steroid Biochemistry and Molecular Biology*, **37**, 899–902.

Redding T.W., Schally A.V., Radulovic S., Milovanovic S., Szepeshazi K. & Isaacs J. (1992) Sustained release formulations of luteinizing hormone-releasing hormone antagonist SB-75 inhibit proliferation and enhance apoptotic cell death of human prostate carcinoma (PC-82) in male nude mice. *Cancer Research*, **52**, 2538–44.

Reinhart J., Mertz L.M. & Catt K.J. (1992) Molecular cloning and expression of cDNA encoding the murine gonadotropin-releasing hormone receptor. *Journal of Biological Chemistry*, **267**, 21281–4.

Reissmann T., Hilgard P., Harleman J.H., Engel J., Comaru-Schally A.M. & Schally A.V. (1992) Treatment of experimental DMBA induced mammary carcinoma with Cetrorelix (SB-75): a potent antagonist of luteinizing hormone-releasing hormone. *Journal of Cancer Research and Clinical Oncology*, **118**, 44–9.

Richardson R.M., Kin C., Benovic J.L. & Hosey M.M. (1993) Phosphorylation and desensitization of human m2 muscarinic cholinergic receptors by two isoforms of the β-adrenergic receptors. *Journal of Biological Chemistry*, **268**, 13650–6.

Rotello R.J., Hocker M.B. & Gerschenson E. (1989) Biochemical evidence for programmed cell death in rabbit uterine epithelium. *American Journal of Physiology*, **134**, 491–5.

Santen R.J., Manni A. & Harvey H. (1986) Gonadotropin-releasing hormone (GnRH) analogs for the treatment of breast and prostatic carcinoma. *Breast Cancer Research and Treatment*, **7**, 129–45.

Schally A.V., Comaru-Schally A.M. & Redding T.W. (1984) Antitumor effects of analogs of hypothalamic hormones in endocrine-dependent cancers. *Proceedings of the Society for Experimental Biology and Medicine*, **175**, 259–81.

Schwanzel Fukuda M., Bick D. & Pfaff D.W. (1989) Luteinizing hormone-releasing hormone (LHRH)- expressing cells do not migrate normally in an inherited hypogonadal (Kallman) syndrome. *Molecular Brain Research*, **6**, 311–26.

Seeburg P.H. & Adelman J.P. (1984) Characterization of cDNA for precursor of human luteinizing hormone releasing hormone. *Nature*, **311**, 666–8.

Segal T., Levy J. & Sharoni Y. (1987) GnRH analogs stimulate phospholipase-C activity in mammary-tumor membranes. *Molecular and Cellular Endocrinology*, **53**, 239–43.

Segal-Abramson T., Giat J., Levy J. & Sharoni Y. (1992) Guanine nucleotide modulation of high affinity gonadotropin-releasing hormone receptors in rat mammary tumors. *Molecular and Cellular Endocrinology*, **85**, 109–16.

Segal-Abramson T., Kitroser H., Levy J., Schally A.V. & Sharoni Y. (1992) Direct effects of luteinizing hormone-releasing hormone agonists and antagonists on MCF-7 mammary cancer cells. *Proceedings of the National Academy of Sciences of the United States of America*, **89**, 2336–9.

Shangold G.A., Murphy S.N. & Miller R.J. (1988) Gonadotrophin-releasing hormone-induced Ca^{2+} transients in single identified gonadotrophs require both intracellular Ca^{2+} mobilisation and Ca^{2+} flux. *Physiological Science*, **85**, 6566–70.

Sharoni Y., Bosin E., Miinster A., Levy J. & Schally A.V. (1989) Inhibition of growth of human mammary tumor cells by potent antagonists of luteinizing hormone-releasing hormone. *Proceedings of the National Academy of Sciences of the United States of America*, **86**, 1648–51.

Smith W.A. & Conn P.M. (1984) GnRH-mediated desensitization of the pituitary gonadotrope is not calcium dependent. *Endocrinology*, **112**, 408–10.

Strader C.D., Sigal I.S. & Dixon R.A.F. (1989) Structural basis of β-adrenergic function. *FASEB Journal*, **3**, 1825–32.

Strader C.D., Sigal I.S., Register R.B., Candelore M.R., Rands E. & Dixon R.A.F. (1987) Identification of residues required for ligand binding to the β-adrenergic receptor. *Proceedings of the National Academy of Sciences of the United States of America*, **84**, 4384–8.

Sumikawa K. & Miledi R. (1988) Repression of nicotinic acetylcholine receptor expression by antisense RNAs and an oligonucleotide. *Proceedings of the National Academy of Sciences of the United States of America*, **85**, 1302–6.

Szende B., Lapis K., Redding T.W., Srkalovic G. & Schally A.V. (1989a) Growth inhibition of MXT mammary carcinoma by enhancing programmed cell death (apoptosis) with analogs of LH-RH and somatostatin. *Breast Cancer Research and Treatment*, **14**, 307–14.

Szende B., Zalatnai A. & Schally A.V. (1989b) Programmed cell death (apoptosis) in pancreatic cancers of hamsters after treatment with analogs of both luteinizing hormone-releasing and somatostatin. *Proceedings of the National Academy of Sciences of the United States of America*, **86**, 1643–7.

Szepeshazi K., Schally A.V., Juhasz A., Nagy A. & Janaky T. (1992) Effect of luteinizing hormone-releasing hormone analogs containing cytotoxic radicals on growth of estrogen-independent MXT mouse mammary carcinoma in vivo. *Anticancer Drugs*, **3**, 109–16.

Thompson M.A., Adelson M.D. & Kaufman L.M. (1991) Lupron retards proliferation of ovarian epithelial tumor cells cultured in serum-free medium. *Journal of Clinical Endocrinology and Metabolism,* **72**, 1036–41.

Tsutsumi M., Zhou W., Millar R.P., Mellon P.L., Roberts J.L., Flanagan C.A., Dong K., Gillo B. & Sealfon S.C. (1992) Cloning and functional expression of a mouse gonadotropin-releasing hormone receptor. *Molecular Endocrinology,* **6**, 1163–9.

Turgeon J.L. & Waring D.W. (1987) Adenosine 3′,5′-monophosphate primes the secretion of follicle-stimulating hormone. *Endocrinology,* **120**, 1602–7.

Vale W., Grant G., Rivier J., Monahan M., Amoss M., Blackwell R., Burgus R. & Guillemin R. (1972) Synthetic polypeptide antagonists of the hypothalamic luteinizing hormone releasing factor. *Science,* **176**, 933.

Walker N.I., Bennett R.E. & Kerr J.R.F. (1989) Cell death by apoptosis during involution of the lactating breast in mice and rats. *American Journal of Anatomy,* **185**, 19–32.

Waxman J.M., Masland S.J., Coomber R.C., Wrigley P.F., Malpas J.S., Powles T. & Lister T.A. (1985) The treatment of postmenopausal women with advanced breast cancer with buserelin. *Cancer Chemotherapy and Pharmacology,* **15**, 171–3.

Waxman J. (1987) Gonadotrophin hormone releasing analogues open new doors in cancer treatment. *British Medical Journal,* **295**, 1084–5.

Wickings E.J., Eidne K.A., Dixson A.F. & Hillier S.G. (1990) Gonadotropin-releasing hormone analogs inhibit primate granulosa cell steroidogenesis via a mechanism distinct from that in the rat. *Biology of Reproduction,* **43**, 305–11.

Wilding G., Chen M. & Gelmann E.P. (1987) LHRH agonists and human breast cancer cells. *Nature,* **329**, 770.

Williamson P., Lang J. & Boyd Y. (1991) The gonadotropin-releasing hormone (GnRH) gene maps to mouse chromosome 14 and identifies a homologous region on human chromosome 8. *Somatic Cell and Molecular Genetics,* **17**, 609–15.

Windle J.J., Weiner R.I. & Mellon P.L. (1990) Cell lines of the pituitary gonadotrope linege derived to targeted oncogenesis in transgenic mice. *Molecular Endocrinology,* **4**, 597–603.

Wojcikiewicz R.J.H., Tobin A.B. & Nahorski S.R. (1993) Desensitization of cell signalling mediated by phosphoinositidase C. *Trends in Pharmcological Science,* **14**, 279–85.

Wong S. K.-F., Parker E.M. & Ross E.M. (1990) Chimeric Muscarinic Cholinergic: β-adrenergic receptors that activate G_s in response to muscarinic agonists. *Journal of Biological Chemistry,* **265**, 6219–24.

Wormald P.J., Eidne K.A. & Millar R.P. (1985) Gonadotropin-releasing hormone receptors in human pituitary: ligand structural requirements, molecular size and cationic effects. *Journal of Clinical Endocrinology and Metabolism,* **61**, 1190–4.

Wyllie A.H. (1980) Glucocorticoid-induced thymocyte apoptosis is associated with endogenous endonuclease activity. *Nature,* **284**, 555–6.

Yang-Feng T.L., Seeburg P.H. & Francke U. (1986) Human luteinizing hormone-releasing hormone gene (LHRH) is located on the short arm of chromosome 8 (region 8p11.2-p21). *Somatic Cell and Molecular Genetics,* **12**, 95–100.

Yano T., Korkut E., Pinski J., Szepeshazi K., Milovanovic S., Groot K., Clarke & Comaru-Schally A.M. (1992) Inhibition of growth of MCF-7 MIII human breast carcinoma in nude mice by treatment with agonists or antagonists of LH-RH. *Breast Cancer Research and Treatment,* **21**, 35–45.

Yoshida S. & Plant S. (1991) A potassium current evoked by growth hormone-releasing hormone in follicular oocytes of *Xenopus Laevis. Journal of Physiology,* **443**, 651–67.

Yoshida S., Plant S., Taylor P.L. & Eidne K.A. (1989) Chloride channels mediate the response to gonadotropin-releasing hormone (GnRH) in *Xenopus* oocytes injected with rat anterior pituitary mRNA. *Molecular Endocrinology,* **3**, 1953–60.

Zeleznick A.J., Ihrig L.L. & Bassett S.G. (1989) Developmental expression of Ca^{++}/Mg^{++} dependent endonuclease activity in rat granulosa and luteal cells. *Endocrinology,* **125**, 2218–20.

6 Cytokines

T. HAMBLIN

INTRODUCTION

Cytokines are molecules produced by cells of the lymphohaemopoietic system (LHS) that are involved in signalling between the cells of that system. Conventionally, antibodies are excluded from this group, even though they form part of the extensive communication that takes place between cells of different lineages.

The LHS may be regarded as the largest and most extensive organ in the body, albeit a fluid and mobile one. It is also the most accessible organ and is consequently the best studied. The cytokines are the hormones that control the function of the LHS, but since the LHS is itself both extensive and mobile, the hormones controlling it do not need to be. With the single and prominent exception of erythropoietin, they are all produced close to their site of action.

Since the LHS is so accessible, it is not surprising that no fewer than 56 cytokines are currently identified, and the number grows weekly. They have been identified from three main lines of investigation. The interferons were first recognized from their interference with viral replication, the haemopoietic growth factors for their effect on the growth of bone marrow colonies in semisolid media and the interleukins from their presence in the supernatant fluid of cultures of lymphocytes in medium containing various mitogens. The names of the various cytokines derive from their mode of discovery but are to some extent accidental. For example, interleukin-3 (IL-3) is an early haemopoietic growth factor, while granulocyte/macrophage colony-stimulating factor (GM-CSF) also stimulates T cell proliferation. In truth, most cytokines are pleiotropic, produced by a variety of cells, and have overlapping and apparently redundant functions.

Table 6.1 lists the most important cytokines according to principal function. I have omitted those whose main function concerns the supporting structure of the bone marrow and blood vessels. Some of these, such as the seven varieties of fibroblast growth factor, and epidermal growth factor, are dealt with elsewhere in this volume. The functions listed in the table are not comprehensive; indeed, for many of the newer cytokines the complete range of activities is simply not known.

THE INTERFERONS

Interferons were first recognized by Isaacs and Lindenmann in 1957. They were described as proteins produced by vertebrate cells in response to virus infection that were able to confer resistance to a wide variety of viruses on cells from the same species. Since their discovery they have emerged as a group of molecules with a variety of activities concerned with the control of growth and differentiation of both haemopoietic and nonhaemopoietic cells.

It is now recognized that there are three types of interferon molecules as described in Table 6.2. (Balkwill, 1989). Interferon-α (IFN-α) is produced by lymphocytes and macrophages. There are at least 15 functional genes clustered on chromosome 9, producing interferons with 90% sequence homology. Type I IFN-αs have 165 or 166 amino acids and are unglycosylated, and type II IFN-αs have 172 amino acids and are glycosylated. The single IFN-β gene is also on chromosome 9 and codes for a protein of 187 amino acids that is secreted by fibroblasts and epithelial cells. Both IFN-α and IFN-β are stimulated by viruses and a variety of other pathogens as well as by double-stranded

Table 6.1. Important Cytokines and Their Functions

Type of Cytokine	Examples
The interferons	Interferon-α, -β and -γ
Haemopoietic growth factors	SCF, GM-CSF, G-CSF, M-CSF, IL-3, IL-5, IL-9, IL-11, LIF, EPO, (IL-1) and (IL-6)
Lymphocytic growth factors	IL-2, IL-4, IL-7, IL-10, IL-12, IL-13, IL-14, LMW-BCGF and TGF-β
Chemokines	IL-8, IP-10, MCP-1, MIP-1, RANTES and MGSA
Multipotent cytokines	IL-1α, IL-1β, IL-1ra, IL-6, TNF-α and TNF-β

Table 6.2. The Interferons

Interferon-α	165/6 aa	T cells B cells Monocytes	Antiviral Enhances NK activity Modulates MHC class I expression Inhibits cell growth Influences differentiation
Interferon-β	166 aa	Fibroblasts	Similar to interferon-α
Interferon-γ	143 aa	T cells NK cells	Similar to interferon-α but also up-regulates MHC class II expression Activates macrophages Induces cytokine secretion and cytokine receptors

RNA. On the other hand, IFN-γ is produced by T cells and natural killer (NK) cells in response to mitogens and specific antigens for which there is pre-existing immunity. It is coded for by a single gene on chromosome 12, and has 166 amino acids.

There are specific receptors for interferons. A 110- to 130-kDa protein coded for by a gene on chromosome 21 acts as a receptor for both IFN-α and IFN-β. The gene for the IFN-γ receptor is located on chromosome 6. When interferons combine with their receptors they induce signals for a number of cellular genes and thus exert multiple regulatory effects on cells. The effects on intracellular proteins are extremely complicated. Perhaps 1% of such proteins are up-regulated by interferon stimulation, with perhaps just as many down-regulated. The majority of genes affected by interferons are responsive to all three types, although some are specifically stimulated or suppressed.

Most of the biological effects of interferons have not been worked out in detail, although some of the antiviral mechanisms are now clear. For example, in the presence of viral double-stranded RNA, interferon induces the synthesis of 2,5′-oligo-adenylate synthetase, which forms 2′,5′-linked oligonucleotides, which activate endogenous endonucleases, which then degrade both messenger and ribosomal RNA (Revel & Chebath, 1986).

The biological effects of interferons are threefold: antiviral, immunomodulatory and control of cell growth and differentiation.

Antiviral Effects

The interferons are extremely potent antiviral agents, acting at 10^{-15} M levels. They are active against a wide variety of viruses and other intracellular parasites, making use of a variety of antiviral mechanisms (Williams & Fish, 1985). As well as antidouble-stranded RNA effect of 2,5′-oligoadenylate synthetase induction, the induction of the *Mx* protein has an anti-influenza effect, the C56 protein protects against the vesicular stomatitis virus and the enzyme indolamine dioxygenase protects against *Toxoplasma gondii*.

Immunomodulatory Effects

Multiple effects of interferon serve to regulate the immune response (Balkwill, 1985a). All interferons up-regulate the expression of class I major histocompatibility (MHC) antigens, which must be expressed if a cell is to be a target of the cytotoxic T cells. In addition, IFN-γ up-regulates MHC class II antigens, even on cells that do not normally express them. These antigens are required for a cell to present antigen to T helper cells and thus trigger the immune response. Induction of MHC class II on tumour cells may be a means of presenting tumour-specific antigens to the immune system.

Interferons increase the numbers of IgG Fc receptors on monocytes and enhance monocyte antibody-dependent cellular cytotoxicity (ADCC). IFN-γ is a macrophage activating factor, enhancing nonspecific cytotoxicity. T cell cytotoxicity is also enhanced. IFN-γ enhances neutrophil ADCC, while all interferons enhance NK activity. IFN-γ up-regulates TNF receptors on many cell lines, and IL-2 receptors on T cells. Finally, IFN-γ is a B cell maturation factor that increases antibody synthesis in the presence of IL-2.

Control of Growth and Differentiation

Interferons induce reversible cytostasis in normal and transformed cells (Taylor-Papadimitriou & Rozengurt, 1985). This effect is mediated in part through the inhibition of cellular proto-oncogenes. Thus, in different systems c-*myc*, c-*mos*, c-*src* and c-H-*ras* are all suppressed by IFN. On the other hand, as has been seen with the immune system, some of the differentiated functions of cells are enhanced.

Applications as Cancer Therapy

Early experiments with animal tumours demonstrated that interferons could inhibit not only virally induced tumours but chemically induced ones as well (Balkwill, 1985b). All of the biological effects detailed above – regulation of cell growth, immunomodulation and virus suppression – may play a part in tumour inhibition. Like the antiviral effect, the antitumour effect is species specific. In murine tumours, a dose–response curve has been demonstrated, with the greatest effect in small tumour masses and in the prevention of metastasis. Human IFNs inhibit the growth of a wide variety of human tumour xenografts in nude mice; however, few regressions are seen and cures are very rare. IFN-α is more active than IFN-γ. Of course in xenografts no effect on host tumour interaction can be assessed.

All three human interferons are now available in recombinant form and have been assessed for antitumour activity. Table 6.3 lists the tumours that have shown clinical response to IFN-α. Although this table correctly demonstrates the broad spectrum of clinical effects, it gives an overoptimistic view of clinical effectiveness, since many of the responses documented are partial or minor.

Hairy Cell Leukaemia (HCL) Almost every patient responds to IFN-α, but complete remissions are rare (Platanias & Golomb, 1993). Those patients with HCL who require treatment do so because of cytopenias, which render the patient susceptible to infections. Low

Table 6.3. Clinical Responses of Tumour Types to Interferons

Interferon-α	
Hairy cell leukaemia	98%
Chronic granulocytic leukaemia	81%
Low-grade lymphoma	42%
Chronic lymphocytic leukaemia	18%
Cutaneous T cell lymphoma	45%
Essential thrombocythaemia	75%
Myeloma	20%
Melanoma	11%
Renal cell carcinoma	17%
Kaposi's sarcoma	48%
Carcinoid	67%
Apudomas	77%
Head and neck (squamous)	90%
Cervical	43%
Interferon-β	
Renal cell carcinoma	11%
Adult T cell leukaemia	50%
Interferon-γ	
Renal cell carcinoma	25%
Adult T cell leukaemia	60%
Chronic granulocytic leukaemia	40%

Source: Modified after Griffiths, Galvani & Cawley, 1989.

doses of IFN-α (2×10^6 U/m^2 subcutaneously three times a week) successfully normalize the blood count over about six months. Most patients eventually relapse when the IFN is stopped but respond well when it is reintroduced. Side effects of malaise and mild fever usually disappear after the first month and are well tolerated.

Lymphomas Advanced low-grade non-Hodgkin's lymphoma responds well to IFN-α at high doses (50×10^6 U/m^2 subcutaneously three times a week) but the toxic effects and cost of such treatment make it very much a last resort when all forms of chemotherapy have failed (Foon & Sherwin, 1984). The same applies for cutaneous T cell lymphoma (Bunn, Foon & Ibide, 1984). IFN-α is ineffective in advanced chronic lymphocytic leukaemia. Low doses produce good responses in stage A diseases (Foon, Bottino & Abrams, 1985), but clinical trials have demonstrated that stage A disease does not need treating.

Chronic Granulocytic Leukaemia Unlike busulphan or hydroxyurea, IFN-α is capable of achieving cytogenetic remission in chronic granulocytic leukaemia (CGL) (although the bcr-abl construct always remains detectable by polymerase chain reaction [PCR]). Between 70 and 80% of patients achieve a complete haematological response on IFN-α (Talpaz et al., 1986), 20 to 40% achieve a major cytogenetic response and 10 to 25% achieve a durable major cytogenetic response. Most patients respond to a dose of 5×10^6 U/m^2 subcutaneously daily, but some have required up to four times this dose. Cytogenetic remission carries with it an improved overall survival. Recent phase III trials have confirmed that patients with haematological responses have an overall survival benefit (Italian Co-operative Study Group, 1994) and it is now clear that IFN-α should be used as a first-line agent in this disease. Phase I/II trials of IFN-α also show a beneficial response in CGL, but although in vitro studies suggest synergism with IFN-γ, there seems to be no clinical benefit to using the drugs in concert (Kurzrock et al., 1987).

Myeloma Although there is no doubt that IFN-α is an effective drug in myeloma, its place in therapy has not yet been established. As a single agent it has little or no value, but early studies suggested that the 'plateau phase' after chemotherapy was longer in patients receiving IFN-α (Mandelli et al., 1990). However, this may have been a statistical artifact because of poor survival in the control group. More recent evidence suggests that the value of IFN-α in prolonging remission is mainly in patients who achieve very low levels of serum paraprotein after, for example, high-dose melphalan (Cunningham et al., 1994).

Kaposi's Sarcoma The original report of the effect of IFN-α in Kaposi's sarcoma gave a response rate of 38%, with the best results being achieved with a dose of 30 $\times$ 10^6 U daily in patients with good immune function (Krown et al., 1983). The median duration of response is 18 months. Recent trials have confirmed the overall response rate.

Melanoma Occasional long-term responses have been reported in melanoma, but although most trials show a response rate of around 15%, they are usually confined to lung, lymph node and soft tissue tumours, and are short lived and in patients with a low tumour burden (Dorval et al., 1986; Kuzmits et al., 1985.)

Renal Cell Carcinoma Occasionally a patient whose primary has been resected and who has small lung secondaries achieves a complete remission. However, for most other patients, a transient partial response in about 15% is the best that can be hoped for (Kirkwood, Ernstoff & Davis, 1985).

Carcinoid and Other APUD Tumours Reductions in tumour markers are commonly seen in these tumours. There is often relief of symptoms, and in 5% of patients objective evidence of response (Erikson et al., 1986).

Papillomata Recurrent laryngeal papillomatosis is a virus-induced condition that is distressing, leading to airways obstruction, and difficult to treat. An encouraging report of 6 of 19 patients achieving a complete response and nine others being left with only minimal residual disease after treatment with 3 $\times$ 10^6 U thrice weekly has been confirmed more recently (McCabe & Clark, 1983) and the value of interferon in this disease remains contentious.

Several reports have suggested good responses to IFN-α in condylomata acuminata, and bladder papillomata respond to intralesional injections (Gall, Hughes & Trofatter, 1983; Eron, Judson & Tucker, 1986). In this last case IFN-α is unlikely to replace simple cautery.

Clinical Trials of IFN-α and IFN-γ Although IFN-γ has been much less evaluated than IFN-α, it shows a similar range of activity. There seems to be little likelihood that it will be a clinically significant agent in cancer. IFN-γ is a more potent immunoregulator than the other interferons but has no greater antitumour activity. The range of responsive tumours is the same.

Side Effects of Interferons All three types of interferon cause 'flu-like' side effects. Fevers, headache, malaise, myalgias and fatigue are almost universal, but usually abate during the first month of treatment. Gastrointestinal effects are rarer, and some patients have disordered liver function tests, neutropenia or thrombocytopenia. At high doses, central nervous system (CNS) effects including disorientation, depression, hallucinations and coma are more common. Occasional patients develop autoantibodies and some become hypothyroid due to immune attack. Some patients develop inactivating antibodies against the interferon.

Summary of Clinical Effectiveness of Interferons in Cancer Interferons have a degree of clinical effectiveness against a group of rare cancers. In general, low-bulk, slow-growing, well-differentiated tumours respond best. IFNs need to be given in low dose over a prolonged period, and responses appear slowly. Their use in combination with chemotherapeutic agents is currently being explored, but at present the IFNs are very minor players in the fight against cancer.

THE REGULATION OF HAEMOPOIESIS

In man around 3 million blood cells are made every second. This is necessary because all types of blood cells have short lifespans and need to be rapidly replenished by the proliferation and differentiation of various precursor cells present in the bone marrow. Such precursors derive from common stem cells, which in the embryo are located first in the yoke sac, then the liver, finally migrating to their adult site in the bone marrow.

Stem cells in the bone marrow are few in number, comprising less than 1 in 10,000 cells, but are capable of almost indefinite self-replication while at the same time being able to differentiate along a wide range of lineages that include erythroid, neutrophil granulocytic, eosinophilic, thrombocytic, mast cell-basophilic, mononuclear phagocytic, B-lymphocytic and various types of T-lymphocytic. Differentiation involves an enormous expansion in cell numbers. Production of cells of these lineages is highly ordered but capable of rapid response to a number of different stimuli. Regulation of haemopoiesis is achieved by the haemopoietic growth factors.

The seminal observation by Bradley and Metcalf (1966) that haemopoietic cells immobilized in agar and supplied with media previously used to sustain the growth on nonhaemopoietic cells would generate colonies of mature neutrophils and macrophages has led to the unravelling of many of the complicated mechanisms of haemopoietic control. Refinements of this work led to the growth of colonies producing other mature elements of peripheral blood, and the term 'colony-stimulating factors' (CSFs) was coined to describe the molecules present in the conditioned medium responsible for stimulating the growth and differentiation of haemopoietic precursors (Metcalf, 1984).

Although much of the important work on haemopoiesis was performed using crude extracts, developments in molecular biology have allowed the production of recombinant forms of the CSFs, which are available for analysis. Four molecules were identified in this way: granulocyte CSF (G-CSF), macrophage CSF (M-CSF), granulocyte-macrophage CSF (GM-CSF) and multi-CSF, now shown to be the same, and usually referred to, as interleukin-3 (IL-3). A consequence of this identity has been the alliance of haematologists, immunologists and molecular biologists in the search for other haemopoietic factors. Thus far IL-5, IL-9 and IL-11 have been identified as such. In addition, stem cell factor (SCF), leukaemia inhibitory factor (LIF), IL-1 and IL-6 all play a part in early haematopoiesis. Finally, erythropoietin, which was discovered in the 1950s, must be numbered among the haemopoietic growth factors, despite strictly being a hormone rather than a cytokine.

These factors, which are summarized in Table 6.4, will now be discussed individually in terms of structure and function and then in a clinical context.

Erythropoietin (EPO) (Krantz, 1991) is the principal controlling factor for erythropoiesis but differs from other haemopoietic growth factors in being produced remote from the bone marrow. The molecule, a 166 amino acid glycoprotein of molecular weight 39 kDa, is secreted mainly by the juxtaglomerular apparatus of the kidney, but lower levels are also produced by the liver and bone marrow macrophages. The primary stimulus for increased EPO production is tissue hypoxia, which is read by the body as anaemia, but of course can be caused by other local and systemic effects. The EPO gene has been mapped to chromosome 7.

The EPO receptor (Youssoufian et al., 1993) is one of a family of cytokine receptors that also include those of IL-3, IL-4, IL-6, IL-7, G-CSF, GM-CSF and the β-subunit of the IL-2 receptor. The EPO receptor gene is found on the short arm of chromosome 19. Interaction of

Table 6.4. The Haemopoietic Growth Factors

SCF	164 aa	Bone marrow stromal cells	Synergizes with other HGFs Mast cell growth factor
LIF	179 aa	Bone marrow stromal cells T cells Macrophages	Synergizes with other HGFs in stimulating early progenitors and megakaryocytes
IL-3	133 aa	T cells	Proliferation of multipotent progenitor cells
GM-CSF	127 aa	Macrophages	Growth and differentiation of multipotent progenitor cells
G-CSF	174 aa	T cells	Differentiation and activation of neutrophils
M-CSF	233 aa or 158 aa	T cells	Growth and development of macrophages Stimulates macrophage functions
IL-5	115 aa	T cells	Growth and differentiation of eosinophils
EPO	165 aa	Kidney	Growth and differentiation of erythroid precursors
IL-9	126 aa	T cells	Synergizes with EPO to promote erythrocyte burst forming units
IL-11	178 aa	Stromal cells	Stimulates megakaryocyte progenitors
(IL-1)	270 aa	Monocytes Macrophages	Synergizes with other HGFs to stimulate early progenitors
(IL-6)	213 aa	Monocytes Macrophages	Synergizes with other HGFs to stimulate early progenitors

EPO with its receptor causes the phosphorylation of several cellular proteins, changes intracellular free calcium levels and alters the expression of c-*myc* and c-*myb* proto-oncogenes.

EPO potentiates the formation of burst-forming units (BFU-E) from the common progenitor cell (CFU-GEMM), and then influences their differentiation through erythroid colony-forming units (CFU-E), erythroblasts of varying degrees of maturity to reticulocytes and erythrocytes (Goldwasser, 1984).

Excessive production of EPO raises the haemoglobin and the haematocrit. The kidney produces excessive quantities of the hormone in a variety of conditions that it interprets as anaemia. These include hypoxia due to right-to-left cardiac shunts, respiratory disease, high-affinity haemoglobin variants, life at high altitudes and renal artery stenosis. There is ectopic production of EPO by a range of tumours which include renal cell carcinoma, cerebellar haemangioblastoma, hepatoma and leiomyoma.

G-CSF is a 24-kDa glycoprotein, α-helical in structure. The 177 amino acid molecule is cleaved from a 207 amino acid precursor. The gene has been mapped to chromosome 17q21-22 close to the break point seen in promyelocytic leukaemia. The proto-oncogenes c-*erb*-B2 and c-*erb*A and the nerve growth factor receptor gene are close by. There is weak sequence homology to the IL-6 gene. The G-CSF receptor consists of a single subunit protein of 150 kDa found on neutrophils and their precursors. There is an extracellular domain similar to the prolactin receptor and a cytoplasmic domain with sequence homology with the IL-4 receptor (Nicola, 1990).

Production of G-CSF is by a variety of cells including monocytes, fibroblasts, activated endothelial cells and bone marrow stromal cells, but not by T lymphocytes. Apart from stimulating granulocytes colony formation, G-CSF also stimulates the growth and differentiation of myeloid leukaemic cell lines, increased neutrophil functions including antibody-dependent cellular cytotoxicity (ADCC), superoxide production and alkaline phosphatase synthesis, and the proliferation and migration of endothelial cells. There is considerable cross-species reactivity (Metcalf & Nicola, 1983; Lopez et al., 1983).

When given to mice, G-CSF has the greatest effect of all cytokines on circulating leukocyte levels, with neutrophils reaching 10 to 15 times control values and monocytes increasing five- to eight-fold (Molineux et al., 1990). There is no effect on red cells or platelets. In man there is a similar effect on neutrophils, but a much smaller effect on monocytes. There is in fact an immediate fall in neutrophils within 5 to 15 minutes of intravenous administration caused by margination within the blood vessels due to rapid changes in affinity of adhesion molecules. At high doses, G-CSF causes increasing levels of neutrophils, which reduce by one half daily when the cytokine is withdrawn. In the marrow there is a 9.4-fold increase in neutrophil production accounted for by an extra 3.2 amplification divisions and the release of newly formed neutrophils after only one day in the marrow instead of the usual four to five days (Lord et al., 1989). In mice there is a 100-fold increase in numbers of circulating multipotent progenitor cells after G-CSF administration (Molineux et al., 1990a); in man the increases are nearer 20-fold (Molineux et al., 1990b; Duhrsen et al., 1988).

M-CSF exists in two forms, as a homodimer formed from two 43-kDa molecules (159 amino acids with varying degrees of glycosylation; 18-kDa and 23-kDa forms also exist), and as a heterodimer formed from the 43-kDa monomer and a 150- to 200-kDa proteoglycan molecule (Kawasaki & Ladner, 1990). It is secreted by monocytes, fibroblasts, epithelial cells and endothelial cells. The M-CSF receptor, which is found on all mononuclear phagocytes, is the product of the c-*fms* proto-oncogene. Both M-CSF and c-*fms* map to chromosome 5q33. Apart from stimulating the formation of macrophage colonies, M-CSF enhances ADCC by monocytes and macrophages, inhibits bone resorption by osteoclasts, stimulates microglial proliferation and regulates placental function.

Mice treated with M-CSF for 7 to 14 days develop an increase in circulating monocytes, promonocytes, and large vacuolated cells resembling macrophages. They also develop anaemia and thrombocytopenia (Shadduck et al., 1987). Given to humans, it has only modest effects on circulating leukocytes.

GM-CSF (Gough & Nicola, 1990) is an 18- to 22-kDa glycoprotein (127 amino acids) secreted by activated T cells, endothelial cells, fibroblasts, mast cells, B cells and macrophages. The gene for GM-CSF has been mapped to the long arm of chromosome 5, closely linked to the genes for IL-3, IL-4, IL-5, M-CSF and c-*fms*. The GM-CSF receptor, which is found on cells of the myelomonocytic lineage, consists of a low-affinity ligand-binding α-subunit and a non–ligand-binding 130-kDa β-subunit that is shared by the IL-3 and IL-5 receptors. Although GM-CSF was initially characterized by its ability to generate neutrophil, monocyte/macrophage and eosinophil colonies, later work has shown it to be one of the most pleiotropic cytokines. It has a proliferative effect on erythroid and megakaryocytic progenitors, and is required for the growth and differentiation of early dendritic cells. It also has proliferative effects on cell lines derived from non-haemopoietic cancers. On mature cells it enhances several functions of neutrophils, eosinophils and macrophages, including superoxide production, leukotriene synthesis, arachidonic acid release, ADCC against tumour cells and phagocytosis. Histamine release from basophils is also increased as is cytokine production by monocytes. Like G-CSF it stimulates the proliferation and migration of endothelial cells, but unlike G-CSF there is no cross-species activity.

Murine GM-CSF significantly increases granulocyte and monocyte levels when given to mice, but these increases are small compared to those of a G-CSF. There was no effect on platelets or red cells (Metcalf et al., 1987). In humans GM-CSF produces a more substantial rise in neutrophils, eosinophils and monocytes. There is little effect on marrow kinetics, but an increased myeloid:erythroid ratio and release of myelocytes into the blood (Lieschke & Burgess, 1992a, 1992b). Animals treated with GM-CSF show an increase in numbers and activation of peritoneal macrophages but no extramedullary haemopoiesis. Effective mobilization of multipotent and committed progenitors occurs with GM-CSF (Socinski et al., 1988), but as with G-CSF this is most effective in the recovery phase following chemotherapy (Siena et al., 1989).

Interleukin-3 (IL-3) is a pleiotropic cytokine derived from activated T cells. It was initially characterized by its ability to induce the production of the enzyme 20-steroid dehydrogenase in cultures of splenic lymphocytes from athymic mice (Ihle, Pepersack & Rebar, 1981), but following purification and cloning was identified with factors that had variously been named mast cell growth factor, P-cell stimulating factor, burst promoting activity, multi-colony stimulating factor, thy-1 inducing factor and WEHI-3 (melanocyte cell line) growth factor (Schrader et al., 1986). Cells other than activated T cells, including thymic epithelial cells, mast cells, keratinocytes and astrocytes have been reported as capable of producing IL-3. The gene for IL-3 maps to the long arm of chromosome 5 (Le Beau et al., 1987) and codes for a 152 amino acid polypeptide with a molecular weight of 15 to 25 kDa depending on glycosylation (Clark-Lewis & Schrader, 1988). It is species specific.

The high-affinity IL-3 receptor comprises a 70-kDa α-subunit and the 130-kD β-subunit used in common with IL-5 and GM-CSF (Kitamura et al., 1991).

IL-3, acting either alone or in concert with other early acting haemopoietic growth factors, supports the proliferation of multipotent progenitors at early stages of their development only, but can synergize with lineage restricted factors in promoting terminal differentiation of haemopoietic progenitors. Among nonhaemopoietic cells, IL-3 stimulates the proliferation of CD4-ve, CD8-ve T cells, skin and gut epithelial cells, basophils and mast cells and follicular lymphoma B cells (Ihle, 1984).

The first in vivo animal experiments were performed with murine IL-3 (Lord et al., 1986). The results were very disappointing, with very modest rises in circulating leukocyte levels. In man there are small rises in neutrophils, monocytes, eosinophila and basophils and sometimes in platelets (Ganser et al., 1990). IL-3 can also mobilize progenitor cells into the circulation.

Interleukin-5 (IL-5) was originally discovered in the mouse as a soluble T cell derived factor involved in B cell maturation and in particular in immunoglobulin secretion (Swain & Dutton, 1982). Coincidentally, it was found to be a differentiation factor for eosinophil polymorphs (Sanderson, Warren & Strath, 1985). In the human, however, it has little or no effect on B cells and seems mainly concerned with eosinophil differentiation (Clutterbuck et al., 1987).

The IL-5 gene maps to the same area of 5q as that for other haemopoietic factors described above (Sutherland et al., 1988), and codes for a 134 amino acid polypeptide with three *N*-glycosylation sites and three cysteines. The biologically active molecule with a molecular weight of 45 to 50 kDa is a homodimer. There is a high degree of species cross reactivity (Sanderson, Campbell & Young, 1988).

The IL-5 receptor is a heterodimer of a 60-kDa α-subunit and the common 130-kDa β-subunit (Devos et al., 1991). In addition to synergizing with other haemopoietic growth factors in the formation of eosinophilic colonies (CFU-Eo), IL-5 is both a chemotactic and activating factor for eosinophils (Lopez et al., 1988).

Interleukin-9 (IL-9) was originally recognized as a cytokine in HTLV-1 conditioned medium by its ability to stimulate the proliferation of the megakaryocytic leukaemic cell line, MO7e (Yang et al., 1989). The gene coding for IL-9 has been mapped to the same band 5q31.1-31.3 as other cytokines referred to above (Kelleher et al., 1991). Chromosomal deletions around this point are common in some forms of myelodysplastic syndrome and acute myeloblastic leukaemia. The gene codes for a 144 amino acid precursor protein that is cleaved to generate the mature 126 amino acid cysteine rich protein with four glycosylation sites. The molecular weight is 14 kDa before glycosylation (Yang et al., 1989). The IL-9 receptor belongs to the haematopoietin receptor superfamily whose molecular characteristics are four conserved cysteine residues and a double tryptophan-serine motif close to the cell membrane (Renauld et al., 1992).

Like IL-5, murine IL-9 has more pleiotropic activity than the human molecule, although this may simply be the result of greater opportunities to study it. Both molecules act in synergy with EPO, IL-3 and GM-CSF to support the production of BFU-E, and acting alone they are capable of sustaining BFU-E in short-term culture (Donahue,

Yang & Clark, 1990; Williams et al., 1990; Bourette et al., 1992; Sonoda et al., 1992). Both human and murine molecules also support the proliferation of T cell lines in vitro and cytotoxic T cell clones also respond to IL-9 (Houssiau et al., 1993). Recent studies suggest that IL-9 is involved with IL-4 in immunoglobulin production by B cells and in IL-6 secretion by mast cells (Dugas et al., 1993). Outside the LHS, IL-9 has a role in the differentiation of hippocampal progenitors in the brain (Merz et al., 1993).

Interleukin-1 (IL-1) and **Interleukin-6** (IL-6) are considered in detail later in this chapter, but mention should now be made of their haematopoietic effects. IL-1 is capable of rescuing mice from otherwise lethal irradiation, which kills principally by haemopoietic suppression. It up-regulates receptors for CSFs and induces proliferation of pluripotent progenitors in the marrow. In addition, IL-1 induces the production of G-CSF by marrow stromal cells and fibroblasts, M-CSF by stromal cells and GM-CSF by fibroblasts and lymphocytes (Ikebuchi et al., 1988).

IL-6 also acts as a growth factor for pluripotent progenitors, enhancing the effect of IL-3, and promotes megakaryocytic maturation and platelet production (Caracciolo, Clar & Rovera, 1989). For completeness we should add that IL-4 also synergizes with haemopoietic cytokines in the stimulation of both primitive and committed progenitors (Rennick et al., 1987).

Interleukin-11 (IL-11) was detected in the culture supernatant of the primate bone marrow stromal cell line PU-34 by its ability to stimulate the IL-6–dependent murine plasmacytoma cell line T1165 in the presence of excess anti–IL-6 antibodies (Paul et al., 1990). The gene for IL-11 maps to chromosome band 19q13 and codes for a 178 amino acid polypeptide after the cleaving of a 21 amino acid signal peptide. There are neither cysteines nor glycosylation sites and the molecular weight is 23 kDa (McKinley et al., 1992). The 19q13 band also contains the BCL-3 gene, which is translocated to 14q in rare cases of chronic lymphocytic leukaemia, but it is difficult to see any connection. The IL-11 receptor is separate from that of IL-6 but shares a common signal transducer subunit with this cytokine, oncostatin M and LIF (Yin et al., 1993).

IL-11 is extremely pleiotropic. It synergizes with IL-3 and IL-4 to shorten the G_0 phase of the cell cycle in early myeloid progenitors and with IL-3 increases the number, size and ploidy of megakaryocytic colonies (Teramura et al., 1992). It has been found to be identical with a factor that inhibits the differentiation of bone marrow adipocytes, and thus may affect the haemopoietic microenvironment by changing yellow marrow to red marrow (Kawashima et al., 1991). In vivo administration causes a rise in platelet counts and promotes CFU-GEMM, CFU-GM, BFU-E and CFU-E in both spleen and bone marrow (Du et al., 1993). Among nonhaemopoietic cells IL-11 stimulates the development of antigen-specific IgG-secreting B cells (Yin, Schendel & Yu-Chung, 1992), but unlike IL-6 it is not stimulatory to myeloma cells. Like IL-6, however, it induces the release of acute-phase reactants from the liver, and like IL-9 it is involved in the differentiation of hippocampal progenitors in the brain (Mehler et al., 1993).

Stem cell factor (SCF) is also known as mast cell growth factor, steel factor and c-*kit* ligand. Mice bearing mutations at one of two loci, dominant white spotting (W) or Steel (Sl), develop profound defects in haemopoiesis, melanocyte production and gametogenesis. The two mutations have been shown to give rise to intrinsic (W) and microenvironmental (Sl) defects. The proto-oncogene c-*kit* (short for kitten, since the feline sarcoma virus contains its sequences) has been mapped to the w locus. A gene coding for a new cytokine has been mapped to the Sl locus. This cytokine has been found to be the ligand for c-*kit*, a transmembrane tyrosine kinase, and identical to the previously described mast cell growth factor (Zsebo et al., 1990; Chabot et al., 1988).

Native SCF has a molecular weight of 30 KDa. It is a noncovalently linked dimer with an analogous structure to that of M-CSF and platelet-derived growth factor (PDGF). Cloning data have suggested a membrane-linked form and a soluble secreted product, the latter comprising the first 164 amino acids of the 185 amino acid extracellular domain of the latter, which has in addition a 27 amino acid transmembrane domain and a 36 amino acid intracellular domain (Martin et al., 1990). Since mice expressing the soluble but not the membrane SCF suffer from similar defects to Steel mice, the membrane-bound cytokine is obviously functionally important.

The SCF receptor is encoded by the proto-oncogene c-*kit*. It is a single 145-kDa polypeptide closely related to the M-CSF and PDGF receptors. The receptor is found on pluripotent stem cells, myeloid and B cell progenitors, erythroid progenitors, mast cells, melanocytes, developing primordial germ cells and embryonal neural tissue (Ogawa et al., 1991).

SCF is produced by marrow stromal cells, fibroblasts and fetal liver cells. Alone it shows very modest effects on early myeloid and lymphoid cells, but it synergizes powerfully with other cytokines. These interactions include: stimulation of the erythroid lineage with EPO; stimulation of early and intermediate myeloid progenitors with IL-3, IL-6, IL-11, GM-CSF and G-CSF; enhancement of megakaryopoiesis with IL-6, IL-3 and IL-11; induction of mast cell proliferation and maturation with IL-3 (Brandt et al., 1992). Among nonhaemopoietic cells interactions include: stimulation of thymocyte proliferation with IL-2 and IL-7, stimulation of early B cell progenitors with IL-7 (Funk, Varas & Witte, 1993), and expansion of primordial germ cells with LIF (Rossi et al., 1993).

Leukaemia inhibitory factor (LIF) (Kurzrock et al., 1991) was first described as a factor additional to GM-CSF and IL-6 that could inhibit proliferation and induce differentiation of the murine myeloid leukaemia cell line M1. It had previously been recognized in a variety of guises: differentiation-stimulating factor (D-factor), differentiation inducing factor (DIF), differentiation inhibiting activity (DIA), differentiation retarding factor (DRF), hepatocyte stimulating factor III (HSF-III), cholinergic neuronal differentiating factor (CNDF), human interleukin for DA cells (HILDA), osteoclast activating factor (OAF) and melanoma derived lipoprotein lipase inhibitor (MLPLI).

The LIF gene has been mapped to chromosome 22q12 (Sutherland et al., 1989) and encodes a mature polypeptide of 179 amino acid residues with a predicted molecular weight of 20 kDa. The native molecule is heavily glycosylated, with a molecular weight of between 38 and 67 kDa (Hilton, Nicola & Metcalf, 1988). LIF expression has been detected in a variety of cells and tissues including activated T cells, monocytes, glial cells, liver fibroblasts, marrow stromal cells, embryonal stem cells, thymic epithelial cells, the uterine endometrial gland, pituitary follicular cells, squamous carcinoma cells and a variety of tumour cell lines. The LIF receptor is a heterodimer, a low-affinity 120-kDa molecule that forms a high-affinity receptor with gp130, the accessory molecule associated with the IL-6, IL-11, oncostatin M, G-CSF, and ciliary neurotrophic factor (CNTF) receptors. In view of structural similarities, and a similar receptor, these cytokines have been grouped into a family (Godard et al., 1992).

Not surprisingly, the functions of LIF resemble those of IL-6 and IL-11. It synergizes with IL-3 to stimulate the production of primitive haemopoietic progenitors and megakaryocyte colonies. When given to mice in vivo it stimulates megakaryocytes in the marrow and platelet numbers in the blood (Metcalf & Nicola, 1991). It also regulates the differentiation and proliferation of certain leukaemic cell lines. Its nonhaemopoietic effects include the IL-6–like effects (Baumann & Wong, 1989) of induction of acute-phase proteins from hepatocytes, the establishment of the cholinergic phenotype in sympathetic neurones and the regulation of bone formation, and its unique effects of induction of myoblast proliferation, inhibition of lipoprotein lipase of activity in adipocytes, inhibition of endothelial cell growth and maintenance of the pluripotent potential of embryonal stem cells. It may be that such is the built-in redundancy of the cytokine system that this last is the only unique effect of LIF, since LIF 'knockout' mice are normal in all respects apart from an inability of the female uterus to implant the blastocyst (Shen & Leder, 1992).

Clinical Importance of Haematopoietic Growth Factors

The clearest and most significant effect of HGFs has been their use in stimulating bone marrow recovery following intensive chemotherapy. The majority of cytotoxic drugs have marrow suppression as their dose-limiting side effect, and deaths following chemotherapy are usually caused by infection or bleeding. Moreover, life in a haematological intensive care unit is extremely expensive. A large body of evidence has now accumulated on the use of G-CSF or GM-CSF in the treatment or prevention of neutropenia in patients with cancer.

With conventional doses of cytotoxic doses both cytokines have shown themselves able to shorten the period of neutropenia and sometimes to abrogate it. Although it is difficult to demonstrate that lives are saved by their use, there are reduced episodes of infection, fewer days in hospital and less antibiotic used (Crawford et al., 1991; Gurney et al., 1992). Whether there are resulting cost savings depends on the pricing of the drugs, which are very expensive. Indeed, they are so expensive that they have not come into routine use in this context. Another bonus for cytokines is that fewer courses of chemotherapy have to be delayed or dosages reduced because of neutropenia. This may benefit those patients in whom dose and schedule intensity is important in curing their tumours.

Many tumours show a dose–response curve for cytotoxic drugs. Since bone marrow suppression is the major dose-limiting side effect with most drugs, treatment with HGFs enables doses to be increased and the schedule shortened until the sensitivity of the next most vulnerable tissue (often the gut) is broached. Several such schedules are currently under investigation in a variety of tumour types. Although clinical responses are often greater, it is too early to evaluate their benefit on prolonging life (Bronchud et al., 1989; De Vries et al., 1991).

An extreme in dose escalation is to use drugs in marrow ablative doses. By re-infusing bone marrow cells harvested and cryopreserved prior to ablative chemotherapy it is possible to restore marrow function within four weeks of treatment in most patients. Such a manoeuvre carries the fancy name of autologous bone marrow transplantation (ABMT), which makes it sound grander than it is. HGFs reduce the period of neutropenia and the use of parenteral antibiotics in ABMT when compared to placebo in randomized controlled trials. Days in hospital are also reduced, but episodes of infection are unchanged. Neither cytokine produces accelerated red cell or platelet recovery (Peters, 1989).

In some patients, ABMT is impossible because of marrow contamination with tumour, marrow fibrosis or previous marrow irradiation. Haemopoietic progenitors circulate in the peripheral blood in small numbers and these increase markedly in the recovery phase after chemotherapy. Sufficient numbers of progenitors can be collected by leucapheresis to rescue patients from ablative chemotherapy in the same way as ABMT. Although this technique was cumbersome in requiring up to five three-hour sessions on a cell separator, there were unexpected benefits. Neutrophil recovery to 0.5×10^9/L took an average of 10 days compared to 24 following ABMT. Even more exciting was the fact that platelet counts recover at the same rate. Moreover, marrow repopulation seemed to be permanent without evidence of late graft failure (Bell, Hamblin & Oscier, 1986). Although less courageous physicians thought it prudent to supplement the blood progenitors with autologous bone marrow, there is now general agreement that this is unnecessary.

The publication of this information seemed to spell the death knell for the commercial exploitation of HGFs. However, it was found that both G-CSF and GM-CSF mobilize progenitor cells into the blood, and when given during the recovery phase from chemotherapy, sufficient numbers can be harvested from a single leucapheresis to support accelerated marrow recovery (Socinski et al., 1988). Multiple leucocytaphereses following HGFs without chemotherapy have generated sufficient progenitor cells for allografting (Russell et al., 1993). At present the mobilization of haemopoietic progenitor cells represents the major use of HGFs.

Another application of HGFs is in the relief of chronic neutropenia. Useful haematological and clinical effects may be achieved outside the sphere of cancer in a variety of congenital neutropenias, moderate aplastic anaemia and the neutropenia associated with zidovudine use in acquired immunodeficiency syndrome (AIDS) (Garavelli, 1992). Myelodysplastic syndrome (MDS) is a clonal disorder of the bone marrow that proceeds to acute leukaemia in about one third of patients, but causes death from cytopenias in at least as many others. Both GM-CSF and G-CSF are capable of raising the neutrophil counts and relieving the tendency to infections in these patients (Vadhan-Raj et al., 1987; Negrin et al., 1989). However, both may also raise the numbers of myeloblasts in blood and marrow. Because of the risk of inducing progression to acute leukaemia the use of HGFs in MDS is limited. Another potential use of G-CSF and GM-CSF is the recruitment of blast cells in acute myeloblastic leukaemia into S phase where they are theoretically more susceptible to killing by cell cycle specific anticancer drugs (Aglietta et al., 1991). Clinical trials to investigate this possibility are proceeding.

The choice between GM-CSF and G-CSF is a difficult one. In clinical trials both seem equally effective, but there has been no head-to-head comparison. Although side effects which include bone pain, fever, myalgia, rashes and minor gastrointestinal symptoms are reportedly greater for GM-CSF than for G-CSF, in truth they are very trivial for both cytokines, and are seldom a reason to withdraw the drug. I suspect that the choice of product will eventually be determined by price.

Because red cells are so much longer lived than are leukocytes or platelets, the demand for an erythrocyte growth factor has been much less. Nevertheless, prolonged transfusion becomes hazardous because of iron overload and sensitization to blood cell antigens. This latter is particularly important in patients with chronic renal failure because of the risk of diminishing the chance of finding a compatible donor for renal transplantation. The only licensed uses of EPO are in chronic renal failure and the anaemia induced by zidovudine in AIDS. Nevertheless, transfusion reactions and the unacceptability of iron chelation therapy have spurred haematologists to explore its use in MDS. Unfortunately, it has shown only minimal benefit, although the combination of EPO and G-CSF produces a clinically useful rise in haemoglobin in 40% of patients (Negrin et al., 1993).

Thrombocytopenia is not benefited by either G-CSF or GM-CSF. The use of circulating stem cells to shorten periods of thrombocytopenia even after nonablative chemotherapy is burgeoning, but a thrombopoietic cytokine would be a welcome addition to the haematologist's armoury.

IL-3, which is currently in phase III clinical trials, stimulates both neutrophil and platelet recovery after marrow suppressive chemotherapy (D'Hondt et al., 1993). It is, however, considerably more toxic than GM-CSF. Most patients have a low-grade fever, bone pain, facial flushing and flu-like symptoms. Debilitating headache is the commonest reason for abandoning treatment. At higher doses the vascular leak syndrome has occurred (Postmus et al., 1992). It is likely that IL-3 will be more useful when used at lower doses in combination with G-CSF or GM-CSF. The fusion protein pIXY 321 (the product of fused IL-3 and GM-CSF genes) has very promising in vitro effects, but initial reports of its clinical use have been disappointing.

IL-6 is another promising cytokine currently in phase II trials that shortens the period of platelet recovery. Side effects are similar to those of other cytokines, with fever predominating. At higher doses a syndrome of weight loss and cachexia may be induced (Lazarus, Winton & Williams, 1993).

IL-11 is currently in phase I/II trials. It appears well tolerated at doses that accelerate recovery of platelet counts after cancer chemotherapy.

A final application for HGFs in cancer treatment is the ex vivo expansion of pluripotent stem cells. These cells may have been derived from cord blood, purged bone marrow, poorly regenerating circulating stem cell harvests or attempts at long-term culture to remove contaminating leukaemia. Many attempts to expand such cells have been made using various cocktails of cytokines. Those employing IL-1, IL-3, IL-6, EPO and SCF have been most successful (Brugger et al., 1993).

Tumour Stimulation by Cytokines

An important caveat on the use of haemopoietic cytokines in cancer therapy must be the potential for tumour cell stimulation. IL-6 stimulates the growth of some sarcomas, carcinomas, EBV transformed cells and myelomas (Kawano et al., 1988; Van Damme et al., 1988; Eustace et al., 1993). GM-CSF stimulates the growth of a number of tumour cell lines including osteogenic sarcoma and adenocarcinoma as well as increasing the number of circulating blast cells in MDS. Indeed, it may act as an autocrine growth factor in some leukaemias (Sporn & Roberts, 1985). IL-3 promotes the proliferation of follicular lymphoma cells (Clayberger et al., 1992). IL-9 may be an autocrine growth factor in Hodgkin's disease (Gruss et al., 1992). Finally, IL-11 and IL-3 have been reported to act synergistically in triggering blast cell proliferation in acute myeloblastic leukaemia (Kobayashi et al., 1993).

THE LYMPHOCYTIC GROWTH FACTORS

If haemopoiesis is complex, lymphopoiesis is even more so. Lymphocytes are the prime source of cytokines, and thus the release of one by one cell type is liable to cause the release of several others in autocrine, paracrine and endocrine reactions. The key to understanding lymphopoiesis is understanding the role of IL-2 in expanding and activating T cells that then become the target of other cytokines that control their functional differentiation. In the mouse, and probably in man, T cells separate into TH1 cells, which secrete a characteristic set of cytokines pushing the system towards cell-mediated immunity, and TH2 cells capable of secreting cytokines that favour humoural immunity (Mossman, 1986). The principal lymphopoietins are listed in Table 6.5.

Interleukin-2 (IL-2) (Waxman & Balkwill, 1992) was first discovered in the supernatants of lymphocytes cultured with phytohaemagglutinin (Morgan, Ruscetti & Gallo, 1976). It was characterized biochemically as a glycoprotein with a molecular weight of 15 to 18 kDa when purified from the T cell leukaemic line, Jurkat. Cloning data have revealed that it is initially translated as a 153 amino acid polypeptide. A 20-residue signal peptide is cleaved to yield the mature cytokine. There is a single 0-glycosylation site on the threonine at position three. Of the three cysteine residues, those at positions 58 and 105 form an essential disulphide link (Taniguchi et al., 1983).

The activities of IL-2 are mediated through a complex receptor system, consisting of at least three components, IL-2Rβ, -α, and -γ (Cosman et al., 1993). The IL-2Rα subunit is a 55-kDa transmembrane glycoprotein previously known as the Tac antigen. Although it binds IL-2 with low affinity, it does not lead to signal transduction except in lymphoid cells, which constitutively express the IL-2Rγ component. This is a 64-kDa transmembrane glycoprotein incapable of binding to IL-2. The 70-kDa β-subunit is also constitutively expressed by lymphoid cells. Alone it acts as an intermediate affinity receptor, again requiring the γ-subunit for signal transduction. Activation of lymphocytes induces the expression of the α component, which then forms an α/β heterodimer that acts as the high-affinity receptor, although still requiring the γ-subunit for signal transduction.

IL-2 is produced by T cells in response to mitogens or antigens presented with appropriate MHC molecules. Its most important activity is to act as an autocrine or paracrine stimulator of T cells expressing the IL-2 receptors. Entry into the G_1 phase of the cell cycle is associated with the expression of IL-2R in certain cells. Stimulation via the high-affinity receptor induces progression into S phase. The ability to produce IL-2 is one of the defining characteristics of TH1 cells. These cells also produce IFN-γ, a potent macrophage activator, in response to IL-2 stimulation.

As well as its effects on T cell growth, IL-2 stimulates the activation growth and tumouricidal effects of natural killer (NK) cells (Grimm et al., 1983). Lymphokine activated killer (LAK) cells are apparently NK cells stimulated by IL-2. IL-2 also augments B cell growth and immunoglobulin production, induces or augments IL-6

Table 6.5. Lymphocytic Growth Factors

IL-2	133 aa	T cells	T cell proliferation and differentiation Activation of NK cells Proliferation and Ig secretion by activated B cells
IL-4	129 aa	T cells	Naive CD4 cells to TH2 Proliferation and differentiation of B cells
IL-7	152 aa	Bone marrow stromal cells	Growth of pre-B and pro-B cells T cell proliferation Generation of cytotoxic T cells
IL-10	160 aa	T cells	Inhibits macrophages Enhances B cell proliferation and Ig secretion
IL-12	179 aa 306 aa dimer	B cells	Growth and activation of NK cells and T cells Naive CD4 cells to TH1
IL-13	132 aa	T cells	Growth and differentiation of B cells Inhibits macrophages
IL-14	468 aa	T cells	Proliferation of activated B cells Inhibits Ig secretion
LMW-BCGF	106 aa	T cells	Growth of activated B cells
TGF-β	112 aa	Fibroblasts	Inhibits proliferation of T and B cells Inhibits NK cell activity

and IFN-γ production (Musso et al., 1992), induces IL-1 and TNF production by macrophages and modulates histamine release by basophils (White et al., 1992).

The in vivo effects of IL-2 have been well studied (Rosenberg et al., 1987). Activation of T cells is signalled by the disappearance of lymphocytes from the peripheral blood, to reappear several hours after the withdrawal of the IL-2 displaying activation markers. High levels of soluble IL-2R are the most useful index of T cell activity.

Activation of T cells initiates several cytokine cascades, and the very apparent clinical effects are probably mediated by macrophage products such as IL-1, IL-6, IFN-γ and TNF-α (Hamblin, 1990). Fever and rigors are usual, together with nausea and vomiting, diarrhoea is common and an exfoliative rash generally occurs if the infusion is prolonged. The serious and life-threatening effects are caused by the vascular leak syndrome. The appearance of activation antigens on vascular endothelial cells is associated with capillary leakiness. Fluid leaking from the vasculature causes hypovolaemia and hypotension. Poor renal blood flow is hazardous to the integrity of the kidneys, while the loss of fluid from the vasculature leads to concomitant peripheral, pulmonary and cerebral oedema. IL-2 infusions have been fatal, but it is hard to disentangle the direct toxic effects of IL-2 from the resuscitive measures taken to counteract the side effects. Albumin infusions into individuals with leaky vasculature and pressor agents to improve the low blood pressure engendered not by a failing heart but by a lack of fluid seem illogical therapeutic endeavours and may make matters worse (Hamblin, 1990).

Experimental studies have demonstrated two separate effects of IL-2 that might have therapeutic benefit. Activation of committed cytotoxic T cells kills immunogenic tumour cells both in vitro and in vivo. On the other hand, non-MHC restricted killing by both NK cells and cytotoxic T cells is also enhanced by IL-2, and, at least in the mouse, is an important mechanism in killing nonimmunogenic tumours (Iigo et al., 1989).

Clinical trials of IL-2 in cancer began in 1982 (Rosenberg et al., 1985). At first there was a concentration of the ex vivo expansion of LAK cells in three to four days' culture with IL-2. Large numbers of peripheral blood mononuclear cells would be harvested by a cell separator, then cultured in roller bottles (later plastic bags). This technique was so cumbersome and expensive that it was extremely unlikely that centres outside the National Institutes of Health (NIH) would take it up. Indeed, for a while the only centre offering this treatment was a private institution in Tennessee. Initial results were promising, particularly in renal cell carcinoma and melanoma. The treatment was extremely toxic, though less so than bone marrow allografting. Less than 10% of patients had complete responses, but some of these were extremely durable, and they occurred in patients for whom there was no other treatment. Attempts to make IL-2 therapy more acceptable and cheaper have included dropping the LAK cells and giving the IL-2 by continuous infusion (West et al., 1987) or subcutaneous injection (Atzpodien et al., 1990).

Despite what are clearly remarkable clinical benefits in a few patients, very few centres are persisting with the drug. A few stalwarts continue with combinations of IL-2 and IFN (Atzpodien et al., 1990) or cytotoxic drugs (Hamblin et al., 1993), but trials of IL-2 as adjuvant immunotherapy following bone marrow transplantation and in acute myeloblastic leukaemia in remission have largely been abandoned.

There remains current interest in tumour infiltrating lymphocytes (TIL) (Rosenberg, Schwarz & Speiss, 1988). In this process, malignant tissue is dissected to tease out infiltrating mononuclear cells, which are cultured with IL-2 for up to 30 days. The cells that are expanded in this system are specifically cytotoxic T cells (mostly CD8+, but occasionally CD4+) rather than NK cells. The cells are then reinfused into the patient with IL-2. Responses of up to 40% of patients with metastatic malignant melanoma have been reported. This technique has only limited application, as up to 70% of cultures fail. However, such cells may be used as vehicles carrying cytokine genes such as TNF for local release in tumour deposits and this idea is a further possible application for IL-2 (Rosenberg et al., 1990).

Interleukin-4 (IL-4) (Paul & O'Hara, 1987) was first described as a B cell growth factor in the supernatant of EL-4 thymoma cells stimulated by phorbol ester. Its effect was distinct from that of IL-2. It induced anti-Ig stimulated B cells to enter S phase. At the same time it was independently discovered as a B cell differentiation factor that induced lipopolysaccharide-activated B cells to produce IgG_1.

IL-4 is a complex glycoprotein of molecular weight 18 to 20 kDa. The secreted protein has 129 amino acid residues with multiple glycosylation sites and six cysteines, all involved in disulphide bonds (Yokota et al., 1986). The production of IL-4 is principally by activated TH2 cells but has also been described by CD8+ T cells and some IL-3 dependent bone marrow cell lines.

The high-affinity IL-4 receptor is a 140-kDa protein with extracellular, transmembrane and cytoplasmic domains. It has significant structural homology with other haemopoietic receptors that are characterized by four conserved cysteine residues and a double tryptophan-serine motif in the extracellular domain close to the transmembrane region (Cosman, 1993).

The biological effects of IL-4 are many and varied (Paul & O'Hara, 1987). Its effects on B cells are most significant. On resting B cells it increases cell size, viability, and surface expression of CD23 and MHC class II. High concentrations induce immunoglobulin class switching to IgE and IgG_4, while low concentrations favour all other isotypes at the expense of these two. On T cells IL-4 promotes the development of thymocytes, is a growth factor for T cell blasts, and enhances the generation of antigen-specific cytotoxic T cells. Macrophage MHC class II expression and CD23 expression are both enhanced. Monocyte cytokine expression and superoxide production is inhibited but macrophage tumouricidal activity and their fusion to form multinucleated giant cells is enhanced (Paul, 1991). There are effects on haemopoietic maturation at primitive and committed progenitor levels in synergy with G-CSF, EPO, IL-1 and IL-11. Mast cell growth is stimulated (Musashi et al., 1991). The expression of various adhesion molecules on endothelial cells is modulated. Fibroblasts may be stimulated to produce colony-stimulating factors. IL-4 induces LAK cell proliferation, and in this activity augments IL-12 but inhibits IL-2 (Naume et al., 1993).

IL-4 may have a potential role in cancer therapy because of observations of the inhibition of growth of some carcinoma cell lines and some B cell lymphomas, its inhibitory effects on terminal differentiation of pre-B cell acute leukaemias and its induction of LAK cells and stimulation of tumour-infiltrating lymphocytes (TIL).

Interleukin-7 (IL-7) was first described as lymphopoetin-1 by Namen and colleagues (1988) and was reported to have precursor B cell growth-promoting activity. The nonglycosylated molecule consists of 177 amino acid residues with a molecular weight of 17.4 kDa. There are six cysteine residues with three potential *N*-glycosylation sites (Goodwin et al., 1989).

Two receptors for IL-7 have been recognized. A high-affinity 75- to 80-kDa receptor is predominately expressed on T cells, while a low-affinity 62- to 70-kDa receptor is found at high levels on B cells and monocytes (Goodwin et al., 1990).

Bone marrow stromal cells and perhaps thymic stromal cells appear to be the only sources of IL-7. Pre-B cells (at the stage of cytoplasmic μ-chains without surface immunoglobulin) are the target for IL-7 stimulation. The main effects are proliferation and differentiation. SCF may be a co-factor (Henney et al., 1989). IL-7 is also a growth and differentiation factor for T cells at the CD3 +ve, CD4 −ve, CD8 −ve, stage of development. IL-7 also has a proliferative effect on mature T cells. This picture remains slightly confused. In some instances IL-7 stimulation requires co-stimulation with a mitogen or a different cytokine such as IL-2 or IL-6, and in some instances it is effective alone. Presumably this reflects the state of prior activation of the T cell (Plum, DeSmedt & Leclercq, 1993). Finally, IL-7 is capable of inducing LAK cells from CD8 +ve T cells, and under special circumstances from CD4 +ve T cells (Hickman et al., 1990).

Injection of IL-7 into mice leads to a three- to five-fold increase in circulating immature B cells, and a 90% reduction of myeloid progenitors in the bone marrow with a 15-fold increase of myeloid progenitors in the spleen (Damia et al., 1992).

Interleukin-10 (IL-10) was initially recognized as a product of TH2 cells that inhibited the production of cytokines by TH1 cells (Fiorentino, Bond & Mosmann, 1989). At the same time it was shown that murine B cell lymphomas produced a cytokine that enhanced mouse thymocyte proliferation in response to IL-2 or IL-4 (Suda et al., 1990). The molecules were shown to be identical. The gene coding for IL-10 has been mapped to chromosome number 1 and codes for a nonglycosylated protein of 160 amino acid residues and molecular weight of 18 kDa (Kim et al., 1992). There is a strong resemblance of part of the gene to an open reading frame sequence in the Epstein-Barr virus (EBV), BCRF1. Possibly the virus has usurped part of the IL-10 gene into its own genome. The viral product shares many of the biological effects of IL-10 (Moore et al., 1990). Characteristics of the IL-10 receptor remain to be defined.

IL-10 is produced by a variety of T cell clones and B cell lines as well as by peripheral blood T cells. It is likely that the suppression of TH1 cytokine inhibition is secondary to the inhibition of macrophage accessory functions, for IL-10 is a potent inhibitor of macrophage function. It suppresses the production of inflammatory cytokines, including TNF, IL-1, IL-6 and IL-8; it up-regulates the production of the IL-1 antagonist; and it suppresses the synthesis of superoxide anion and reactive oxygen and nitrogen intermediates. It down-regulates MHC class II expression and thus antigen-presenting capacity. On the other hand, IL-10 enhances B cell viability, proliferation of Ig production and MHC class II expression, and is a growth factor for thymocytes and mast cells as well as enhancing the development of cytotoxic T cells. It is easy to see the value of this gene to the EBV (Moore et al., 1993).

IL-10 is thought to have clinical applications as an anti-inflammatory agent, while IL-10 antagonist, may have a role as anti-EBV agents, especially in EBV-associated tumours.

Interleukin-12 (IL-12) is a pleiotropic cytokine identified in the supernatant of cultured EBV-transformed RPMI-8866 cells (Kobayashi et al., 1989). It is a 75-kDa glycoprotein heterodimer. The smaller subunit (p35) has sequence homology to IL-6 and G-CSF, while the disulphide-linked larger unit (p40) resembles the soluble IL-6R. The two subunits are, respectively, 197 and 306 amino acid residues in length. It is suggested that p35 is responsible for ligand binding and p40 for signal transduction (Wolf et al., 1991). A high-affinity IL-12 receptor has been identified on mitogen activated CD4 +ve and CD8 +ve T cells and on CD56 +ve NK cells (Desai et al., 1992).

IL-12 promotes the growth of activated NK, CD4 +ve and CD8 +ve T cells, increases both ADCC and NK cell cytotoxicity and contributes to macrophage activation through IFN-γ synthesis by these cells. It is a moot point as to whether IL-12 is solely responsible for the development of LAK cells, as a product of IL-2 stimulated cells. IL-12 seems to have a major role in favouring the development of TH1 cells and may be the major determinant in IFN-γ production (Trinchieri, 1993).

The major clinical potentials for IL-12 are in the treatment of AIDS and cancer. Mononuclear cells from HIV-infected patients produce much reduced amounts of IL-12, and this is thought to favour a TH2-like profile of immune function with hypergammaglobulinaemia and defects in cell-mediated immunity. Clinical trial are beginning to see if IL-12 could reverse that tendency. Preclinical experiments suggest that IL-12 is a more potent anticancer agent than IL-2. Phase I trials are beginning shortly (Hall, 1994).

Interleukin-13 (IL-13) was discovered by a primarily molecular approach (Minty et al., 1993). The ligation of the CD28 antigen on T lymphocytes by a surface antigen B7 on activated B cells and monocytes is a key step in the activation of T lymphocytes and the accumulation of lymphokine mRNAs. Anti-CD28 was used to induce the mRNA and differential screening of an organized subtracted cDNA library revealed the gene coding for IL-13. The gene has been mapped to chromosome 5q23-31 close to the gene for IL-4. The gene codes for a 132 amino acid protein with an 18 amino acid signal peptide. The molecular weight of the recombinant protein is 9 kDa, but there are many *N*-glycosylation sites.

IL-13 is strongly inhibitory to monocytes, down-regulating the production of inflammatory cytokines such as IL-6, IL-1, IL-8, TNF-α and MIP-2. It shares this effect with IL-4 and IL-10. It also increases the proliferation of B cells, up-regulating CD23, and synergizes with IL-2 in the production of IFN-γ by NK cells without inhibiting LAK generation.

Suggestions on its therapeutic utility are as an anti-inflammatory agent, as an inhibitor of HIV replication and as an adjunct to IL-2 therapy of cancer.

THE CHEMOKINES

The chemokines (Table 6.6) are a superfamily of small, inducible, secreted, pro-inflammatory cytokines characterized by four conserved cysteine residues that chemoattract and activate different leukocyte subsets (Oppenheim et al., 1991). In the C-X-C or α subfamily, which includes IL-8, MGSA, β-thromboglobulin, platelet factor 4 and IP-10, the first two cysteines are separated by a variable amino acid, while in the β subfamily the first two cysteines are adjacent (C-C). This includes RANTES, MIP-1α, MIP-1β, MCP-1 and I-309. The genes for the α subfamily all map to chromosome 4q, and those for the β subfamily to 17q. In general the former act on neutrophils and the latter on monocytes and T lymphocytes.

Interleukin-8 (IL-8) (Schall, 1991) is a 10-kDa peptide produced by LPS-stimulated mononuclear leucocytes. The molecule has four variants 77, 72, 70 or 69 amino acids long, thought to be derived by postsecretory enzymatic cleavage. There are four cysteine residues that participate in disulphide bridges, and no sites for *N*-glycosylation. It is believed to exist in solution as a dimer. It exerts its activity through two high-affinity receptors. Type I receptors bind only IL-8, while type II also bind to MGSA and MIP-2. IL-8 is produced by a number of cells, including T-lymphocytes, monocytes, fibroblasts, epithelial cells, chondrocytes, keratinocytes and mesothelial cells. In vitro effects include neutrophil chemotaxis, augmentation of lysozymal enzyme release and up-regulation of surface receptors. Recently, it has been shown to inhibit adhesion to endothelial cells. In vivo administration induces neutrophil chemotaxis, and experimental animals show transient granulocytopenia followed by granulocytosis when IL-8 is given intravenously. Injection elsewhere causes the accumulation of granulocytes at the site of injection.

Melanoma growth-stimulating activity (MGSA) (Oppenheim et al., 1991) is also known as GROα. The gene was discovered in Chinese hamster embryo fibroblasts using subtractive hybridization techniques with normal and tumourigenic cells. It was independently cloned from a melanoma cell line. The genes for MIP-2α and MIP-2β show 90% and 86% sequence homology, respectively. The mature peptide has 73 amino acid residues without glycosylation. Gene expression occurs in monocytes, fibroblasts, melanocytes, mammary epithelial cells and endothelial cells in response to PDGF, IL-1 or TNF. In certain tumour cell lines it is expressed constitutively.

MGSA is ten times as potent as IL-8 as a granulocyte attractant, but less active in activation and neutrophil degranulation. It has modest stimulatory activity for melanoma cell lines and down-regulates

Table 6.6. Chemokines

IL-8	69 aa	Monocytes	Chemotaxis of neutrophils T cells and basophils Activates neutrophils Increases neutrophil adhesion
MGSA	73 aa	Monocytes	Chemotaxis and neutrophils Growth factor for melanoma cells
IP-10	77 aa	Monocytes	Chemotaxis monocytes and T cells Promotes T cell adhesion
MCP-1	76 aa	Monocytes	Chemotaxis monocytes Monocyte adhesion and cytokine production
MIP-1α	66 aa	T cells	Chemotaxis monocytes T cells, eosinophils Inhibits stem cell growth
MIP-1β	69 aa	T cells	Chemotaxis monocytes T cells Adhesion of T cells Inhibits effect of MIP-1 on stem cell growth
RANTES	68 aa	T cells	Chemotaxis monocytes T cells, eosinophils Chemotaxis, activation of basophils

the expression of types I and III collagen by synovial fibroblasts. It binds to the IL-8 type II receptor and to a distinct MGSA receptor.

RANTES (*r*egulated upon *a*ctivation, *n*ormal *t* *e*xpressed and *s*ecreted) (Baggiolini & Dahinden, 1994) is an 8.4-kDa peptide expressed by circulating T cells and by T cell clones in culture, but not by T cell lines. It has the interesting property of being down-regulated by T cell activation. It is a 68 amino acid peptide with four cysteines and no *N*-glycosylation sites. It causes migration of monocytes and CD4 +ve T cells.

Monocyte chemotactic protein 1 (MCP-1) (Miller & Krangel, 1991), also known as monocyte chemotactic and activating factor (MCAF), is an 8.4-kDa glycoprotein originally isolated from culture supernatants of glioma cells and myelomonocytic cells. It is secreted by monocytes, fibroblasts and endothelial cells when activated by IL-1 or TNF. The mature protein has 76 amino acid residues and is variably glycosylated. Two additional monocyte chemoattractants with 62% and 72% sequence homology, respectively, have been recognized and named MCP-2 and MCP-3. MCP-1 has been shown to attract monocytes both in vitro and in vivo. In addition, it induces superoxide anion generation and release of lysosomal enzymes, modulation of adhesion factors and the release of cytokines. It attracts and activates basophils and is the most potent factor for basophil histamine release. MCP-1 is cytostatic for some tumour cell lines.

Macrophage inflammatory protein (MIP-1) (Oppenheim et al., 1991) is the name given to two closely related chemokines released from LPS-stimulated macrophages. Despite their original description as neutrophil attractants, neither recombinant protein exhibits this activity in vitro. Rather, they both (like other C-C cytokines) act as monocyte chemoattractants. MIP-1α also attracts B cells, cytotoxic T cells and T helper cells; MIP-1β is less potent and attracts mainly CD4 +ve T cells. MIP-1α suppresses haemopoiesis but may be antagonized in this effect by MIP-1β. MIP-1α, but not MIP-1β, attracts and degranulates eosinophils.

The chemokines clearly are important mediators of inflammation that have not yet reached the clinic. It remains to be seen whether they can be used to modify the effector response against cancer.

MULTIPOTENT CYTOKINES

This group of cytokines is so pleiotropic that it is difficult to categorize. They are involved in inflammation, haemopoiesis and resistance to cancer. I have listed them in Table 6.7.

Table 6.7. Multipotent Cytokines

IL-1α	159 aa	Monocytes	Wide variety effects on inflammatory and immune systems Synergizes with haemopoietic growth factors
IL-1β	153 aa	Monocytes	Similar to IL-1α
IL-1ra	152 aa	Monocytes	Inhibits IL-1 by binding IL-1 receptors
IL-6	184 aa	T cells	Activates haemopoietic progenitors Maturation of megakaryocytes Growth and differentiation of B cells and T cells Production of acute-phase reactants
TNF-α	157 aa	Monocytes	Immunostimulant Mediator of inflammatory process Activator of almost everything
TNF-β	171 aa	Lymphocytes	Similar to TNF-α
TGF-β	112 aa	Platelets	Stimulatory and inhibitory effects on many cell types
Oncostatin-M	195 aa	Monocytes	Production of acute-phase reactants Endothelial cell activation Suppression of tumour cell lines

Transforming growth factor beta (TGF-β) is a stable multifunctional polypeptide growth factor. Specific receptors for this protein are found on virtually all mammalian cells and it is capable of acting both as a proliferative and antiproliferative agent. It is dealt with in detail elsewhere in this volume.

Interleukin-1 (IL-1) (Dinarello, 1991) is the name that designates two separate proteins, IL-1α and IL-1β. They are the products of different genes but recognize the same receptors and have overlapping functions. The pleiotropic nature of IL-1 is evident in the plethora of alternative names: lymphocyte activating factor, endogenous pyrogen, leukocytic endogenous mediator, mononuclear factor, catabolin, osteoclast activating factor, hemopoietin-1, melanoma growth inhibition factor, tumour inhibitory factor-2, mitogenic protein, helper peak-1, T cell replacing factor III, B cell activating factor and B cell differentiating factor.

IL-1α and IL-1β are structurally related polypeptides with 25% sequence homology. Both are initially synthesized as 30- to 32-kDa propeptides of 270 and 269 amino acids, respectively. C-terminal cleavage of 159 and 153 amino acids reveals the mature polypeptides, which both have molecular weights of 17 kDa. A membrane-bound form of IL-1 has been identified on the surface of macrophages, endothelial cells, dendritic cells and fibroblasts, but the significance of its presence and the mode of secretion of IL-1 remain controversial.

An inhibitor of IL-1 has also been cloned. This molecule, known as IL-1 receptor antagonist (IL-1ra), binds to the IL-1 receptor with similar affinity to IL-1 but has no stimulatory activity. IL-1ra is induced in monocytes by the same signals that induce IL-1α and IL-1β; namely IgG, LPS, phorbol ester and zymosan.

Two distinct receptors bind both types of IL-1. Both are members of the immunoglobulin superfamily. An 80-kDa membrane-bound receptor protein (type I) is found on T cells, fibroblasts, keratinocytes, endothelial cells, dendritic cells, synovial cells, chondrocytes and hepatocytes. Type II receptors are found on B cells, neutrophils and bone marrow cells. The major difference in the two receptors is in the size of the cytoplasmic domain: 213 amino acids for type I and only 29 for type II. In general, IL-1α binds better to the type I receptor, and IL-1β to the type II receptor. It appears that only type I receptors are capable of signal transduction on ligand binding. A possible role for the type II receptor is to be shed as a soluble IL-1 binding protein to act as an antagonist (Sims et al., 1993).

The widespread distribution of IL-1 receptors is reflected in its many and varied activities (Dinarello & Wolff, 1993). In general it produces the spectrum of effects that we associate with inflammation.

There is a multifactorial stimulation of haemopoiesis as described previously, particularly to produce inflammatory cells. Hepatocytes are stimulated to produce acute-phase reactant proteins, while albumin synthesis is reduced. There is a general increase in the manufacture of prostaglandins, particularly by fibroblasts, endothelial cells and smooth muscle cells. There is stimulation of the production of insulin, corticotropin releasing factor and adrenocorticotropin. Fever is induced, and there is a tendency to induce slow-wave sleep. In preparation for the healing process that follows tissue injury, both osteoblasts and osteoclasts are activated to facilitate bone remodelling, collagenase is secreted by a number of different types of cell and endothelial cells and fibroblasts are activated to induce angiogenesis.

Stimulation of the immune system is a major effect. The differentiation and proliferation of Pre-B and B cells and the induction of Ig secretion are all direct or indirect effects. T cells are activated by co-stimulation with other cytokines, the induction of IL-2 receptors and the synthesis of cytokines. Natural killer activity is also enhanced.

The very pleiotropy of IL-1 will limit its therapeutic use. Indeed, the dose-limiting side effects of other cytokines are in part due to IL-1 induction. In small doses it may have a role in encouraging bone marrow recovery after chemotherapy. There is perhaps more promise for IL-2ra. Strategies may be contemplated that would use this agent to reduce the toxicity of IL-2 or IL-12 therapy.

Interleukin-6 (IL-6) was first described as a 26-kDa protein produced by fibroblastoid cells on stimulation with double-stranded RNA, cyclohexamide or virus (Billiau, 1987). Because of its weak antiviral activity it was first known as interferon-2. Among its other synonyms are monocyte derived human B cell growth factor, B cell stimulating factor 2, plasmacytoma growth factor, T cell activation factor, cytolytic T cell differentiation factor and hepatocyte stimulating factor, and the cells capable of producing it with appropriate stimulation include monocytes, endothelial cells, retinal pigment epithelial cells, fibroblasts, hepatocytes, keratinocytes, astrocytes, osteoblasts, bone marrow stromal cells, Sertoli cells, activated T and B cells, myelomas, melanomas, glioblastomas and bladder and renal carcinomas. Its range of target cells is almost as large and includes T and B cells, fibroblasts, myeloid progenitor cells and hepatocytes (Wong & Clark, 1988).

The gene for IL-6 codes for a 213 amino acid polypeptide containing a signal sequence of 14 residues. There are two disulphide bonds, and both *O*- and *N*-glycosylation sites. Unusually for cytokines, the degree of glycosylation affects function. This, and the tendency for variable phosphorylation at exposed serine sites, may account for IL-6 molecules from different origins behaving differently in the same assay system (Wong & Clark, 1988).

IL-6 exerts its biological activity through a high-affinity receptor complex consisting of an 80-kDa membrane-bound glycoprotein that binds with low affinity, and a 130-kDa glycoprotein that is required for high-affinity binding and for signal transduction. The smaller component has two subdomains, one showing structural similarity with the immunoglobulin superfamily, and one showing the four conserved cysteine residues with a double tryptophan–serine motif close to the cell membrane typical of the haemopoietin superfamily of receptors. The larger component is the gp130 molecule common to the LIF, oncostatin M, CNTF and IL-11 receptors (Hirano et al., 1990).

Like IL-1, IL-6 plays a major role in the mediation of the inflammatory and immune responses caused by infection or injury. In particular, IL-6 is involved in the induction of B cell differentiation, the generation of acute-phase reactants in the liver, growth promotion of myeloma and hybridoma cells, IL-2 production and IL-2R induction in T cells as well as their proliferation and differentiation, enhancement of IL-3 dependent haemopoiesis and particularly megakaryopoiesis, inhibition of melanoma, myeloid leukaemia and breast carcinoma cell lines, stimulation of certain sarcoma and carcinoma cell lines, proliferation of Kaposi's sarcoma cells, the induction of renal mesangial cell growth, promotion of keratinocyte growth and neuronal differentiation (Hirano et al., 1990).

IL-6 transgenic mice develop a massive plasmacytosis, a thrombocytosis and mesangioproliferative glomerulonephritis (Suematsu et al., 1989). The plasmacytosis is polyclonal. Nevertheless, IL-6 seems to be an important autocrine or paracrine stimulant in multiple myeloma, and anti–IL-6 antibodies have entered therapeutic trials in myeloma (Klein et al., 1991). Inhibition of IL-6 activity may play a future part in controlling myeloma and Kaposi's sarcoma as well as mesangioproliferative glomerulonephritis and certain autoimmune diseases. IL-6 has entered clinical trials as a stimulus to platelet recovery after cytotoxic drugs.

Oncostatin M (OSM) is a pleiotropic cytokine affecting the growth and differentiation of a variety of normal and tumour cells. It was originally discovered in the culture supernatant of phorbol ester stimulated U937 human histiocytic lymphoma cells. A 28-kDa glycoprotein from this soup was found to inhibit the growth of A375 human melanoma cells (Zarling et al., 1986).

The gene for OSM has been mapped to chromosome 22q12 close to the gene for LIF. Both the gene and the protein show structural similarities to LIF, G-CSF, IL-6 and CNTF, which have a four-helix bundle structure similar to that of growth hormone. The gene codes for a 252 amino acid peptide with a 25 amino acid signal sequence that is cleaved to form a procytokine which then undergoes C-terminal processing to form the 196 amino acid mature cytokine (Rose & Bruce, 1991).

OSM is able to bind directly to the gp130 subunit used by the LIF, IL-6, CNTF and IL-11 receptors, but this does not result in signal transduction. It is able to use the complete LIF receptor and probably an OSM-specific component that links to gp130 (Davis et al., 1993).

OSM is secreted by macrophages and activated T cells. Its effects are numerous. It inhibits the growth of a number of tumour cell lines, but is stimulatory to Kaposi's sarcoma cells, human erythroleukaemia cells and normal fibroblasts (Miles et al., 1992; Nair et al., 1992). It induces an increase of low-density lipoprotein receptor expression on hepatocytes – a property useful in lowering the serum cholesterol (Grove et al., 1991; Richards et al., 1992). OSM has important effects on vascular endothelial cells, modulating cellular morphology and stimulating the release of plasminogen activator and several cytokines including IL-6, G-CSF and GM-CSF (Brown et al., 1991, 1993). Like IL-1 and IL-6, it stimulates hepatocytes to release acute-phase reactants (Richards et al., 1992).

Currently, several therapeutic applications for OSM are contemplated. It may be that its suppression of tumour cell lines in vitro may translate into a clinically useful tumour suppressive effect. The possibility of synergistic effects with IL-6 and TGF-α is also being explored.

Tumour necrosis factor (TNF) is the product of nearly a century of research into the phenomenon of tumour regression during infection, but in real life it probably has more to do with the control of the inflammatory process than with cancer. William Coley, a New York surgeon, began his research in the 1890s after reading of a patient with a sarcoma who was cured after an episode of erysipelas (Coley, 1906). Coley's toxin, a filtrate of bacterial cultures, was sometimes successful systemic treatment for cancer. Interest in it waned with the introduction of radiotherapy and chemotherapy, although it became clear that a factor in the serum of animals treated with bacterial endotoxin would induce tumour necrosis when injected into tumour-bearing animals. Carswell et al. (1975) named this substance 'tumour necrosis factor'. Another cytotoxic factor produced by activated T lymphocytes was shown to have similar activity and was named lymphocytotoxin (Granger & Williams, 1968) and was later designated TNF-β. Slightly later, a factor that causes wasting in rabbits chronically infected with *Trypanosomia brucei* and called cachectin was shown to be identical to TNF-β (Beutler & Cerami, 1988).

The genes for both TNF-α and TNF-β were cloned in 1984 (Pennica et al., 1984; Gray et al., 1984) and as expected the recombinant proteins were toxic for tumour cells in vitro and caused tumour necrosis in vivo. Unfortunately, they were extremely toxic, causing a syndrome similar to toxic shock, and death in small doses.

The genes for both molecules map to chromosome 6q. TNF-α is an *N*-glycosylated polypeptide of 157 amino acids with a molecular weight of 17 kDa. TNF-β is a 171 amino acid peptide with a molecular weight of 25 kDa. Both molecules circulate as trimers. A membrane form of TNF-β is found on the surface of monocytes and has lytic activity and possibly a role in cell communication (Kreigler et al., 1988).

Two distinct receptors for TNF have been identified and virtually every cell type has one or both. Both can bind to either type of TNF, and both belong to a family of receptors that includes nerve growth factor receptor, CD27, CD30 and CD40. They differ in their intracellular domains. It is suggested that the 75-kDa type A receptor mediates proliferative and regulatory signals, while the 55-kDa type B receptor is responsible for the lytic activity (Tartaglia & Goeddel, 1992).

In view of their ubiquitous receptors, it is hardly surprising that the TNFs should have so many activities (Vassalli, 1992). Their overall effect is to gear up the body to face invasion and damage, in this respect resembling IL-1, which is their universal companion in the fight. Through the release of HGFs they stimulate the bone marrow; activate and differentiate macrophages; cause neutrophils to degranulate and release leukotrienes and stimulate lymphocytes to divide, fibroblasts to release collagenase, chondrocytes to resorb proteoglycans, osteoclasts to resorb bone and muscle cells to increase their metabolism. Glucose metabolism is facilitated and lipid stores prevented from being reconstituted. It triggers all known mediators of inflammation.

When given systemically, TNF causes a transient fever, leukocytosis, raised acute-phase reactants and hypertriglyceridaemia. High doses produce the features of septic shock: hypotension, hypothermia, hypoglycaemia, acidosis, hepatic and bowel necrosis and acute interstitial pneumonitis. TNF clearly plays a part in the systemic effects of severe infections and also in certain parasitical infections and autoimmune diseases. Toxic as it is to patients, it is more toxic to microbial invaders, and gene knockout animals would be unlikely to survive.

The role of TNF in cancer is much less promising than had been hoped for. Clinical trials of TNF have produced minimal effect and maximal toxicity. Studies are currently underway to examine the possibility of transfecting TNF into cultured TIL cells and re-infusing these to home on the tumour and release TNF locally (Rosenberg et al., 1990).

CONCLUSION

In isolating the cytokines, we have uncovered one of the chief mechanisms by which cells live, grow and have their being. While other factors such as addressins, inhibins and adhesion factors are clearly important, the chemical messengers given us an insight into the complexities of life. One is struck by the built-in redundancies of function and the multiplicities of activities in each individual molecule. It is also apparent that they are tested in highly artificial environments, mostly in unglycosylated forms. Moreover, although it is necessary to exclude other cytokines from the soup in order to pin down particular actions, this very act of definition is highly artificial. In vivo, there are usually several different molecules interacting at the same time; some agonists and some antagonists. It is likely that, like people, they behave differently in each other's company from how they behave on their own.

Nevertheless, despite all these caveats, we are beginning to get an impression of how cells grow and interact. Without doubt these new discoveries will aid our understanding of cancer and influence our treatment strategies. Do not be gulled into what the theologians call a 'realized eschatology'. The 'last things' are yet to be discovered. I do not doubt that between the time of completing this chapter and its publication many more cytokines will have been discovered and many more reactivities identified.

ACKNOWLEDGMENTS

I have only quoted a minute fraction of the cytokine literature, relying on reviews for most of the older information. However, I would not have been able to start writing this chapter without the minireviews published anonymously in the Genzyme and R & D Systems catalogues. There is no obvious way to acknowledge this in the references, so I do so here.

REFERENCES

Agglietta M., DeFelice L., Stacchini A. & Petti M.C. (1991) Effect of haematopoietic group factors on the proliferation of acute myeloid and lymphoid leukaemias. *Leukaemia*, **5**, 979–84.

Atzpodien J., Korfer A., Franks C.R., Poliwodea H. & Kirchner H. (1990) Home therapy with recombinant interleukin-2 and interferon-α2b in advanced human malignancies. *Lancet*, **335**, 1509–12.

Baggiolini M. & Dahinden C.A. (1994) CC Chemokines in allergic inflammation. *Immunology Today,* **15**, 127–33.

Balkwill F.R. (1985a) The regulatory role of interferons in the human immune response. In J. Taylor-Papadimitriou (Ed.) *Interferons, their impact in biology and medicine,* pp. 61–80. Oxford Medical Publications, Oxford.

Balkwill F.R. (1985b) Antitumour effects of interferons in animals. *Interferon: in vivo & clinical studies,* **4**, 23–45.

Balkwill F.R. (1989) *Cytokines in cancer therapy.* Oxford University Press, Oxford.

Baumann H. & Wong G.G. (1989) Hepatocyte stimulating factor III share structural and functional identity with leukemia inhibitory factor. *Journal of Immunology,* **143**, 1163–7.

Bell A.J., Hamblin T.J. & Oscier D.G. (1986) Circulating stem cell autografts. *Bone Marrow Transplantation,* **1**, 103–10.

Beutler B. & Cerami A. (1988) Tumour necrosis, cacchexia, shock, and inflammation a common mediator. *Annual Review of Biochemistry,* **57**, 505–18.

Billiau A. (1987) Interferon $\alpha 2$ as a promoter of growth and differentiation of B cells. *Immunology Today,* **8**, 84–7.

Bourette R.P., Royet J., Mouchiroud G., Schmitt E. & Blanchet J.P. (1992) Murine interleukin 9 stimulated the proliferation of mouse erythroid progenitor cells and favours the erythroid differentiation of multipotent FDCP-mix cells. *Experimental Hematology,* **20**, 868–73.

Bradley T.R. & Metcalf D. (1966) The growth of mouse bone marrow cells *in vitro. Australian Journal of Experimental Biology and Medical Science,* **4**, 287–300.

Brandt J., Briddel R.A., Srour E.F., Leemhuis T.B. & Hoffman R. (1992) Role of c-*kit* ligand in the expansion of human hematopoietic progenitor cells. *Blood,* **79**, 634–41.

Bronchud M., Howell A., Crowther D., Hopwood P., Souza L. & Dexter T.M. (1989) The use of granulocyte colony stimulating factor to increase the intensity of treatment with doxorubicin in patients with advanced breast cancer and ovarian cancer. *British Journal of Cancer,* **60**, 121–5.

Brown T.J., Liu J., Brashern-Stein C. & Shoyab M. (1993) Regulation of granulocyte colony stimulating factor and granulocyte macrophage colony stimulating factor expression by Oncostatin M. *Blood,* **82**, 33–7.

Brown T.J., Rowe J.M., Liu J. & Shoyab M. (1991) Regulation of IL-6 expression by oncostatin M. *Journal of Immunology,* **147**, 2175–80.

Brugger W., Mocklin W., Heimfeld S., Berenson R.J., Mertelsmann R. & Kanz L. (1993) Ex vivo expansion of enriched peripheral blood CD34+ progenitor cells by stem cell factor, interleukin-1α (IL-1α), IL-6, IL-3, interferon-γ, and erythropoietin. *Blood,* **81**, 2579–84.

Bunn P.A., Foon K. & Ibide D. (1984) Recombinant leukocyte A interferon: an active agent in advanced T cell lymphomas. *Annals of Internal Medicine,* **101**, 484–7.

Caracciolo D., Clar S.C. & Rovera G. (1989) Human interleukin 6 supports granulocytic differentiation of haematopoietic progenitor cells and acts synergistically with GM-CSF. *Blood,* **73**, 666–70.

Carswell E.A., Old L.J., Kassel R.J., Green S., Fiore N. & Williamson B. (1975) An endotoxin induced serum factor that causes necrosis of tumours. *Proceedings of the National Academy of Sciences of the United States of America,* **72**, 3666–70.

Chabot B., Stephenson D.A., Chapman V.M., Besmer P. & Bernstein A. (1988) The proto-oncogene c-*kit* encoding a transmembrane tyrosine kinase receptor maps to the mouse W locus. *Nature*, **335**, 88–9.

Clark-Lewis I. & Schrader J.W. (1988) Molecular structure and biological activities of P-cell stimulating factor (interleukin-3). In J.W. Schrader (Ed.) *Lymphokines*, Vol. 15, pp. 1–37. Academic Press, San Diego.

Clayberger C., Luna-Fineman S., Lee J.E., Pillai A., Campbell M., Levy R. & Krensky A.M. (1992) Interleukin 3 is a growth factor for human follicular B cell lymphoma. *Journal of Experimental Medicine*, **175**, 371–6.

Cosman D. (1993) The hematopoietin receptor superfamily. *Cytokine*, **5**, 95–106.

Clutterbuck E.J., Shields J., Gordon J., Campbell H.D., Young I.G. & Sanderson C.J. (1987) Recombinant human interleukin 5 is an eosinophil differentiation factor but has no activity in standard human B cell growth factor assays. *European Journal of Immunology*, **17**, 1743–50.

Crawford J., Ozer H., Stoller R., Johnson D., Lyman G., Tabbara I., Kris M., Grous J., Piccozi V. & Rausch G. (1991) Reduction by granulocyte colony stimulating factor of fever and neutropenia induced by chemotherapy in patients with small cell lung cancer. *New England Journal of Medicine*, **325**, 164–70.

Cunningham D., Paz-Arez L., Gore M.E., Malpas J., Hickish T., Nicolson M., Meldrum M., Viner C., Milan S., Selby P.J., Norman A., Raymond J. & Powles R. (1994) High dose melphalan for multiple myeloma: long term follow up data. *Journal of Clinical Oncology*, **12**, 764–8.

Damia G., Komschilies K.L., Faltyneck C.R., Ruscetti F.W. & Wiltrout R.H. (1992) Administration of recombinant human interleukin-7 alters the frequency and number of myeloid progenitor cells in the bone marrow and spleen of mice. *Blood*, **79**, 1121–9.

Davis S., Aldrich T.H., Stahl N., Pan L., Taga T., Kishimoto T., Ip N.W. & Yancopoulos G.D. (1993) LIFR beta, and gp130 as heterodimerizing signal transducers of the tripartite CNTF receptor. *Science*, **260**, 1805–8.

Desai B.B., Quinn P.M., Wolitzky A.G., Mongini P.K., Chizzonite R. & Gately M.K. (1992) IL-12 receptor. II. Distribution and regulation of receptor expression. *Journal of Immunology*, **148**, 3125–32.

Devos R., Plaetinck G., Van der Heyden J., Cornelis S., Vanderkerckhove J., Fiers W. & Tavernier J. (1991) Molecular basis of a high affinity murine interleukin-5 receptor. *EMBO Journal*, **10**, 2133–7.

De Vries E.G.E., Biesma B., Willemse P.H., Mulder M.H., Stern A.C., Aalders J.G. & Vellenga E. (1991) A double blind placebo controlled study with granulocyte-macrophage colony stimulating factor during chemotherapy for ovarian carcinoma. *Cancer Research*, **51**, 116–22.

D'Hondt V., Weynants P., Humblet Y., Guillaume T., Canon J.L., Beaudin H., Duprez P., Longueville J., Mull R., Chatelain C. & Symany M. (1993) Dose dependent interleukin-3 stimulation of thrombopiesis and neutropoiesis, in patients with small cell lung cancer before and following chemotherapy: a placebo controlled randomized study. *Journal of Clinical Oncology*, **11**, 2063–71.

Dinarello C.A. (1991) Interleukin-1 and interleukin-1 antagonists. *Blood*, **77**, 1627–52.

Dinarello C.A. & Wolff S.M. (1993) The role of interleukin-1 in disease. *New England Journal of Medicine*, **328**, 106–13.

Donahue R.E., Yang Y.C. & Clark S.C. (1990) Human P40 T cell growth factor (interleukin-9) erythroid colony formation. *Blood*, **75**, 2271–5.

Dorval T., Palangie T., Jouve M., Garcia-Giralt E., Israel L., Falcoff E., Schurab D. & Pouillart D. (1986) Clinical phase II trial of recombinant DNA interferonα2b in patients with metastatic malignant melanoma. *Cancer*, **58**, 215–8.

Du X.X., Neben T., Goldman S. & Williams D.A. (1993) Effects of recombinant human interleukin 11 on haematopoietic reconstitution in transplant mice: acceleration of recovery of peripheral blood neutrophils and platelets. *Blood*, **81**, 27–34.

Dugas B., Renauld J.C., Pene J., Bonnefoy J.Y., Peti-Frere C., Braquet P., Bousquet J., Van Snick J. & Mencia-Huerta J.M. (1993) Interleukin-9 potentiates the interleukin-4 induced immunoglobulin (IgM, IgG and IgE) production by normal human B lymphocytes. *European Journal of Immunology*, **23**, 1687–92.

Duhrsen U., Villeval J.L., Boyd J., Kannourakis G., Morstyn G. & Metcalf D. (1988) Effects of recombinant human granulocyte colony stimulating factor on hemopoietic progenitor cells in cancer patients. *Blood*, **72**, 2074–81.

Erikson B., Oberg K., Alm G., Karlsson A., Lundquist G., Anderson T., Wilandr E. & Wide L. (1986) Treatment of malignant endocrine pancreatic tumours with human leucocyte interferon. *Lancet*, **2**, 1027–30.

Eron L.J., Judson F. & Tucker S. (1986) Interferon therapy for condylomata acuminata. *New England Journal of Medicine*, **315**, 1059–64.

Eustace D., Han X., Gooding R., Rowbottom A., Riches P. & Heyderman E. (1993) Interleukin 6 (IL-6) functions as an autocrine growth factor in cervical carcinomas in vitro. *Gynecological Oncology*, **50**, 15–9.

Fiorentino D.F., Bond M.W. & Mosmann T.R. (1989) Two types of mouse T helper cell. IV Th2 clones secrete a factor that inhibits cytokine production by Th1 clones. *Journal of Experimental Medicine*, **170**, 2081–95.

Foon K., Bottino G. & Abrams P. (1985) Phase II trial of recombinant leukocyte A IFN in advanced chronic lymphatic leukaemia. *American Journal of Medicine*, **78**, 216–20.

Foon K. & Sherwin S.A. (1984) Treatment of advanced non-Hodgkin's lymphoma with recombinant IFN-α. *New England Journal of Medicine*, **311**, 1148–52.

Funk P.E., Varas A. & Witte P.L. (1993) Activity of stem cell factor and IL-7 in combination on normal bone marrow B lineage cells. *Journal of Immunology*, **150**, 748–52.

Gall S.A., Hughes C.E. & Trofatter K. (1983) Interferon for therapy of condylomata acuminata. *American Journal of Obstetrics and Gynecology*, **153**, 157–63.

Ganser A., Lindemann A., Seipelt G., Oltmann O.G., Herrman F., Eder M., Frisch J., Schulz G., Mertelsmann R. & Hoelzer D. (1990) Effects of recombinant interleukin-3 in patients with normal haematopoiesis and in patients with bone marrow failure. *Blood*, **76**, 666–76.

Godard A., Heymann D., Raher S., Anegon I., Peyrat M.A., Le Mauff B., Mouray E., Gregoire M., Virdee K. & Soulilou J.P. (1992) High and low affinity receptors for human interleukin for DA cells/leukemia inhibitory factor on human cells. Molecular characterization and cellular distribution. *Journal of Biological Chemistry*, **267**, 3214–22.

Goldwasser E. (1984) Erythropoietin and its mode of action. *Blood Cells*, **10**, 147–62.

Goodwin R.G., Lupton S., Schmierer A., Hjerrild K.J., Jerzy R., Clevenger W., Gillis S., Cosman D. & Namen A.E. (1989) Human interleukin-7: molecular cloning and growth factor activity on human and murine B-lineage cells. *Proceedings of the National Academy of Sciences of the United States of America*, **86**, 302–6.

Goodwin R.G., Friend D., Ziegler S.F., Jerzy R., Falk B.A., Gimpel S., Cosman D., Dower S.K., March C.J. & Namen A.E. (1990) Cloning of the human and murine interleukin-7 receptors: demonstration of a soluble form and homology to a new receptor superfamily. *Cell*, **60**, 941–51.

Gough N.M. & Nicola N.A. (1990) Granulocyte-macrophage colony-stimulating factor. In T.M. Dexter, J.M. Garland & N.G. Testa (Eds.) *Colony stimulating factors: molecular and cellular biology*, pp. 111–53. Marcel Dekker, New York.

Granger G.A. & Williams T.W. (1968) Lymphocyte cytotoxicity *in vitro*: activation and release of a cytotoxic factor. *Nature*, **218**, 1253–4.

Gravelli P.L. (1992) Efficacy of granulocyte colony stimulating factor (G-CSF) on neutropenia in zidovudine treated patients with AIDS and ARC: a preliminary report. *Haematologica*, **77**, 293–4.

Griffiths S.D., Galvani D.W. & Cawley J.C. (1989) The interferons. In T.J. Hamblin (Ed.) *Immunotherapy of Disease*, pp. 43–69. Kluwer Academic Publishers, Dordrecht.

Grimm E.A., Ramsay K.M., Mazumder A., Wilson D.J., Djeu J.Y. & Rosenberg S.J. (1983) Lymphokine activated killer cell phenomenon. II. Precursor phenotype is serologically distinct from peripheral T lymphocytes, memory thymus derived lymphocytes, and natural killer cells. *Journal of Experimental Medicine*, **157**, 884–97.

Grove R.I., Mazzucco C.E., Radka S.F., Shoyab M. & Kiener P.A. (1991) Oncostatin M upregulates low density lipoprotein receptors in HepG2 cells by a novel mechanism. *Journal of Biological Chemistry*, **266**, 18194–9.

Gruss H.J., Brach M.A., Drexler H.G., Bross K.J. & Herrmann F. (1992) Interleukin 9 is expressed by primary and cultured Hodgkin and Reed-Sternberg cells. *Cancer Research*, **52**, 1026–31.

Gurney H., Anderson H., Radford J., Potter M.R., Swindell R., Syeward W., Kamthan A., Chang J., Weiner J. & Thatcher N. (1992) Infection risk in patients with small cell lung cancer receiving intensive chemotherapy and recombinant human granulocyte-macrophage colony stimulating factor. *European Journal of Cancer*, **28**, 105–12.

Hall S.S. (1994) IL-12 holds promise against cancer, glimmer of AIDS hope. *Science*, **263**, 1685–6.

Hamblin T.J. (1990) Interleukin 2: side effects are acceptable. *British Medical Journal*, **300**, 275–6.

Hamblin T.J., Sadullah S., Williamson P., Stevenson J., Oskam R., Palmer P. & Franks C.R. (1993) A phase III study of recombinant interleukin 2 and 5-fluorouracil chemotherapy in patients with metastatic colon cancer. *British Journal of Cancer*, **68**, 1186–9.

Henney C.S. (1989) Interleukin 7: effects on early events in lymphopoiesis. *Immunology Today*, **10**, 170–3.

Hickman C.J., Crim J.A., Mostowski J.S. & Siegel J.P. (1990) Regulation of human cytotoxic T lymphocyte development by IL-7. *Journal of Immunology*, **145**, 2415–20.

Hilton D.J., Nicola N.A. & Metcalf D. (1988) Purification of a murine inhibitory factor from Krebs ascites cells. *Analytical Biochemistry*, **173**, 359–67.

Hirano T., Akira S., Taga T. & Kishimoto T. (1990) Biological and clinical aspects of interleukin 6. *Immunology Today*, **11**, 443–9.

Houssiau F.A., Renauld J.C., Stevens M., Lehmann F., Lethe B., Coulie P.G. & Van Snick J. (1993) Human T cell lines and clones respond to IL-9. *Journal of Immunology*, **150**, 2634–40.

Ihle J.N. (1984) Biochemical and biological properties of interleukin-3: a lymphokine mediating the differentiation of a lineage of cells that includes prothymocytes and mastlike cells. In S. Gillis & F.P. Inman (Eds.) *Contempory topics in molecular immunology*, Vol. 10, pp. 93–119. Plenum Press, New York.

Ihle J.N., Pepersack L. & Rebar L. (1981) Regulation of T-cell differentiation: in vitro induction of 20 alfa hydroxysteroid dehydrogenase in splenic lymphocytes from athymic mice by a unique lymphokine. *Journal of Immunology*, **126**, 2184–9.

Iigo M., Nakajima K., Nakajima Y. & Hoshi A. (1989) Effects of interleukin-2 and interferon A/D treatment on lymphocytes from tumour bearing mice. *British Journal of Cancer*, **59**, 883–8.

Ikebuchi K., Ihle J.N., Hirai Y., Wong G.G., Clark S.C. & Ogawa M. (1988) Synergistic factors for stem cell proliferation: further studies of the target stem cells and the mechanism of stimulation by interleukin-1, interleukin-6 and granulocyte colony stimulating factor. *Blood*, **72**, 2007–14.

Isaacs A. & Lindenmann J. (1957) Virus interference, I the Interferon. *Proceedings of the Royal Society of London. Series B*. 256–67.

Italian Co-operative Study Group on Chronic Myelod Leukemia. (1994) Interferon alfa-2a as compared with conventional chemotherapy for the treatment of chronic myeloid leukemia. *New England Journal of Medicine*, **330**, 820–5.

Kawano M., Hirano T., Matsuda T., Taga T., Horli Y., Iwato K., Asaoku H., Tang B., Tanabe O. & Tanaka H. (1988) Autocrine generation and requirement of BSF-2/IL-6 for human multiple myelomas. *Nature*, **332**, 83–5.

Kawasaki E.S. & Ladner M.B. (1990) Molecular biology of macrophage colony-stimulating factor. In T.M. Dexter, J.M. Garland & N.G. Testa (Eds.) *Colony stimulating factors: molecular and cellular biology*, pp. 155–176. Marcel Dekker, New York.

Kawashima I., Ohsumi J., Mita-Honjo K., Shimoda-Tikano K., Ishikawa H., Sakakibara S., Miyadai K. & Takiguchi Y. (1991) Molecular cloning of cDNA encoding adipogenesis inhibitory factor and identity with interleukin 11. *FEBS Letters*, **283**, 199–202.

Kelleher K., Bean K., Clark S.C., Leung W.H., Yang-Feng T.L., Chen J.W., Lin P.F., Luo W. & Yang Y.C. (1991) Human interleukin-9: genomic sequence, chromosomal location, and sequences essential for its expression in human T-cell leukemia virus (HTLV)-1-transformed human T cells. *Blood*, **77**, 1436–41.

Kim J.M., Brannan C.I., Copeland N.G., Jenkins N.A., Khan T.A. & Moore K.W. (1992) Structure of the mouse IL-10 gene and chromosomal localisation of the mouse and human genes. *Journal of Immunology*, **148**, 3618–23.

Kirkwood, J.M., Ernstoff M.S. & Davis C.A., (1985) Comparison of intramuscular and intravenous recombinant α-2 interferon in melanoma and other cancers. *Annals of Internal Medicine*, **103**, 32–6.

Kitamura T., Sato N., Arai K. & Miyajima A. (1991) Expression cloning of the human IL-3 receptor cDNA reveals a shared beta subunit for the human IL-3 and GM-CSF receptors. *Cell*, **66**, 1165–74.

Klein B., Wijdenes J., Zhang X.G., Jourdan M., Boiron J.M., Brochier J., Liautard J., Merlin M., Clement C. & Morel-Fournier B. (1991) Murine anti-interleukin-6 monoclonal antibody therapy for a patient with plasma cell leukemia. *Blood*, **78**, 1198–204.

Kobayashi M., Fitz L., Ryan M., Hewick R.M., Clark S.C., Loudon R., Sherman F., Perussia B. & Trinchieri G. (1989) Identification and purification of natural killer cell stimulatory factor (NKSF), a cytokine with multiple biologic effects on human lymphocytes. *Journal of Experimental Medicine*, **170**, 827–46.

Kobayashi S., Teramura M., Sugawara I., Oshimi K. & Mizoguchi H. (1993) Interleukin-11 acts as an autocrine growth factor for human megakaryoblastic cell lines. *Blood*, **81**, 889–93.

Krantz S.B. (1991) Erythropoietin. *Blood*, **77**, 419–34.

Krown S., Real F.X., Cunningham-Rundles S., Myskowski P., Koziner B., Fein S., Mittleman A., Oettgen H. & Safai B. (1983) Preliminary observations on the effect of recombinant leukocyte A interferon in homosexual man with Kaposi's sarcoma. *New England Journal of Medicine*, **308**, 1071–6.

Kreigler M., Perez C., DeFay K., Albert I. & Lu S.D. (1988) A novel form of TNF/cachectin is a cell surface cytotoxic transmembrane protein: ramifications for the complex physiology of TNF. *Cell*, **53**, 43–53.

Kurzrock R., Estrov Z., Wetzler M., Guttermann J.U. & Talpaz M. (1991) LIF: not just a leukemia inhibitory factor. *Endocrine Reviews*, **12**, 208–17.

Kurzrock R., Talpaz M., Kantarjian H., Walters R., Saks S., Trujillo J.M. & Gutterman J.U. (1987) Therapy of chronic myelogenous leukaemia with recombinant interferon α. *Blood*, **70**, 943–7.

Kuzmits R., Kokoschka G.M., Micksche M., Ludwig H. & Flener R. (1985) Phase II results with recombinant interferon: renal cell carcinoma and malignant melanoma. *Oncology*, **42**(Suppl. 1), 26–32.

Lazarus H.M., Winton E.F. & Williams S.F. (1993) Phase-I study of human interleukin-6 after autologous bone marrow transplantation in patients with poor prognosis breast cancer. *Blood*, **82**(Suppl. 1), 173a.

Le Beau M.M., Epstein M.D., O'Brien S.J., Neinhuis A.W., Yang Y.C., Clark S.C. & Rowley J.D. (1987) *Proceedings of the National Academy of Sciences in the United States of America*, **84**, 5913–7.

Lieschke G.J. & Burgess A.W. (1992a) Granulocyte colony stimulating factor and granulocyte macrophage colony stimulating factor (Part 1). *New England Journal of Medicine*, **327**, 28–35.

Lieschke G.J. & Burgess A.W. (1992b) Granulocyte colony stimulating factor and granulocyte macrophage colony stimulating factor (Part 2). *New England Journal of Medicine*, **327**, 99–106.

Lopez A.F., Nicola N.A., Burgess A.W., Metcalf D., Battye F.L., Sewell W.A. & Vadas M.A. (1983) Activation of granulocyte cytotoxic function by purified mouse colony-stimulating factors. *Journal of Immunology*, **131**, 2938–8.

Lopez A.F., Sanderson C.J., Gamble J.R., Campbell H.D., Young I.G. & Vadas M.A. (1988) Recombinant eosinophil 5 is a selective activator of human eosinophil function. *Journal of Experimental Medicine*, **167**, 219–24.

Lord B.I., Bronchud M.H., Owens S., Chang J., Howell A., Souza L. & Dexter T.M. (1989) The kinetics of human granulopoiesis following treatment with granulocyte colony-stimulating factor *in vivo*. *Proceedings of the National Academy of Sciences of the United States of America*, **86**, 9499–503.

Lord B.I., Molineux G., Testa N.G., Kelly M., Spooncer E. & Dexter T.M. (1986) The kinetic responses of haemopoietic precursor cells, *in vivo*, to highly purified recombinant interleukin 3. *Lymphokine Research*, **5**, 97–104.

McCabe B.F. & Clark K.F. (1983) Interferon-α and laryngeal papillomatosis. *Annals of Otology, Rhinology and Laryngology*, **92**, 2–7.

McKinley D., Wu Q., Yang-Feng T. & Yang Y.C. (1992) Genomic sequence and chromosomal location of human interleukin-11 gene (IL-11). *Genomics*, **13**, 814–19.

Mandelli F., Avvisati G., Amadori S., Boccadoro M., Gernone A., Lauta V.M., Dammaco F. & Pileri A. (1990) Maintenance treatment with recombinant interferon alpha-2b in patients with multiple myeloma responding to conventional induction chemotherapy. *New England Journal of Medicine*, **322**, 1430–4.

Martin F.H., Suggs S.V., Langley K.E., Lu H.S., Ting J., Okino K.H., Morris C.F., McNeice I.K. Jacobsen F.W., Mendiaz E.A., Birkett N.C., Smith K.A., Johnson M.J., Parker V.P., Flores J.C., Patel A.C., Fisher E.F., Erjavec H.O., Herrera C.J., Wypych J., Sachdev R.K., Pope J.A., Leslie I., Wen D., Lin C.H., Cupples R.L. & Zsebo K.M. (1990) Primary structure and functional expression of rat and human stem cell factor DNAs, *Cell*, **63**, 203–11.

Merz H., Houssiau F.A., Orscheschek K., Renauld J.C., Fliedner A., Herin M., Noel H., Kadin M., Mueller-Hermelink H.K. & Van-Snick J. (1991) Interleukin-9 expression in human malignant lymphomas: unique association with Hodgkin's disease and large anaplastic lymphoma. *Blood*, **78**, 1311–7.

Metcalf D. (1984) *The hemopoietic colony stimulating factors*. Elsevier, Amsterdam.

Metcalf D, Begley C.G., Williamson D.J., Nice E.C., DeLamater J., Mermod J.J., Thatcher D., & Schmidt A. (1987) Hemopoietic responses in mice injected with purified recombinant murine GM-CSF. *Experimental Hematology*, **15**, 1–9.

Metcalfe D. & Nicola N.A. (1983) Proliferative effects of purified granulocyte colony-stimulating factor (G-CSF) on normal mouse hemopoietic cells. *Journal of Cellular Physiology*, **116**, 198–206.

Metcalf D., Hilton D & Nicola N.A. (1991) Leukemia inhibitory factor can potentiate murine megakaryocyte production in vitro. *Blood*, **77**, 2150–3.

Miles S.A., Martinez-Maza O., Rezai A., Magpantay L., Kishimoto T., Nakamura S., Radka S.F. & Linsley P.S. (1992) Oncostatin M as a potent mitogen for AIDS-Kaposi's sarcoma derived cells. *Science*, **255**, 1432–4.

Miller M.D. & Krangel M.S. (1992) The human cytokine I-109 is a monocyte chemoattractant. *Proceedings of the National Academy of Sciences of the United States of America*, **89**, 2950–4.

Minty A., Chalon P., Derocq J.M., Dumont X., Guillemot J.C., Kaghad M., Labit C., Leplatois P., Liauzun P., Miloux B., Minty C., Casellas B., Loison G., Lupker J., Shire D., Ferrara P. & Caput D. (1993) Interleukin-13 is a new human lymphokine regulating inflammatory and immune responses. *Nature*, **362**, 248–50.

Molineux G., Pojda Z. & Dexter T.M. (1990a) A comparison of hematopoiesis in normal and splenectomized mice treated with granulocyte colony stimulating factor. *Blood*, **75**, 563–9.

Molineux G., Podja Z., Hampson I.N., Lord B.I. & Dexter T.M. (1990b) Transplantation potential of peripheral blood stem cells induced by granulocyte colony stimulating factor. *Blood,* **76**, 2153–8.

Moore K.W., Vieirs P., Fiorentino D.F., Trounstine M.L., Khan T.A. & Mosmann T.R. (1990) Homology of cytokine synthesis inhibitory factor (IL-10) to the Epstein Barr virus gene BCRFI. *Science,* **248**, 1230–4.

Moore K.W., O'Garra A., De Waal-Malefyt R., Vieira P. & Mosmann T.R. (1993) Interleukin-10. *Annual Review of Immunology,* **11**, 165–90.

Morgan D.A., Ruscetti F.W. & Gallo R. (1976) Selective in vitro growth of T lymphocytes from normal human bone marrows. *Science,* **193**, 1007–8.

Musso T., Espinoza-Delgado I., Pulkki K., Gusella G.L., Longo D.L. & Varesio L. (1992) IL-2 induces IL-6 production in human monocytes. *Journal of Immunology,* **148**, 795–800.

Nair B.C., DeVico A.L., Nakamura S., Copeland T.D., Chen Y., Patel A., O'Neil T., Oroszlan S., Gallo R.C. & Sarngadharan M.G. (1992) Identification of a major growth factor for AIDS-Kaposi's sarcoma cells as oncostatin M. *Science,* **255**, 1430–2.

Namen A.E., Schmierer A.E., March C.J., Overall R.W., Park L.S., Urdall D. & Mochizuki D.Y. (1988) B cell precursor growth promoting activity. Purification and characterisation of a growth factor active on lymphocyte precursors. *Journal of Experimental Medicine,* **167**, 988–1002.

Namen A.E., Lupton S., Hjerrild K., Wignall J., Mochizuki D.Y., Schmierer A., Mosley B., March C.J., Urdall D. & Gillis S. (1988) Stimulation by B cell progenitors by cloned murine interleukin-7. *Nature,* **333**, 571–3.

Negrin R.S., Haeuber D.H., Nagler A., Olds L.C., Donlon T., Souza L.M. & Greenberg P.L. (1989) Treatment of myelodysplastic syndromes with recombinant human granulocyte colony stimulating factor. A phase I/II trial. *Annals of Internal Medicine,* **110**, 976–84.

Negrin R.S., Stein R., Vardiman J., Doherty K., Cornwell J., Krantz S. & Greenberg P.L. (1993) Treatment of anemia of myelodysplastic syndromes using recombinant human granulocyte colony stimulating factor in combination with erythropoietin. *Blood,* **82**, 737–43.

Nicola N.A. (1990) Granulocyte colony-stimulating factor. In T.M. Dexter, J.M. Garland & M.G. Testa (Eds.) *Colony stimulating factors: molecular and cell biology,* pp. 77–109. Marcel Dekker, New York.

Ogawa M., Matsuzaki Y., Nishikawa S. Hayashi S.I., Kunisada T., Sudo T., Kina T., Nakauchi H. & Nishikawa S.I. (1991) Expression and function of c-*kit* in hemopoietic progenitor cells. *Journal of Experimental Medicine,* **174**, 63–71.

Oppenheim J.J., Zachariae C.O.C., Mukaida N. & Matsushima K. (1991) Properties of the novel proinflammatory supergene "intercrine" cytokine family. *Annual Review of Immunology,* **9**, 617–48.

Paul S.R., Bennett F., Calvetti J.A., Kelleher K., Wood C.R., O'Hara R.M., Jr., Leary A.C., Sibley B., Clark S.C., Williams D.A. & Yang Y.C. (1990) Molecular cloning of a cDNA encoding interleukin 11, a stromal cell derived lymphopoietic and hematopoietic cytokine. *Proceedings of the National Academy of Sciences of the United States of America,* **87**, 7512–6.

Paul W.E. & O'Hara J. (1987) B cell stimulatory factor 1 interleukin 4. *Annual Review of Immunology,* **5**, 429–59.

Peters W.P. (1989) The effect of human recombinant colony stimulating factors on hematopoietic reconstitution following autologous bone marrow transplantation. *Seminars in Hematology,* **26**, 18–23.

Platanias L.C. & Golomb H.M. (1993) Hairy cell leukaemia. *Clinical Haematology*, **6**, 887-98.

Plum J., De Smedt M. & Leclercq G. (1993) Exogenous IL-7 promotes the growth of CD− CD4− Cd8− CD44+ CD25+/− precursor cells and blocks the differentiation pathway of TCR-alpha beta cells in fetal thymus organ culture. *Journal of Immunology*, **150**, 2706–16.

Postmus P.E., Gietema J.A., Damsma O., Biesma B., Limburg P.C., Vellenga E. & de Vries E.G. (1992) Effects of recombinant interleukin-3 in patients with relapsed small lung cancer treated with chemotherapy: a dose finding study. *Journal of Clinical Oncology*, **10**, 1131–40.

Renauld J.C., Druez C., Kermouni A., Houssiau F., Uyttenhove C., Van Roost E. & Van Snick J. (1992) Expression cloning of the murine and human interleukin-9 receptor cDNAs. *Proceedings of the National Academy of Sciences of the United States of America*, **89**, 5690–4.

Rennick D., Yang G., Muller-Seiberg C., Smith C., Arai N. & Takabe Y. (1987) Interleukin-4 (B cell stimulatory factor 1) can enhance or antagonise the factor dependent growth of haemopoietic progenitor cells. *Proceedings of the National Academy of Sciences of the United States of America*, **84**, 6889–93.

Revel M. & Chebath J. (1986) Interferon-activated genes. *Trends in Biochemical Sciences*, **11**, 166–70.

Richards C.D., Brown T.J., Shoyab M., Baumann H. & Gauldie J. (1992) Recombinant oncostatin M stimulates the production of acute phase proteins in HepG2 cells and rat primary hepatocytes in vitro. *Journal of Immunology*, **148**, 1731–6.

Rose T.M. & Bruce A.G. (1991) Oncostatin M is a member of the cytokine family that includes leukemia inhibitory factor, granulocyte colony stimulating factor and interleukin 6. *Proceedings of the National Academy of Sciences of the United States of America*, **88**, 8641–5.

Rosenberg S.A., Aebersold P., Cornetta K., Kasid A., Morgan R.A., Moen R., Karson E.M., Lotze M.T., Yang J.C., Topalian S.L., Merino M.J., Kulver K., Miller A.D., Blaese R.M. & Anderson R.F. (1990) Gener transfer into humans – immunotherapy of patients with advanced melanoma, using tumour infiltrating lymphocytes modified by retroviral gene transduction. *New England Journal of Medicine*, **323**, 570–8.

Rosenberg S.A., Lotze M.T., Muul L.M., Leitman S., Chang A.E., Ethinghausen S.E., Matory Y.L., Skibber J.M., Shilani E., Vetto J.T., Seipp C.A., Simpson C. & Reichert C.M. (1985) Special report: observations on the systemic administration of autologous lymphokine activated killer cells and recombinant interleukin-2 to patients with metastatic cancer. *New England Journal of Medicine*, **313**, 1485–92.

Rosenberg S.A., Schwarz S.L., & Spiess P.J. (1988) Combination immunotherapy for cancer: synergistic antitumour interactions of interleukin-2, alfa interferon and tumour infiltrating lymphocytes. *New England Journal of Medicine*, **319**, 1676–80.

Rossi P., Dolci S., Albanesi C., Grimaldi P., Ricca R. & Geremia R. (1993) Follicle stimulating hormone induction of Steel factor (SLF) mRNA in mouse Sertoli cells and stimulation of DNA synthesis in spermatogonia by soluble SLF. *Developmental Biology*, **155**, 68–74.

Russell N.H., Hunter A., Rogers S., Hanley J. & Anderson D. (1993) Peripheral blood stem cells as an alternative to marrow for allogeneic transplantation. *Lancet*, **341**, 1482.

Sanderson C.J., Campbell H.D. & Young I.G. (1988) Molecular biology of eosinophil differentiation factor (interleukin-5) and its effects on human and mouse B cells. *Immunological Reviews*, **102**, 29–50.

Sanderson C.J., Warren D.J. & Strath M. (1985) Identification of a lymphokine that stimulates eosinophil differentiation in vitro, its relationship to IL-3, and functional properties of eosinophils produced in cultures. *Journal of Experimental Medicine*, **162**, 60–74.

Schall T.J. (1991) Biology of RANTES/SIS cytokine family. *Cytokine*, **3**, 165–83.

Shadduck R.K., Waheed A., Boegel F., Pigoli G., Porcellini A. & Rizzoli V. (1987) The effect of colony stimulating factor-1 *in vivo*. *Blood Cells*, **13**, 49–63.

Schrader J.W. (1986) The panspecific hemopoietin of activated T lymphocytes (interleukin-3). *Annual Review of Immunology*, **4**, 205–30.

Shen M.M. & Leder P. (1992) Leukemia inhibitory factor is expressed by the preimplantation uterus and selectively blocks primitive ectoderm formation in vitro. *Proceedings of the National Academy of Sciences of the United States of America*, **89**, 8240–4.

Siena S., Bregni M., Brando B., Ravagnani F., Bonadonna G. & Giammi A.M. (1989) Circulation of CD34+ hematopoietic stem cells in the peripheral blood of high dose cyclophosphamide treated patients: enhancement by intravenous recombinant human granulocyte macrophage colony stimulating factor. *Blood*, **74**, 1905–14.

Sims J.E., Gayle M.A., Slack J.L. Alderson M.R., Bird T.A., Giri J.G., Collota F., Re F., Mantovani A. & Shanebeck K. (1993) Interleukin-1 signalling occurs exclusively via the type I receptor. *Proceedings of the National Academy of Sciences of the United States of America*, **90**, 6155–9.

Socincki M.A., Cannistra S.A., Elias A., Antman K.H., Schnipper L. & Griffin J.D. (1988) *Lancet*, **1**, 1194–8.

Tartaglia L.A. & Goeddel D.V. (1992) Two TNF receptors. *Immunology Today*, **13**, 151–3.

Sonada Y., Maekawa T., Kuzuyama Y., Clark S.C. & Abe T. (1992) Human interleukin-9 supports formation of a subpopulation of erythroid bursts that are responsive to interleukin-3. *American Journal of Hematology*, **41**, 84–91.

Sporn, M.B. & Roberts A.B. (1985) Autocrine growth factors and cancer. *Nature*, **313**, 745–7.

Suda T., O'Garra A., MacNeil I., Fischer M., Bond M.W. & Zlotnik A. (1990) Identification of a normal thymocyte growth promoting factor derived from B cell lymphomas. *Cellular Immunology*, **129**, 228–40.

Sutherland G.R., Baker E., Callen D.F., Campbell H.D., Young I.G., Sanderson C.J., Garson O.M., Lopez A.F. & Vadas M.A. (1988) Interleukin 5 is at 5q31 and is deleted in the 5q- syndrome. *Blood*, **71**, 1150–2.

Vadhan-Raj S., Keating M., LeMaistre A., Hittleman W.N., McCredie K., Trujillo J.M., Broxmeyer H.E., Henney C. & Gutterman J.U. (1987) Effects of recombinant human granulocyte-macrophage colony stimulating factor in patients with myelodysplastic syndromes. *New England Journal of Medicine*, **317**, 1545–52.

Sutherland G.R., Baker E., Fernandez K.E., Callen D.F., Goodwin R.G., Lupton S., Namen A.E., Shannon M.F. & Vadas M.A. (1989) *Human Genetics*, **82**, 371–2.

Swain S. & Dutton R.W. (1982) Production of a B cell growth promoting activity, (DL)BCGF, from a cloned T cell line and its assay in the BCL1 B cell tumor. *Journal of Experimental Medicine*, **156**, 1821–34.

Taniguchi T., Matsui H., Fujitas T., Takaoka C., Kashima N., Yoshimoto R. & Hamuro J. (1983) Structure and expression of a cloned cDNA for human interleukin-2. *Nature*, **302**, 305–10.

Taylor-Papadimitriou J. & Rozengurt E. (1985) Interferons as regulators of cell growth and differentiation. In J. Taylor-Papadimitriou (Ed.) *Interferons, their impact in biology and medicine*, pp. 81–98. Oxford Medical Publications, Oxford.

Teramura M., Kobayashi S., Hoshino S., Oshimi K. & Mizoguchi H. (1992) Interleukin 11 enhances human megakaryocytopoiesis in vitro. *Blood*, **79**, 327–31.

Trinchieri G. (1993) Interleukin 12 and its role in the general of TH1 cells. *Immunology Today*, **14**, 335–7.

Van Damme J., Van Beeumen J., Decock B., Van Snick J., De lay M. & Billiau A. (1988) Separation and comparison of two monokines with lymphocyte activating factor activity: IL-1 beta and hybridoma growth factor (HGF). Identification of leukocyte derived HGF as IL-6. *Journal of Immunology*, **140**, 1534–41.

Vassalli P. (1992) The pathophysiology of tumour necrosis factors. *Annual Review of Immunology*, **10**, 411–52.

Waxman J. & Balkwill F. (1992) *Interleukin-2*. Blackwell Scientific Publications, Oxford.

West W.H., Tauer K.W., Yannelli J.R., Marshall G.D., Orr D.W., Thurman G.B. & Oldham R.K. (1987) Continuous infusion recombinant interleukin-2 in adoptive immunotherapy of advanced cancer. *New England Journal of Medicine*, **316**, 898–905.

White M.V., Igarashi Y., Emery B.E., Lotze M.T. & Kaliner M.A. (1992) Effects of in vivo administration of interleukin-2 (IL-2) and IL-4, alone and in combination, on ex vivo human basophil histamine release. *Blood*, **79**, 1491–5.

Williams B.R.G. & Fish E.N. (1985) Interferon and viruses: *in vitro* studies. In J. Taylor-Papadimitriou (Ed.) *Interferons, their impact in biology and medicine*, pp. 40–60. Oxford Medical Publications, Oxford.

Williams D.E. Morrisey P.J., Mochizuki D.Y., de Vries P., Anderson D., Cosman D., Boswell H.S., Cooper S., Grabstein K.H. & Broxmeyer H.E. (1990) T cell growth factor P-40 promotes the proliferation of myeloid cell lines and enhances erythroid burst formation by normal murine bone marrow cells in vitro. *Blood*, **76**, 906–11.

Wolf S.F., Temple P.A., Kobayashi M., Young D., Dicig M., Lowe L, Dzialo R., Fitz L. Ferenz C. & Hewick R.M. (1991) Cloning of cDNA for natural killer cell stimulatory factor, a heterodimeric cytokine with multiple biologic effects on T and natural killer cells. *Journal of Immunology*, **146**, 3074–81.

Wong G.C. & Clark S.C. (1988) Multiple actions of interleukin 6 within a cytokine network. *Immunology Today*, **9**, 137–9.

Yang Y.C., Ricciardi S., Ciarletta A., Calvetti J., Kelleher K. & Clark S.C. (1989) Expression cloning of cDNA encoding a novel human haematopoietic growth factor: human homologue of murine T-cell growth factor P40. *Blood*, **74**, 1880–4.

Yin T., Schendel P. & Yu-Chung Y. (1992) Enhancement of in vitro and in vivo antigen specific antibody responses by interleukin 11. *Journal of Experimental Medicine*, **175**, 211–6.

Yokota T., Otsuka T., Mossmann T., Banchereau J. DeFrance T., Blanchard D., De Vries J.E., Lee F. & Arai K. (1986) Isolation and characterisation of a human interleukin cDNA clone, homologous to mouse B cell stimulatory factor 1, that expresses B cell and T cell stimulating activities. *Proceedings of the National Academy of Sciences of the United States of America,* **83**, 5894–98.

Youssoufian H., Longmore G., Neumann D., Yoshimoura A. & Lodish H.F. (1993) Structure, function, and activation of the erythropoietin receptor. *Blood,* **81**, 2223–36.

Zarling J.M., Shoyab M., Marquardt H., Hanson M.B., Lioubin M.N. & Todaro D.J. (1986) Oncostatin M – a growth regulator produced by differentiated histiocytic lymphoma cells. *Proceedings of the National Academy of Sciences of the United States of America,* **83**, 9739–43.

Zsebo K.M., Williams D.A., Geissler E.N., Broudy V.C., Martin F.H., Atkins H.L., Hsu R.Y., Birkett N.C., Okino K.H., Modock D.C., Jacobson F.W., Langley K.E., Smith K.A. Takeishi T., Cattanach B.M., Galli S.J. & Suggs S.V. (1990) Stem cell factor is encoded at the *S1* locus of the mouse and is the ligand for the c-*kit* tyrosine kinase receptor. *Cell,* **63**, 213–24.

PART 2

The Prevention of Endocrine-Dependent Tumours

7 Familial Cancer

AUDREY D. GODDARD AND DONALD M. BLACK

INTRODUCTION

Neoplastic transformation involves the accumulation of mutations in genes that become oncogenic through the acquisition of a dominant function (the proto-oncogenes) and in genes that must be inactivated for the initiation and progression of malignancy (recessive oncogenes or tumour suppressors). Tumour suppressor genes were first identified as the target of inactivating mutations in inherited cancer, while mutation of the dominantly acting oncogenes has been associated with somatic alteration in the developing tumour. However, recent identification of germline mutation of proto-oncogenes and site-specific mutations in presumed tumour suppressor genes in familial cancers blurs this distinction.

Almost all cancers occur in both familial and sporadic forms. Families affected with an inherited genetic predisposition to one or multiple forms of cancer are rare and typically have an autosomal dominant mode of inheritance (Knudson, 1986; Li, 1990). The prototypical inherited cancer syndrome is familial retinoblastoma (RB), and the epidemiological study of this tumour and mathematical modeling of the age of onset in the familial versus sporadic cases led Knudson in 1971 to propose the now classic 'two-hit' theory for inherited cancers. Two rate-limiting mutational events were proposed; the first mutation is either germinal (in heritable retinoblastoma) or somatic (in nonfamilial cases), and the second event is always somatic. We now know that in certain heritable cancers, the first mutation inactivates a single allele of a tumour supressor gene and the rate-limiting second mutation is the loss of the remaining normal allele. The predisposing inherited lesions are proposed to be recessive, resulting in the loss of function of one copy of a gene that remains latent until the normal allele is inactivated.

This 'two-hit' hypothesis also fits the epidemiological data for familial cancers other than retinoblastoma, including neuroblastoma, pheochromocytoma, and Wilms' tumor (WT) (Breslow et al., 1988; Knudson & Strong, 1972a, 1972b). A broader version of this model can also be applied to cancers that require the accumulation of more than two mutations before expression of the fully malignant phenotype. Colorectal carcinoma occurs in both familial and sporadic forms; however, the epidemiological data for colorectal cancer suggests the accumulation of approximately six independent mutational events (Armitage & Doll, 1954). Comparison of the age of diagnosis for sporadic colorectal cancer with that in familial disease implied that one or two fewer mutations were necessary in those patients carrying an inherited mutation (Ashley, 1969). The epidemiological analysis of colorectal cancer, retinoblastoma and other tumours suggests that inactivation of a single allele of a tumour suppressor locus followed by somatic inactivation of the remaining allele, with or without the requirement for alterations in other dominant or recessive oncogenes, is a common mechanism in the development of human malignancy. This model suggests that some familial cancers result from recessive mutations that increase the risk of malignancy above that of the normal population by producing target cells requiring one less mutation to initiate malignancy.

The inherited cancer syndromes imply the presence of human genes that play a role in the maintenance of the balance between cell death, differentiation and division. Mutation of these genes perturbs this equilibrium, thereby predisposing to neoplastic changes. To date, eight genes that can predispose to cancer when mutated in the germline have been identified and an additional six loci have been assigned a chromosomal region (Table 7.1) and are currently the subjects of extensive cloning efforts.

LOCALIZATION OF PREDISPOSING GENES

Chromosomal Abnormalities

The 'two-hit' hypothesis for inactivation of tumour suppressor genes was first confirmed in retinoblastoma through the rare patients who carry germline interstitial deletions of chromosome 13 (Yunis, Zuniga & Ramirez, 1981). A second conclusion could be drawn from the observation of these deletions in retinoblastoma patients. A specific chromosomal abnormality associated with a disease may indicate

Table 7.1. Inherited Cancer Syndromes

Syndrome	Location	Allele Loss	Gene (Function)
Beckwith-Wiedemann	11p15	Yes paternal disomy	?*IGF2* (growth factor)
Breast cancer, early-onset Breast/ovarian carcinoma	17q12–q21	Yes	BRCA (unknown function)
Breast cancer, early-onset	13q12–13	Yes	?
Dysplastic naevus syndrome[a]	1p36		?
Familial adenomatous polyposis	5q21–22	Yes	*APC* (unknown function)
Familial melanoma[b]	9p21		?
Gorlin[c]	9q		?
Hereditary nonpolyposis colorectal cancer	2p15–16	No	? (DNA replication)
Li-Fraumeni	17p	Yes	*TP53* (transcriptional regulation)
Multiple endocrine neoplasia type 1	11q13	Yes	?
Multiple endocrine neoplasia type 2A	10q11.2	No	*RET* (tyrosine kinase receptor)
Multiple endocrine neoplasia type 2B	10q11.2	No	? *RET*
Neurofibromatosis type I[d]	17q11.2	Yes	*NF1* (GTPase-activating protein)
Neurofibromatosis type II	22q12	Yes	*NF2* (cytoskeletal-membrane link)
Non-hereditary polyposis coil	2p22	No	MSH2 (DNA repair)
Non-hereditary polyposis coli	3p21	?	MLH1 (DNA repair)
Retinoblastoma	13q14	Yes	*RB1* (transcriptional regulation)
von Hippel-Lindau	3p25–p26	Yes	*VHL* (unknown function)
WAGR	11p13	Yes	*WT1* (transcriptional regulation)

[a]Dysplastic naevus syndrome (Bale et al., 1989; Gruis et al., 1990).
[b]Familial melanoma (Cannon-Albright et al., 1992).
[c]Gorlin syndrome (Gailani et al., 1992).
[d]MEN-1 (Larsson et al., 1988).

a potential candidate region in which gene(s) affected by the predisposing lesion reside. Since mutations of the same genes are believed to be involved in the development of both inherited and sporadic tumors, this is true for both rare constitutional chromosomal abnormalities and the more frequently observed tumour-specific chromosomal aberrations.

Allele Loss

The most common chromosomal mechanisms that lead to the loss of the second allele include mitotic recombination and loss of the chromosome carrying the normal allele with or without duplication of the chromosome bearing the mutant allele (Cavenee et al., 1983; Dryja et al., 1984). A direct result of these mechanisms is the loss of DNA in the tumour. Assay for the tumour-specific loss of genetic material requires the identification of locus-specific polymorphic markers (restriction fragment length polymorphisms (RFLPs), variable number tandem repeats (VNTRs), and di- and trinucleotide repeats (microsatellites)) in the DNA of constitutional cells. The observation of only one variant in the tumour (homozygous or hemizygous), when two forms are present in constitutional cells (heterozygous), is indicative of loss of genetic material. Loss of heterozygosity (LOH) in tumour cells affecting a limited genomic region has been used to suggest the presence of tumour suppressor genes in a wide variety of tumours.

Genetic Linkage

The collection of informative pedigrees segregating the disease is an initial step in determining the chromosomal region to which the predisposing gene maps. The inheritance of the cancer susceptibility can be followed through a family and linkage to other markers assessed. Linkage to protein polymorphisms or to the expression of genetically controlled phenotypes has been largely superseded by the use of RFLPs, VNTRs and microsatellites. The combination of linkage analysis with the knowledge of disease-associated cytogenetic abnormalities and LOH can result in a reasonably restricted region for analysis. The task of searching the whole genome for genetic linkage has been very labour intensive. However, the development of a high-density genetic map of the human genome, based on microsatellites and the intensive genotyping methods used to develop the map, should make genomic searches more feasible.

MOLECULARLY CHARACTERIZED FAMILIAL CANCER GENES

The genes responsible for familial cancer cloned to date (see Table 7.1) have been isolated by two strategies. A positional cloning approach based on a knowledge of the genes' location in conjunction with overlapping deletions and/or translocations was used to identify the majority of the familial cancer genes, and these are *APC, NF1, NF2, RB1, VHL* and *WT1*. An approach based on the joint knowledge of chromosomal position and candidate genes in that region led to the implication of *TP53* in Li-Fraumeni syndrome and *RET* in multiple endocrine neoplasia type 2A (MEN-2A), and a suggestion that *IGF2* is involved in Beckwith-Wiedemann syndrome.

Functionally, these loci are components of cellular pathways transducing regulatory signals. Biochemically, they act at multiple points in the transduction of external signals to the nucleus, including growth factor and receptor interactions; membrane and cytosolic signal transduction components; and in the nucleus, regulators of transcription, DNA replication and cell division.

Nuclear Genes

Three familial cancers are known to result from mutations in genes encoding nuclear transcription factors. These cancers vary considerably in their genetics and phenotypes. Retinoblastoma results from the mutation of a single gene (*RB1*) on chromosome 13q14. Inheritance of a mutant *RB1* allele predisposes to retinoblastoma (Friend et al., 1986) and a limited repertoire of second tumours (Friend et al., 1987). Wilms' tumour occurs in a simple familial form, and as one phenotypic manifestation of three distinct growth abnormality syndromes, the WAGR, Denis-Drash and Beckwith-Wiedemann syndromes. No candidate gene nor even chromosomal position has been proposed for familial Wilms' tumour; however, the gene at chromosome 11p13, which is the target for alterations in WAGR and Denis-Drash syndromes, has been identifed (*WT1*) (Bonetta et al., 1990; Call et al., 1990; Gessler et al., 1990) and the insulin-like growth factor 2 (*IGF2*) at 11p15 is a candidate for the gene altered in Beckwith-Wiedemann syndrome. Li-Fraumeni syndrome is characterized by an autosomal dominant predisposition to cancers in multiple tissues, and mutations of the *TP53* gene on chromosome 17p13 have been found in a subset of these families (Malkin et al., 1990; Srivastava et al., 1990a).

The Retinoblastoma Susceptibility Locus (RB1) There are only about 15 cases of familial retinoblastoma in the United Kingdom per annum, and the vast majority of cases are sporadic. A ubiquitous distribution (Goddard et al., 1988; Lee et al., 1987) implies that the *RB1* product has an important role in the development and maintenance of a broad range of tissues. In some cancers, such as retinoblastoma and osteosarcoma, inactivation of *RB1* initiates the malignant process, while in other tumours aberrations in *RB1* contribute to the progression of the tumour.

pRB is a transcription factor involved in the regulation of the cell cycle. Alteration in the level of phosphorylation of pRB during the cell cycle regulates its activity (Buchkovich, Duffy & Harlow, 1989; Chen et al., 1989; DeCaprio et al., 1989; Mihara et al., 1989). pRB is inactivated at the G_1/S boundary by phosphorylation by $p34^{cdc2}$ kinase (Lin et al., 1991). It remains in the inactive state throughout G_2 and M and is reactivated by dephosphorylation as the cell reenters G_1. In its unphosphorylated form, pRB binds to proteins required for the transition from G_1 to S phase, modulating their activity. A number of nuclear proteins interact with pRB (Defeo-Jones et al., 1991; Huang et al., 1991; Kaelin et al., 1991). Four of these have been identified: the transcription factor E2F/DRTF (Bagchi, Weinmann & Raychaudhuri, 1991; Bandara & La Thangue, 1991; Bandara et al., 1991; Chellappan et al., 1991; Chittenden, Livingston & Kaelin, 1991); a protein with E2F-like activity (Ap12) (Helin et al., 1992; Kaelin et al., 1992; Shan et al., 1992); the oncoprotein c-*myc* (Rustgi, Dyson & Bernards, 1991); and p48, a protein with homology to a negative regulator of *ras* cyclic-AMP pathway in yeast (Qian et al., 1993).

The ubiquitous role of pRB in the regulation of the cell cycle is enigmatic, considering that inheritance of a mutant allele predisposes to retinoblastoma, to a lesser extent osteosarcoma, and even more rarely other tumours. However, *RB1* mutations occur at high frequency in these tumours as part of their malignant progression (Goddard & Solomon, 1993). A limited number of cells, including retinoblasts and osteoblasts, may be particularly dependent on pRB-dependent regulation of the G_1/S checkpoint in the cell cycle. In other cell types, with redundant regulatory pathways, loss of the pRB is only effective in conjunction with mutational disruption of other pathways, such as that regulated by p53, and, therefore, mutation of *RB1* is seen in later stages of malignancy.

TP53 Mutations and Li-Fraumeni Syndrome While somatic mutations in *TP53* are implicated in the progression of more than 30 types of human malignancy (Caron de Fromentel & Soussi, 1992;

Hollstein et al., 1991), germline mutations in *TP53* predispose to an autosomal dominant predisposition to cancer of the breast, brain, bone, soft tissues, haematopoietic system, and adrenal cortex in Li-Fraumeni syndrome (Malkin et al., 1990; Srivastava et al., 1990a).

Like pRB, p53 is an ubiquitously expressed transcription factor (El-Deiry et al., 1992; Fields & Jang, 1990) that appears to be involved with the progression of the cell through the G_1/S checkpoint in the cell cycle. Both proteins are the target of inactivation by the oncoproteins of DNA tumour viruses through the formation of stable inactive complexes (DeCaprio et al., 1988; Egan, Bayley & Branton, 1989; Imai et al., 1991; Lane & Harlow, 1982; Lane & Crawford, 1979; Linzer & Levine, 1979; Ludlow et al., 1989; Ludlow et al., 1990; McCormick et al., 1981; Sarnow et al., 1982; Whyte et al., 1988). The fact that viruses have developed mechanisms to circumvent the regulatory functions of both of these two proteins implies that while they both regulate the cell cycle at the same checkpoint they most likely affect different pathways.

p53 appears to accomplish its regulatory role by interacting with other proteins, including heat shock proteins, the oncoprotein *MDM2* (Oliner et al., 1993), and the product of the *WT1* locus (Maheswaran et al., 1993). This latter interaction between *WT1* and p53 modulates both proteins' ability to affect the expression of their respective targets (Maheswaran et al., 1993). p53 is regulated during the cell cycle by both phosphorylation (Bischoff et al., 1990), and via the interaction between p53 and *MDM2* (Oliner et al., 1993). Overexpression of *MDM2* in tumours occurs in the absence of p53 mutations, suggesting that the two are alternative mechanisms that serve the purpose of inactivating p53 (Leach et al., 1993; Reifenberger et al., 1993). A more specific role for p53 may be to restrict the cell's entry into S phase and replication of DNA after exposure to DNA-damaging agents until DNA repair is complete (Kastan et al., 1992; Kuerbitz et al., 1992; Lane, 1992; Lee & Bernstein, 1993).

The presence of a single mutant *TP53* allele can result in a dominant-negative phenotype (Herskowitz, 1987) by the formation of inactive p53 oligomers between mutant and wild-type proteins (Green, 1989). Point mutations leading to inactivation of wild-type p53 and its oligomerization partners may be more transforming than deletion of the entire allele or point mutations that affect only the function of the p53 molecule carrying the mutation (i.e., some Li-Fraumeni syndrome (Srivastava et al., 1992), and hepatocellular carcinoma (Bressac et al., 1991; Hsu et al., 1991) mutations). In support of this is the observation of the mild phenotype of mice, which are heterozygous for a null *TP53* allele (Donehower et al., 1992).

Wilms' Tumor and 11p13 Wilm's tumour, or nephroblastoma, is the commonest solid pediatric tumour, affecting 1 in 10,000 children, usually during the first five years of life. Most cases are sporadic and unilateral, but about 7% are bilateral and a further 1% show family clustering (Breslow et al., 1988). The WAGR syndrome is characterized by Wilms' tumour, aniridia, genitourinary abnormalities, mental retardation and constitutional deletion of the 11p13 region (Miller, Fraumeni & Manning, 1964; Riccardi et al., 1978). In Denys-Drash syndrome (Denys et al., 1967; Drash et al., 1970; Miller et al., 1964), Wilms' tumour occurs in association with pseudohermaphroditism and progressive renal failure and point mutations of *WT1* (Pelletier et al., 1991).

The *WT1* locus encodes a nuclear transcription factor related to the EGR and Krox family of transcription factors (Call et al., 1990; Gessler et al., 1990), which are activated during the G_0 to G_1 transition in growth-stimulated cells (Chavrier et al., 1988). *WT1* binds to the same DNA sequence as EGR-1 (Rauscher et al., 1990), causing transcriptional repression (Madden et al., 1991). Binding to p53 induces *WT1* to act as a trancriptional activator (Maheswaran et al., 1993). These data suggest that *WT1*, like p53 and *RB1*, is involved in cell cycle control. However, the narrow expression profile of *WT1* in the developing fetal kidney and gonads (Pritchard-Jones et al., 1990; van Heyningen et al., 1990) suggests that *WT1* most likely exerts its effect in a very limited repertoire of cell types and is involved in the differentiation process of these tissues, while p53 and pRB function in all cell types.

While the loss of normal *WT1* function can contribute to tumourigenesis, WT1 does not always function as a classic tumour suppressor. Like p53, a dysfunctional *WT1* protein can produce more severe abnormalities than a reduction in the level of the protein due to deletion of a single allele, potentially by sequestering proteins (such as p53) in inactive complexes or by altering the profile of target genes recognized.

Hereditary Nonpolyposis Colorectal Cancer and DNA Replication The majority of hereditary nonpolyposis colorectal cancer families are linked to a locus on chromosome 2p (Loci) (Peltomäki et al., 1993) and 3p (Lindbolm et al., 1993). Precancerous lesions and invasive colorectal tumours from these patients consistently show instability of microsatellite and monotonic sequences throughout the genome, indicating that the predisposing allele is associated with a greatly decreased genetic stability (Aaltonen et al., 1993; Ionov et al., 1993; Thibodeau, Bren & Schaid, 1993). The DNA mismatch repair genes MSH2 (Fish et al., 1993; Leach et al., 1993) and MLH1 (Bronner et al., 1994; Papadopoulos et al., 1994) have recently been identified as the NHPPC genes on chromosomes 2p and 3p, respectively.

pRB, p53 and *WT1* modulate the expression of factors that are necessary for the cell to enter S phase and replicate DNA. p53 has the ability to monitor DNA damage and restrict the replication of DNA until the damage has been repaired or if damage is too severe to trigger apoptosis. *FCC* may act in this pathway of DNA repair and replication by either failing to detect DNA damage, perhaps by acting in the p53 pathway or by inducing mutations during replication.

Cytoplasmic Proteins in Familial Cancer

A growing number of tumour suppressor loci encode proteins that are localized in the cytoplasm. Proposed functions for these proteins include the physical linkage of integral membrane proteins to the cytoskeleton (*NF2*), cytoskeletal organization (*APC*), cell-cell or cell-matrix interactions (*DCC, VHL*) and cytoplasmic signalling (*NF1, VHL*). In general, these classes of proteins would be expected to be involved in determination of cell shape and organization, motility and anchorage, reorganization of the cytoplasm during cell division and extra- and intracellular communication.

Colorectal Carcinoma Familial adenomatous polyposis (FAP) and Gardner syndrome (GS) patients inherit dominant mutations at the *APC* locus and develop precancerous hyperproliferative lesions (Groden et al., 1991; Miyoshi et al., 1992; Nishisho et al., 1991). About 70 FAP patients in the United Kingdom go on to develop colorectal cancers each year. Three chromosomal regions frequently undergo LOH, and these are 5q, 17p and 18q (Vogelstein et al., 1988). 5q is the site of the predisposing genetic lesion in FAP and GS, and 5q allele loss is observed in colorectal cancer, suggesting the inactivation of a tumour suppressor locus. Mutation of *APC* occurs in early adenomas (Powell et al., 1992), indicating that inactivation of *APC* is a key step in the early stages of colorectal cancer. Dysplastic benign adenomas show LOH at 5q (Rees et al., 1989; Vogelstein et al., 1988), indicating the contribution to progression of complete inactivation of *APC*. Further progression to the carcinoma stage correlates with LOH affecting 18q and 17p (Vogelstein et al., 1988). In addition, activation of the dominantly acting oncogene *ras* appears to be associated with the transition from early- to late-stage adenomas (Bos et al., 1987; Forrester et al., 1987).

APC encodes a 300-kDa cytoplasmic protein (Smith et al., 1993) that has homology to myosins and keratins in regions predicted to form coiled-coil structures (Groden et al., 1991; Kinzler et al., 1991). The *APC* protein can form homo-oligmers via interactions of these aminoterminal sequences (Su et al., 1993). The potential to form inactive oligmers suggests that a single mutant *APC* molecule could function in a dominant negative fashion, reminiscent of p53 and *WT1*. *APC* may be involved in cell adhesion through interaction with β-catenin (Rubenfeld et al., 1993; Su et al., 1993), disruption of which is manifested in transformed cells.

The two other tumour suppressor loci implicated in colorectal cancer have been identified as *DCC* (Fearon et al., 1990) and *TP53* (Vogelstein et al., 1988). *DCC* on 18q is inactivated in the later stages of colorectal cancer development. It encodes a 190-kDa transmembrane phosphoprotein with homology to the neural cell adhesion molecules (Fearon et al., 1990), molecules which play a role in cell–cell adhesion and communication. Inactivation of *DCC* may disrupt normal interactions between cells or between cells and the extracellular matrix, thereby providing a growth advantage. No colon cancer families have been identified that show linkage to *DCC* and no germline *DCC* mutations have been identified.

Neurofibromatosis Type I Neurofibromatosis type I (*NF1*) is one of the commonest autosomal dominant conditions predisposing to cancer seen in man, affecting about 1 in 2,000. Mutations in the *NF1* gene predispose to the multiple benign abnormalities and tumours of *NF1* (Ponder, 1990). *NF1* is a tumour suppressor gene that maps to band q11.2 on human chromosome 17 (Ponder, 1990). LOH on proximal 17q is observed in *NF1*-associated tumours (Glover et al., 1991; Xu et al., 1992) and inactivating mutations are seen in the germline of familial patients and in tumours (Cawthon et al., 1990; Viskochil et al., 1990; Wallace et al., 1990). Benign neurofibromas and schwannomas remain heterozygous for the *NF1* region, suggesting that in a similar fashion to *APC*, reduced levels of the encoded protein may result in a growth advantage and complete loss may be involved in the progression of the benign lesion (Ponder, 1990).

The *NF1* gene encodes a protein called neurofibromin with homology to the yeast IRA proteins (inhibitory regulators of the *ras*-cAMP pathway) and mammalian p120^{GAP} (*ras*-GTPase-activating protein) (Buchberg et al., 1990; Xu et al., 1990b), which suggests that *NF1* may have a role in the *ras* signalling pathway. The neurofibromin catalytic domain was able to compensate for *ira1* and *ira2* mutants of *S. cerivisiae*, and stimulate *ras*-GTPase activity (Ballester et al., 1990;

Martin et al., 1990; Xu et al., 1990a). Growth stimulatory signals induce *ras* to exchange GDP for GTP, switching it from an inactive to an active state. The GAP proteins may serve two functions in the *ras* signalling cycle (Hall, 1990). GAPs may release their own downstream signal (Adari et al., 1988; Cales et al., 1988; Yatani et al., 1991) and then enhance *ras*·GTP-GTPase activity (Trahey & McCormick, 1987), thus both transducing the signal from and regulating the levels of the effector complex. Loss of neurofibromin would increase the levels of activated *ras* and inactivate one pathway through which $p21^{ras}$·GTP communicates. Multiple *ras* signalling routes are present in most cells (Bollag & McCormick, 1992; Bollag & McCornick, 1991). An increase in *ras*·GTP coupled with loss of one signalling pathway could result in overstimulation of the remaining pathways. Mutation of *NF1* does not appear to occur with *ras*-activating mutations (DeClue et al., 1992), like *TP53* and *MDM2,* neurofibromin and *ras* are alternative targets leading to the accumulation of active *ras*·GTP.

Neurofibromatosis Type II The suppressor gene predisposing to neurofibromatosis type II (*NF2* or *SCH*) may also play a role in the maintenance of the normal phenotype through regulation of membrane/cytoplasm organization or signalling. *NF2* encodes a protein known as merlin or schwannomin, with homology to the erthyrocyte band 4.1 family, suggesting that it functions, similarly to *APC* and *DCC,* in the cytoplasm, perhaps as a link between membrane proteins and the cytoskeleton (Rouleau et al., 1993; Trofatter et al., 1993). Other members of this family are phosphorylated in response to growth factors and may be involved in mediating signal transduction via modulation of cell–cell or cell–matrix interactions.

von Hippel-Lindau Syndrome The gene responsible for von Hippel-Lindau syndrome has recently been identified by positional cloning (Latif et al., 1993). This gene (*VHL*) is the target of mutation in von Hippel-Lindau–associated tumours and sporadic renal cell carcinomas. A putative role in signal transduction or cell adhesion is inferred by the homology of an acid repeat domain to the procyclic surface membrane protein of *Trypanosoma brucei.*

Receptors and Growth Factors

It may be expected that the inactivation of a receptor for a growth inhibitory factor, or the reduction in such a factor itself, could be implicated in inherited predisposition to cancer. Mutation of a tyrosine kinase receptor (*RET*) in multiple endocrine neoplasia type 2A

(MEN-2A) could be the first example of this model. Overexpression of a growth factor (IGF2) has been implicated in Wilms' tumour.

Multiple Endocrine Neoplasia Type 2A and the *RET* Oncogene MEN-2A is a dominantly inherited cancer syndrome affecting tissue of neuroectodermal origin. Between 20 and 30 cases of medullary thyroid cancer in the United Kingdom occur annually in MEN-2 families. Like hereditary nonpolyposis colon cancer, linkage of MEN-2A to a chromosomal region (10q11.2) has not been supported by LOH for probes in the same region, suggesting that inactivation of a suppressor allele was not the mechanism predisposing to this cancer syndrome. The recent report of germline mutations in the proto-oncogene *RET* in MEN-2A (Mulligan et al., 1993) has confirmed this theory. A high percentage of mutations in *RET* affect conserved cysteine residues in the extracellular domain of the receptor. Such alterations could alter the conformation of the protein and affect *RET* signal transduction or even ligand specificity or affinity. *RET* is distantly related to the cadherin family (Schneider, 1992). Cadherins are transmembrane molecules that mediate homophillic Ca^{2+}-dependent cell–cell adhesion. The *RET* ligand could be a target molecule on another cell, contact with which could signal cell–cell or cell–matrix interaction. Alteration of *RET* could reduce a growth inhibitory signal, leading to enhanced growth potential of cells expressing half normal/half wild-type *RET*. Alternatively, constitutive activation of *RET* tyrosine kinase activity could lead to growth stimulation of the cell in the absence of ligand.

RET is structurally rearranged in 25% of papillary thyroid carcinomas by the replacement of 5′ *RET* sequences with other expressed sequences (Fusco et al., 1987). These rearrangements tend to produce dominant phenotypes in transfection assays.

Beckwith-Wiedemann Syndrome and Insulin-like Growth Factor 2 Beckwith-Wiedemann syndrome is associated with rearrangements of the 11p15 region, including trisomy and paternal uniparental disomy of 11p15 and leads to multiorgan developmental abnormalities, including an increased risk of Wilms' tumour (Henry et al., 1991; Sotelo-Avila & Gooch, 1976). Familial Beckwith-Wiedemann syndrome is a rare autosomal dominant trait showing incomplete penetrance and is linked to 11p15 (Koufos et al., 1989; Ping et al., 1989). Tumour-specific allele loss affecting 11p15 in Wilms' tumour (Henry et al., 1989; Koufos et al., 1989; Reeve et al., 1989) is unusual in that it is almost always the maternally derived allele that is lost (Henry et al., 1991). This observation is suggestive of an imprinting affect in which the maternally and paternally derived alleles of a gene or genes in the region are not functionally equivalent. Thus, in the case of Beckwith-Wiedemann syndrome, LOH does not appear to point to the presence of a tumour supressor gene.

Insulin-like growth factor II (*IGF2*) maps to this region and is differentially imprinted in the mouse with higher levels of expression from the paternal allele (DeChiara, Robertson & Efstratiadis, 1991). The loss of maternal sequences coupled with duplication of the paternal counterpart in Wilms' tumour results in higher levels of *IGF2* in the tumour. Indirect evidence that *IGF2* overexpression plays a role in Beckwith-Wiedemann syndrome is supported by constitutively altered *IGF2* expression in Beckwith-Wiedemann syndrome patients (Weksberg et al., 1993). Also, *IGF2* imprinting is relaxed in Wilms' tumour without LOH and expression occurs from both maternal and paternal alleles (Ogawa et al., 1993; Rainier et al., 1993), suggesting that overexpression plays a role in the aetiology of Wilms' tumour perhaps via the overstimulation of the cellular growth through an autocrine mechanism. Other loci in this chromosomal region, such as H19 (Ferguson-Smith et al., 1993) may also be involved through alterations in imprinting.

BREAST AND OVARIAN CANCER

Genetics

Breast cancer currently affects 1 in 12 women in the United Kingdom. Each year there are about 25,000 new cases. Over half of the women diagnosed with breast cancer eventually die from the disease. The incidence of breast cancer is increasing and this trend is likely to continue for some time, as no major environmental cause of breast cancer has been identified and there is no known way of substantially reducing the risk.

Most breast cancer cases are not inherited. However, about 6% of cases are due to an inherited susceptibility. This means that 1 in 200 women get breast cancer because they have inherited a mutation in a susceptibility gene. There are therefore about 150,000 women in the United Kingdom who carry a breast cancer susceptibility mutation. Such carriers have a greater than 80% lifetime risk of developing breast cancer, whereas noncarriers have a less than 10% chance of getting the disease (Bishop & Easton, 1993; Claus, Risch & Thompson, 1991).

Ovarian cancer is about one fifth as common as breast cancer, with over 5000 new cases each year. At the moment, the vast majority of women diagnosed as having ovarian cancer die from this disease. About 5% of ovarian cancer cases are thought to be due to an inherited susceptibility (Schildkraut, Risch & Thompson, 1989). Interestingly, the risk of ovarian cancer is increased in relatives of women with breast cancer and vice versa. This suggests the existence of genes that predispose to both breast and ovarian cancer.

Breast cancer cases, and probably ovarian cancer cases, that are due to an inherited susceptibility are usually at an age. More than one third of cases diagnosed before the age of 30 are estimated to be due to familial breast cancer. This contribution is reduced to about 1% of cases diagnosed after the age of 80 (Claus, Risch & Thompson, 1990). However, it should be noted that in all age groups, the majority of breast cancer cases are sporadic and do not occur as a result of an inherited susceptibility. This fact is very important in trying to genetically map the breast cancer susceptibility genes.

Susceptibility Genes

The p53 gene is commonly mutated in sporadic forms of breast and ovarian cancer. Additionally, germline p53 mutations predispose women to many tumour types, including breast cancer (Malkin et al., 1990; Srivastava et al., 1990b). It is estimated that about 1% of breast cancer susceptibility is due to germline mutation in the p53 gene.

The gene responsible for the majority of hereditary breast cancer was mapped in 1990 by Mary-Clare King and her colleagues at the University of California, Berkeley (Hall et al., 1990). This gene maps to the long arm of human chromosome 17 and has been called *BRCA1* (Hall et al., 1992). It has been demonstrated that the *BRCA1* gene is responsible for almost all families with a susceptibility to breast and ovarian cancer from a study involving over 200 families (Easton et al., 1993). About half of these with only breast cancer are estimated to be due to the *BRCA1* gene (Easton et al., 1993). This is likely to be an underestimate, as small families that have one or more sporadic breast cancer cases will show no evidence of *BRCA1* linkage, even though the majority of affected women in these families may have inherited *BRCA1* mutations. The actual contribution *BRCA1* makes to breast cancer susceptibility and the involvement of this gene in sporadic disease cannot be fully determined until the *BRCA1* gene has been identified. However, it is probable that over 100,000 women in the United Kingdom carry germline *BRCA1* mutations. Female carriers have a risk of developing either breast or ovarian cancer of about 60% by age 50, rising to over 80% by age 70 (Easton et al., 1993).

The Hunt for *BRCA1*

Since the report of breast cancer linkage to chromosome 17, many researchers have been involved in the hunt for this gene. *BRCA1* was eventually identified by a positional cloning strategy in summer 1994 (Miki et al., 1994; Futreal et al., 1994). The gene is transcribed to give a 7.8kb mRNA in many tissues. The *BRCA1* transcript has a large open reading frame encoding an 1863 amino acid protein. The function of the *BRCA1* gene product is unknown, although the protein contains a RING-finger motif, which is believed to be involved in protein-protein interactions. *BRCA1* germline mutations have been detected in over 80 families (Shattuck-Eidens et al., 1995). The majority of these are loss of function mutations, indicating that *BRCA1* is a tumour suppressor gene. Somatic *BRCA1* mutations have been identified in five ovarian epithelial tumours (Boyd, 1995), but to date, none have been reported in breast tumours.

BRCA2

A second early-onset breast cancer susceptibility locus, *BRCA2* has been mapped to 13q12-q13 (Wooster et al., 1995). *BRCA2* is believed to be responsible for all the large families, showing high penetrance susceptibility to breast cancer, which are not linked to *BRCA1*.

Allele Loss in Breast and Ovarian Cancer

LOH studies have shown that chromosome 17 markers are lost at significant frequencies in sporadic breast and ovarian cancer (Black & Solomon, 1993). Losses are seen in over 80% of late-stage ovarian adenocarcinomas (Foulkes et al., 1993) and in 30 to 40% of breast carcinomas (Sato et al., 1990).

Analysis of breast and ovarian tumours from families in which the disease is linked to *BRCA1* also show LOH with chromosome 17 markers. The alleles that are linked to the disease in these families are retained in the tumours and the wild-type alleles are lost (Kelsell et al., 1993; Smith et al., 1992). This results in the tumours being homozygous or hemizygous for the *BRCA1* mutation. This observation suggests that *BRCA1* is a recessively acting tumour suppressor gene. However, it is possible that the observed loss is not directed at *BRCA1*, as there are many other putative tumour suppressor genes on chromosome 17. Interestingly, when chromosome 17 LOH is observed in ovarian tumours, the entire chromosome is almost always lost. Additionally, there does not seem to be any peak of allele loss in the

BRCA1 region. It is therefore unclear if BRCA1 actually is a tumour suppressor gene.

PROSTATE CANCER

Genetics

Prostate cancer is the third most frequently diagnosed cancer and the second most frequent cause of death due to cancer in men in the United Kingdom. Approximately 12,000 males are diagnosed annually and about 8,500 die from this disease. Nearly one third of all men over 50 years have latent or incidental prostate cancer, which is usually revealed at autopsy. The frequency increases substantially with each decade of life from 10 to 20% for men in their fifties, to 50 to 75% in those in their nineties. Thus, the number of cases is likely to increase steadily over the next decade as the population ages. It is apparent that the cases of clinically manifest prostate cancer represents only a small fraction, about 10%, of the latent prostate cancer. Life-threatening prostate cancer results from the progression of a subset of these common, small, latent lesions.

Like breast cancer, the majority of prostate cancer is sporadic, but some family clustering indicates that there is also a genetic susceptibility to the disease. It has recently been shown that about 10% of prostate cancer cases can be explained by the inheritance of genes giving an autosomal dominant susceptibility (Carter et al., 1992). In a similar fashion to breast cancer, there is an age effect, with over 40% of cases diagnosed before the age of 55 having a genetic origin. Male carriers of the susceptibility genes have a greater than 80% risk of the disease by age 85, as opposed to a less than 5% risk for noncarriers. Additionally, families in Iceland, with an inherited susceptibility to breast cancer, also show increased frequencies of prostate cancer (Tulinius et al., 1992).

Allele Loss in Prostate Cancer

LOH studies have found losses on chromosomes 7, 8p, 10q, 11p and 16q (Bergerheim et al., 1991; Kunimi et al., 1991). The 8p locus is additionally the fourth most frequent loss seen in colon cancer after chromosomes 18 (*DCC*), 5q (*APC*) and 17p (p53). Chromosome 16q is the most frequent site of loss seen in breast cancer, indicating that the same tumour suppressor gene may be involved in diverse tumour types. Once the chromosome 8p colon cancer and the 16q breast cancer tumour suppressor genes have been identified, it will be interesting to see if they are indeed mutated in prostate tumours, and if they are, is there any correlation with tumour progression?

The chromosome 10q loss seems to be specific to prostate cancer. This has been delineated by LOH studies to the 10q23-qter interval. Unfortunately, the amount of cytogenetic information on prostate cancer is relatively sparse when compared with that on other common adenocarcinomas. Nevertheless, cytogenetic analyses of prostate tumours have revealed frequent alterations involving the long arm of chromosome 10. Interestingly, chromosomal breaks seem to cluster at 10q24, so this may be the site of the 10q prostate cancer tumour suppressor gene.

CONCLUSIONS

Tumour suppressor genes have diverse functions, acting as growth factors, receptors, cytoplasmic organizers, signal transducers and nuclear factors. Tumour suppressors appear to regulate unrestricted growth by transducing inhibitory growth signals or limiting the efficacy of stimulatory signals. Investigation of the mechanisms through which the tumour suppressor genes act has resulted in a functional link with the dominant oncogenes. The retinoblastoma gene regulates two known proto-oncogenes, c-*fos* (through *E2F*) and c-*myc* (via *E2F* and through direct interaction). The Wilms' tumour suppressor gene, *WT1*, may also inhibit the expression of early response genes through binding to the same DNA sequence as the EGR-1 transcription factor. Neurofibromin potentiates *ras* by stimulating GTPase activity and, possibly, by acting as a downstream effector molecule. In multiple endocrine neuroplasia type 2A, the target of predisposing germline mutations is a dominant oncogene of the tyrosine kinase receptor family, and in hereditary nonfamilial polyposis coli a dominant alteration is expected in a DNA repair or replication gene.

The division between dominant and recessive mutations becomes blurred in some cases. For example, the oligomerization of p53 can lead to the formation of nonfunctional complexes between mutant and wild-type proteins. Other tumour suppressor products with the potential for protein–protein interactions, such as *APC* and *WT1*, may also act in this dominant-negative fashion. The introduction of a normal allele of a tumour suppressor locus into cells lacking any normal product from that locus has unequivocally demonstrated the dominant effects of wild-type *RB1* and p53 (Baker et al., 1990; Bookstein et al., 1990; Huang et al., 1988; Takahashi et al., 1991).

A number of loci that predispose to cancer are expected to be identified within the next few years, including those for breast cancer, melanoma, nonpolyposis-associated colon cancer, multiple endocrine neoplasia type 1 and Gorlin syndrome.

REFERENCES

Aaltonen L.A., Peltomaki P., Leach F.S., Sistonen P., Pylkkanen L., Mecklin J.P., Jarvinen H., Powell S.M., Jen J., Hamilton S.R., Petersen G.M., Kinzler K.W., Vogelstein B. & de la Chapelle A. (1993) Clues to the pathogenesis of familial colorectal cancer [see comments]. *Science,* **260**, 812–16.

Adari H., Lowly D.R., Willumsen B.M., Der C.J. & McCormick F. (1988) Guanosine triphosphatase activating protein (GAP) interacts with the p21 *ras* effector binding domain. *Science,* **240**, 518–21.

Armitage P. & Doll R. (1954) The age distribution of cancer and a multi-stage theory of carcinogenesis. *British Journal of Cancer,* **8**, 1–12.

Ashley D.J.B. (1969) Colonic cancer arising in polyposis coli. *Journal of Medical Genetics,* **6**, 376–8.

Bagchi S., Weinmann R. & Raychaudhuri P. (1991) The retinoblastoma protein copurifies with E2F-I, an E1A-regulated inhibitor of the transcription factor E2F. *Cell,* **65**, 1063–72.

Baker S.J., Markowitz S., Fearon E.R., Wilson J.K. & Vogelstein B. (1990) Suppression of human colorectal carcinoma cell growth by wild-type p53. *Science,* **249**, 912–15.

Bale S.J., Dracopoli N.C., Tucker M.A., Clark W.H., Fraser M.C., Stanger B.Z., Green P., Donis-Keller H., Houseman D.E. & Greene M.H. (1989) Mapping the gene for hereditary cutaneous malignant melanoma-dysplastic naevus to chromosome 1p. *New England Journal of Medicine,* **320**, 1367–72.

Ballester R., Marchuk D., Boguski M., Saulino A., Letcher R., Wigler M. & Collins F. (1990) The NF1 locus encodes a protein functionally related to mammalian GAP and yeast IRA proteins. *Cell,* **63**, 851–9.

Bandara L. & La Thangue N.B. (1991) Adenovirus E1a prevents the retinoblastoma gene product from complexing with a cellular transcription factor. *Nature,* **351**, 494–7.

Bandara L.R., Adamczewski J.P., Hunt T. & La Thangue N.B. (1991) Cyclin A and the retinoblastoma gene product complex with a common transcription factor. *Nature,* **352**, 249–51.

Bergerheim U.S.R., Kunimi K., Collins V.P. & Ekman P. (1991) Deletion mapping of chromosomes 8, 10, and 16 in human prostatic carcinoma. *Genes, Chromosomes and Cancer,* **3**, 215–20.

Bischoff J.R., Friedman P.N., Marshak D.R., Prives C. & Beach D. (1990) Human p53 is phosphorylated by p60-cdc2 and cyclin B-cdc2. *Proceedings of the National Academy of Sciences of the United States of America,* **87**, 4766–70.

Bishop D.T. & Easton D.F. (1993) Preface to the breast cancer linkage consortium papers. *American Journal of Human Genetics,* **52**, 677.

Black D.M. & Solomon E. (1993) The search for the familial breast-ovarian cancer gene. *Trends in Genetics,* **9**, 22–6.

Bollag G. & McCormick F. (1992) NF is enough of GAP. *Nature,* **356**, 663–4.

Bollag G. & McCormick F. (1991) Differential regulation of rasGAP and neurofibromatosis gene product activities. *Nature,* **351**, 576–9.

Bonetta L., Kuehn S.E., Huang A., Law D.J., Kalikin L.M., Koi M., Reeve A.E., Brownstein B.H., Yeger H., Williams B.R.G. & Fenberg A.P. (1990) Wilms tumor locus on 11p13 defined by multiple CpG island-associated transcripts. *Science*, **250**, 994–7.

Bookstein R., Shew J.Y., Chen P.L., Scully P. & Lee W.-H. (1990) Suppression of tumorigenicity of human prostate carcinoma cells by replacing a mutated *RB* gene. *Science*, **247**, 712–15.

Bos J.L., Fearon E.R., Hamilton S.R., Verlaan-de Vries M., van Boom J.H., van der Eb A.J. & Vogelstein B. (1987) Prevalence of ras gene mutations in human colorectal cancers. *Nature*, **327**, 293–7.

Breslow N., Beckwith J.B., Ciol M. & Shaples K. (1988) Age distribution of Wilms' tumor: report from the National Wilms' Tumor Study. *Cancer Research*, **48**, 1653–7.

Bressac B., Kew M., Wands J. & Ozturk M. (1991) Selective G to T mutations of p53 gene in hepatocellular carcinoma from southern Africa. *Nature*, **350**, 429–31.

Bronner C.E., Baker S.M., Morrison P.T., Warren G., Smith L.G., Lescoe M.K., Kane M., Earabino C., Lipford J. & Lindblom A. (1994) Mutation in the DNA mismatch repair gene homologue hHLHl is associated with hereditary non-polyposis colon cancer. *Nature*, **368**, 258–61.

Buchberg A.M., Cleveland L.S., Jenkins N.A. & Copeland N.G. (1990) Sequence homology shared by neurofibromatosis type-1 gene and IRA-1 and IRA-2 negative regulators of the RAS cyclic AMP pathway. *Nature*, **347**, 291–4.

Buchkovich K., Duffy L.A. & Harlow E. (1989) The retinoblastoma protein is phosphorylated during specific phases of the cell cycle. *Cell*, **58**, 1097–105.

Cales C., Hancock J.F., Marshall C.J. & Hall A. (1988) The cytoplasmic protein GAP is implicated as the target for regulation by the *ras* gene product. *Nature*, **332**, 548–51.

Call K.M., Glaser T., Ito C.Y., Buckler A.J., Pelletier J., Haber D.A., Rose E.A., Kral A., Yeger H., Lewis W.H., Jones C. & Houseman D.E. (1990) Isolation and characterization of a zinc finger polypeptide gene at the human chromosome 11 Wilms' tumor locus. *Cell*, **60**, 509–20.

Cannon-Albright L.A., Goldgar D.E., Meyer L.J., Lewis C.M., Anderson D.E., Fountain J.W., Hegi M.E., Wiseman R.W., Petty E.M., Bale A.E., Olopafe O., Diaz M., Kwiatkowski D., Piepkorn M., Zone J. & Skolnick M.H. (1992) Assignment of a locus for familial melanoma, MLM, to chromosome 9p13-p22. *Science*, **258**, 1148–52.

Caron de Fromentel C. & Soussi T. (1992) TP53 tumor suppressor gene: a model for investigating human mutagensis. *Genes, Chromosomes and Cancer*, **4**, 1–15.

Carter B.S., Beaty T.H., Steinberg G.D., Childs B. & Walsh P.C. (1992) Mendelian inheritance of familial prostate cancer. *Proceedings of the National Academy of Sciences of the United States of America*, **89**, 3367–71.

Cavenee W.K., Dryja T.P., Phillips R.A., Benedict R., Gallie B.L., Murphree A.L., Strong L.C. & White R.L. (1983) Expression of recessive alleles by chromosomal mechanisms in retinoblastoma. *Nature*, **305**, 779–84.

Cawthon R.M., Weiss R., Xu G.F., Viskochil D., Culver M., Stevens J., Robertson M., Dunn D., Gesteland R., O'Connell P. & White R. (1990) A major segment of the neurofibromatosis type 1 gene: cDNA sequence, genomic structure, and point mutations. *Cell*, **62**, 193–201.

Chavrier P., Zerial M., Lemaire P., Almendral J., Bravo R. & Charnay P. (1988) A gene encoding a protein with zinc fingers is activated during G0/G1 transition in cultured cells. *EMBO Journal*, **7**, 2–35.

Chellappan S.P., Hiebert S., Mudryj M., Horowitx J.M. & Nevins J.R. (1991) The E2F transcription factor is a cellular target for the RB protein. *Cell*, **65**, 1053–61.

Chen P.-L., Scully P., Shew J.-Y., Wang J.Y.J. & Lee W.-H. (1989) Phosphorylation of the retinoblastoma gene product is modulated during the cell cycle and cellular differentiation. *Cell*, **58**, 1193–98.

Chittenden T., Livingston D.M. & Kaelin W.G.J. (1991) The T/E1A-binding domain of the retinoblastoma product can interact selectively with sequence-specific DNA-binding protein. *Cell*, **65**, 1073–82.

Claus E.B., Risch N. & Thompson W.D. (1991) Genetic analysis of breast cancer in the cancer and steroid hormone study. *American Journal of Human Genetics*, **48**, 232–242.

Claus E.B., Risch N.J. & Thompson D.W. (1990) Age at onset as an indicator of familial risk of breast cancer. *American Journal of Epidemiology*, **131**, 961–72.

DeCaprio J.A., Ludlow J.W., Figge J., Shew J.-Y., Huang C.-M., Lee W.-H., Marsilio E., Paucha E. & Livingston D.M. (1988) SV40 large tumor antigen forms a specific complex with the product of the retinoblastoma susceptibility gene. *Cell*, **54**, 275–83.

DeCaprio J.A., Ludlow J.W., Lynch D., Furukawa Y., Griffen J., Piwnica-Worms H., Huang C.-M. & Livingston D.M. (1989) The product of the retinoblastoma susceptibility gene has properties of a cell cycle regulatory element. *Cell*, **58**, 1085–95.

DeChiara T.M., Robertson E.J. & Efstratiadis A. (1991) Paternal imprinting of the mouse insulin-like growth factor II gene. *Cell*, **64**, 849–59.

DeClue J.E., Papageorge A.G., Fletcher J.A., Diehl S.R., Ratner N., Vass W.C. & Lowy D.R. (1992) Abnormal regulation of mammalian p21ras contributes to malignant tumor growth in von Recklinghausen (type 1) neurofibromatosis. *Cell*, **69**, 265–73.

Defeo-Jones D., Huang P.S., Jones R.E., Haskell K.M., Vuocolo G.A., Hanobik M.G., Hube H.E. & Oliff A. (1991) Cloning of cDNAs for cellular proteins that bind to the retinoblastoma gene product. *Nature*, **352**, 251–4.

Denys P., Malvaux P., van den Berghe H., Tanghe W. & Proesmans W. (1967) Association d'un syndrome anatomo-pathologique de pseudohermaphrodisme masculin, d'une tumeur de Wilms, d'une nephropathie parenchymateuse et d'un mosaicisme XX/XY. *Archives de Francaise Pediatirque*, **24**, 729–39.

Donehower L.A., Harvey M., Slagle B.L., McArthur M.J., Montgomery C.A.J., Butel J.S. & Bradley A. (1992) Mice deficient for p53 are developmentally normal but susceptible to spontaneous tumours. *Nature*, **356**, 215–21.

Drash A., Sherman F., Hartmann W.H. & Blizzard R.M. (1970) A syndrome of pseudohermaphroditism, Wilms' tumor, hypertension and degenerative renal disease. *Journal of Pediatrics*, **76**, 585–93.

Dryja T.P., Cavenee W., White R., Rapaport J.M., Petersen R., Albert D.M. & Bruns G.A.P. (1984) Homozygosity of chromosome 13 in retinoblastoma. *New England Journal of Medicine*, **310**, 550–3.

Easton D.F., Bishop D.T., Ford D., Cockford G.P. & Breast Cancer Linkage Consortium. (1993) Genetic linkage analysis in familial breast and ovarian cancer – results from 214 families. *American Journal of Human Genetics*, **52**, 678–701.

Egan C., Bayley S.T. & Branton P.E. (1989) Binding of the Rb1 protein to E1A products is required for adenovirus transformation. *Oncogene*, **4**, 383–8.

El-Deiry W.S., Kern S.E., Pietenpol J.A., Kinzler K.W. & Vogelstein B. (1992) Definition of a consensus binding site for p53. *Nature Genetics*, **1**, 45–49.

Fearon E.R., Cho K.R., Nigro J.M., Kern S.E., Simons J.W., Ruppert J.M., Hamilton S.R., Preisinger A.C., Thomas G., Kinzler K.W. & Vogelstein B. (1990) Identification of a chromosome 18q gene that is altered in colorectal cancers. *Science*, **247**, 49–56.

Ferguson-Smith A., Sasaki H., Cattanach B. & Surani A. (1993) Parental-origin-specific epigenetic modification of the mouse *H19* gene. *Nature*, **362**, 751–5.

Fields S. & Jang S.K. (1990) Presence of a potent transcription activating sequence in the p53 protein. *Science*, **249**, 1046–49.

Fishel R., Lescoe M.K., Rao M.R.S., Copeland N.G., Jenkins N.A., Garber J., Kane M. & Kolodner R. (1993) The human mutator gene homolog MSH2 and its association with hereditary nonpolyposis colon cancer. *Cell*, **75**, 1027–38.

Forrester K., Almoguera C., Han K., Grizzle W.E. & Perucho M. (1987) Detection of high incidence of K-ras oncogenes during human colon tumourigenesis. *Nature*, **327**, 298–303.

Foulkes W.D., Black D.M., Stamp G.W.H., Solomon E. & Trowsdale J. (1993) Very frequent loss of heterozygosity throughout chromosome 17 in sporadic ovarian carcinoma. *International Journal of Cancer*, **54**, 220–5.

Friend S.H., Bernards R., Rogelj S., Weinberg R.A., Rapaport J.M., Alberts D.M. & Dryja T.P. (1986) A human DNA segment with properties of the gene that predisposes to retinoblastoma and osteosarcoma. *Nature*, **323**, 643–6.

Friend S.H., Horowitz J.M., Gerber M.R., Wang X.-F., Bogenmann E., Li F.P. & Weinberg R.A. (1987) Deletions of a DNA sequence in retinoblastomas and mesenchymal tumors: organization of the sequence and its encoded protein. *Proceedings of the National Academy of Sciences of the United States of America*, **84**, 9059–63.

Fusco A., Grieco M., Santoro M., Berlingieri M.T., Pilotti S., Pierotti M.A., Della Porta G. & Vecchio G. (1987) A new oncogene in human thyroid papillary carcinomas and their lymph-nodal metastases. *Nature*, **328**, 170–2.

Futreal P.A., Liu Q., Shattuck-Eidens D., Cochran C., Harshman K., Tartigian S., Michelle Bennett L., Haugen-Strano A., Swensen J., Miki Y., Eddington K., McClure M., Frye C., Ding W., Gholami Z., Terry L., Jhanwar S., Berchuck A., Inglehart J.D., Marks J., Bollinger D.G., Barrett J.C., Skolnick M.H., Kamb A. & Weisman R. (1994) BRCA1 mutations in primary breast and ovarian carcinomas. *Science*, **266**, 120–2.

Gailani M.R., Bale S.J., Leffell D.J., DiGiovanna J.J., Peck G.L., Poliak S., Drum M.A., Pastakia B., McBride O.W., Kase R., Greene M., Mulvihill J.J. & Bale A.E. (1992) Developmental defects in Gorlin syndrome related to a putative tumor suppressor gene on chromosome 9. *Cell*, **69**, 111–7.

Gessler M., Poustka A., Cavenee W., Neve R.L., Orkin S.H. & Bruns G.A. (1990) Homozygous deletion in Wilms tumours of a zinc-finger gene identified by chromosome jumping. *Nature*, **343**, 774–8.

Glover T.W., Stein C.K., Legius E., Andersen L.B., Brereton A. & Johnson S. (1991) Molecular and cytogenetic analysis of tumors in von Recklinghausen neurofibromatosis. *Genes, Chromosomes and Cancer*, **3**, 62–70.

Goddard A.D., Balakier H., Canton M., Dunn J., Squire J., Reyes E., Becker A., Phillips R.A. & Gallie B.L. (1988) Infrequent genomic rearrangement and normal expression of the putative RB1 gene in retinoblastoma tumors. *Molecular and Cellular Biology*, **8**, 2082–8.

Goddard A.D. & Solomon E. (1993) Genetic aspects of cancer. *Advances in Human Genetics*, **21**, 321–76.

Green M.R. (1989) When the products of oncogenes and anti-oncogenes meet. *Cell*, **56**, 1–3.

Groden J., Thliveris A., Samowitz W., Carlson M., Gelbert L., Albertsen H., Joslyn G., Stevens J., Spirio L., Robertson K., Sargeant L., Krapcho K., Wolff E., Burt R., Hughes J.P., Warrington J., McPherson J., Wasmuth J., Le Pasilier D., Abderrahim H., Cohen D., Leppert M. & White R. (1991) Identification and characterization of the familial adenomatous polyposis coli gene. *Cell*, **66**, 589–600.

Gruis N.A., Bergman W., Franks R.R., Bale J.J., Tucker M.A. & Dracopoli N.C. (1990) Locus for susceptibility to melanoma on chromosome 1p. *New England Journal of Medicine*, **322**, 853–4.

Hall A. (1990) The cellular functions of small GTP-binding proteins. *Science*, **249**, 635–40.

Hall J.M., Friedman L., Guenther C., Lee M.K., Weber J.L., Black D.M. & King M.C. (1992) Closing in on a breast-cancer gene on chromosome-17q. *American Journal of Human Genetics*, **50**, 1235–42.

Hall J.M., Lee M.K., Newman B., Morrow J.E., Anderson L.A., Huey B. & King M.-C. (1990) Linkage of early-onset familial breast cancer to chromosome 17q21. *Science*, **250**, 1684–9.

Helin K., Lees J.A., Vidal M., Dyson N., Harlow E. & Fattaey A. (1992) A cDNA encoding a pRB-binding protein with properties of the transcription factor E2F. *Cell*, **70**, 337–50.

Henry I., Bonaiti-Pellié C., Chehensse V., Beldjord C., Schwartz C., Utermann G. & Junien C. (1991) Uniparental paternal disomy in a genetic cancer-predisposing syndrome. *Nature*, **351**, 665–7.

Henry I., Grandjouan S., Couillin P., Barichard F., Huerre J.C., Glaser T., Philip T., Lenoir G., Chaussain J.L. & Junien C. (1989) Tumor-specific loss of 11p15.5 alleles in del11p13 Wilms tumor and in familial adrenocortical carcinoma. *Proceedings of the National Academy of Sciences of the United States of America*, **86**, 3247–51.

Herskowitz I. (1987) Functional inactivation of genes by dominant negative mutations. *Nature*, **329**, 219–22.

Hollstein M., Sidransky D., Vogelstein B. & Harris C.C. (1991) p53 mutations in human cancers. *Science*, **253**, 49–53.

Hosking L., Trowsdale J., Nicolai H., Solomon E., Foulkes W., Stamp G., Singer E. & Jeffreys A. (1995) A somatic BRCA1 mutation in an ovarian tumour. *Nature Genetics*, **9**, 343–4.

Hsu I.C., Metcalf R.A., Sun T., Welsh J.A., Wang N.J. & Harris C.C. (1991) Mutational hotspot in the p53 gene in human hepatocellular carcinomas. *Nature*, **350**, 427–8.

Huang H.-J.S., Yee J.-K., Shew J.-Y., Chen P.-L., Bookstein R., Friedmann T., Lee E.Y.-H.P. & Lee W.-H. (1988) Suppression of the neoplastic phenotype by replacement of the RB gene in human cancer cells. *Science*, **242**, 1563–6.

Huang S., Lee W.-H. & Lee E.Y.-H.P. (1991) A cellular protein that competes with SV40 T antigen for binding to the retinoblastoma gene product. *Nature*, **350**, 160–2.

Imai Y., Matsushima Y., Sugimura T. & Terada M. (1991) Purification and characterization of human papillomavirus type 16 E7 protein with preferential binding capacity to the underphosphorylated form of retinoblastoma gene product. *Journal of Virology*, **65**, 4966–72.

Ionov Y., Peinado M.A., Malkhosyan S., Shibata D. & Perucho M. (1993) Ubiquitous somatic mutations in simple repeated sequences reveal a new mechanism for colonic carcinogenesis. *Nature*, **363**, 558–61.

Kaelin W.G., Krek W., Sellers W.R., DeCaprio J.A., Ajchenbaum F., Fuchs C.S., Chittenden T., Li Y., Farnham P.J., Blanar M.A., Livingston D.M. & Flemington E.K. (1992) Expression cloning of a cDNA encoding a retinoblastoma-binding protein with E2F-like properties. *Cell*, **70**, 351–64.

Kaelin W.G.J., Pallas D.C., DeCaprio J.A., Kaye F.J. & Livingston D.M. (1991) Identification of cellular proteins that can interact specifically with the T/E1A-binding region of the retinoblastoma gene product. *Cell*, **64**, 521–32.

Kastan M.B., Zhan Q., el, D.W., Carrier F., Jacks T., Walsh W.V., Plunkett B.S., Vogelstein B. & Fornace A.J. (1992) A mammalian cell cycle checkpoint pathway utilizing p53 and GADD45 is defective in ataxia-telangiectasia. *Cell*, **71**, 587–97.

Kelsell D.P., Black D.M., Bishop D.T. & Spurr N.K. (1993) Genetic analysis of the BRCA1 region in a large breast/ovarian family: refinement of the minimal region containing BRCA1. *Human Molecular Genetics*, **2**, 1823–8.

Kinzler K.W., Nilbert M.C., Su L.-K., Vogelstein B., Bryan T.M., Levy D.B., Smith K.J., Preisinger A.C., Hedge P., McKechnie D., Finniear R., Markham A., Groffen J., Boguski M.S., Altschul S.F., Horii A., Ando H., Miyoshi Y., Miki Y., Nishisho I. & Nakamura Y. (1991) Identification of FAP locus genes from chromosome 5q21. *Science*, **253**, 661–5.

Knudson A.G. (1971) Mutation and cancer: statistical study of retinoblastoma. *Proceedings of the National Academy of Sciences of the United States of America*, **68**, 820–3.

Knudson A.G. (1986) Genetics of human cancer. *Annual Review of Genetics*, **20**, 231–51.

Knudson A.G. & Strong L.C. (1972a) Mutation and cancer: a model for Wilms' tumor of the kidney. *Journal of the National Cancer Institute*, **48**, 313–24.

Knudson A.G. & Strong L.C. (1972b) Mutation and cancer: neuroblastoma and pheochromocytoma. *American Journal of Human Genetics*, **24**, 514–32.

Koufos A., Grundy P., Morgan K., Aleck K.A., Hadro T., Lampkin B.C., Kalbakji A. & Cavenee W.C. (1989) Familial Weidemann-Beckwith syndrome and a second Wilms tumor locus both map to 11p15.5. *American Journal of Human Genetics*, **44**, 711–19.

Kuerbitz S.J., Plunkett B.S., Walsh W.V. & Kastan M.B. (1992) Wild-type p53 is a cell cycle checkpoint determinant following irradiation. *Proceedings of the National Academy of Sciences of the United States of America*, **89**, 7491–5.

Kunimi K., Bergerheim U.S.R., Larsson I.-L., Ekman P. & Collins V.P. (1991) Allelotyping of human prostatic adenocarcinoma. *Genomics,* **11**, 530–6.

Lane D. & Harlow E. (1982) Two different viral transforming proteins bind the same host tumor antigen. *Nature,* **298**, 517.

Lane D.P. (1992) p53, guardian of the genome. *Nature,* **358**, 15–16.

Lane D.P. & Crawford L.V. (1979) T antigen bound to a host protein in SV40-transformed cells. *Nature,* **278**, 261–3.

Larsson C., Skogseid B., Oberg K., Nakamura Y. & Nordenskjold M. (1988) Multiple endocrine neoplasia type 1 gene maps to chromosome 11 and is lost in insulinoma. *Nature,* **332**, 85–7.

Latif F., Tory K., Gnarra J., Yao M., Duh F.M., Orcutt M.L., Stackhouse T., Kuzmin I., Modi W., Geil L., Schmidt L., Zhou F., Li H., Wei M.H., Chen F., Glenn G., Choyle P., Walther M.M., Weng Y., Duan D.R., Dean M., Glavac D., Richards F.M., Crossey P.A., Ferguson-Smith M.A., Le Paslier D., Chumakov I., Cohen D., Chinault A.C., Maher E.R., Linehan W.M., Zbar B. & Lerman M.I. (1993) Identification of the von Hippel-Lindau disease tumor suppressor gene. *Science,* **260**, 1317–20.

Leach F.S., Nicolaides N.C., Papadopoulos N., Liu B., Jen J., Parsons R., Peltomäki P., Sistonen P., Aaltonen L.A., Nyström-Lahti M., Guan X.-Y., Zhang J., Meltzer P.S., Yu J.-W., Kao F.-T., Chen D.J., Cerosaletti K.M., Fournier, R.E.K., Todd S., Lewis T., Leach R.J., Naylor S.L., Weissenbach J., Mecklin J.-P., Järvinen H., Petersen G.M., Hamilton S.R., Green J., Jass J., Watson P., Lynch H.T., Trent J.M., de la Chapelle A., Kinzler K.W. & Vogelstein B. (1993) Mutuations of muts homolog in hereditary non-polyposis colorectal cancer. *Cell,* **75**, 1215–25.

Leach F.S., Tokino T., Meltzer P., Burrell M., Oliner J.D., Smith S., Hill D.E., Sidransky D., Kinzler K.W. & Vogelstein B. (1993) *p53* mutation and *MDM2* amplification in human soft tissue sarcomas. *Cancer Research,* **53**, 2231–4.

Lee J.M. & Bernstein A. (1993) p53 mutations increase resistance to ionizing radiation. *Proceedings of the National Academy of Sciences of the United States of America,* **90**, 5742–6.

Lee W.-H., Bookstein R., Hong F., Young L.-J., Shew J.-Y. & Lee E.Y.-H.P. (1987) Human retinoblastoma susceptibility gene: cloning, identification, and sequence. *Science,* **235**, 1394–9.

Li F.P. (1990) Familial cancer syndromes and clusters. *Current Problems in Cancer,* **14**, 73–114.

Lin B.T., Gruenwald S., Morla A.O., Lee W.H. & Wang J.Y. (1991) Retinoblastoma cancer suppressor gene product is a substrate of the cell cycle regulator cdc2 kinase. *EMBO Journal,* **10**, 857–64.

Lindblom A., Tannergard P., Werelius B. & Nordenskjold M. (1993) Genetic mapping of a second locus predisposing to hereditary non-polyposis colon cancer. *Nature Genetics,* **5**, 279–82.

Linzer D.I.H. & Levine A.J. (1979) Characterization of a 54K dalton cellular SV40 tumor antigen present in SV40-transformed cells and uninfected embyonal carcinoma cells. *Cell,* **17**, 43–52.

Ludlow J.W., DeCaprio J.A., Huang C.-M., Lee W.-H., Paucha E. & Livingston D.M. (1989) SV40 large T antigen binds preferentially to an underphosphorylated member of the retinoblastoma susceptibility gene family product. *Cell,* **56**, 57–65.

Ludlow J.W., Shon J., Pipas J.M., Livingston D.M. & DeCaprio J.A. (1990) The retinoblastoma susceptibility gene product undergoes cell cycle-dependent dephosphorylation and binding to and release from SV40 large T. *Cell*, **60**, 387–96.

Madden S.L., Cook D.M., Morris J.F., Gashler A., Sukhatme V.P. & Rauscher F.J. (1991) Transcriptional repression mediated by the WT1 wilms-tumor gene-product. *Science*, **253**, 1550–3.

Maheswaran S., Park S., Bernard A., Morris J.F., Rauscher F.J., Hill D.E. & Haber D.A. (1993) Physical and functional interaction between WT1 and p53 proteins. *Proceedings of the National Academy of Sciences of the United States of America*, **90**, 5100–4.

Malkin D., Li F.P., Strong L.C., Fraumeni J.F., Nelson C.E., Kim D.H., Kassel J., Gryka M.A., Bischoff F.Z., Tainsky M.A. & Friend S.H. (1990) Germ line p53 mutations in a familial syndrome of breast cancer, sarcomas, and other neoplasms. *Science*, **250**, 1233–8.

Martin G.A., Viskochil D., Bollag G., McCabe P.C., Crosier W.J., Haubruck H., Conroy L., Clark R., O'Connell P., Cawthon R.M., Innis M.A. & McCormick F. (1990) The GAP-related domain of the neurofibromatosis type 1 gene product interacts with ras p21. *Cell*, **63**, 843–9.

McCormick F., Clark R., Harlow E. & Tjian R. (1981) SV40 antigen binds specifically to a cellular 53K protein in vitro. *Nature*, **292**, 63–5.

Merajen S.D., Pham T.M., Caduff R.F., Chen M., Poy E.L., Cooney K.A., Weber B.L., Collins F.S., Johnston C. & Frank T.S. (1995) Somatic mutations in the BRCA1 gene is sporadic ovarian tumours. *Nature Genetics*, **9**, 439–43.

Mihara K., Cao X.-R., Yen A., Chandler S., Driscoll B., Murphree A.L., T'Ang A. & Fung Y.-K.T. (1989) Cell cycle-dependent regulation of phosphorylation of the human retinoblastoma gene product. *Science*, **246**, 1300–3.

Miki Y., Swensen J., Shattuck-Eidens D., Futreal P.A., Harshman K., Tartigian S., Liu Q., Cochran C., Michelle-Bennett L., Ding W., Bell R., Rosenthal J., Hussey C., Tran T., McClure M., Frye C., Hattier T., Phelps R., Haugen-Strano A., Katcher H., Yakumo K., Gholami Z., Shaffer D., Stone S., Bayer S., Wang C., Bogden R., Dayananth P., Ward J., Tonin P., Narod S., Bristow P.K., Norris F.H., Helvering L., Morrison P., Rosteck P., Lai M., Barrett J.C., Lewis C., Newhausen S., Cannon-Albright L., Goldgar D., Weisman R., Kamb A. & Skolnick M.H. (1994) A strong candidate for the breast and ovarian cancer susceptibility gene BRCA1. *Science*, **266**, 66–71.

Miller R.W., Fraumeni J.F.J. & Manning M.D. (1964) Association of Wilms' tumor with aniridia, hemihypertrophy and other congenital malformations. *New England Journal of Medicine*, **270**, 922–7.

Miyoshi Y., Ando H., Nagese H., Nishisho I., Horii A., Miki Y., Mori T., Utsunomiya J., Baba S., Petersen G., Hamilton S.R., Kinzler K.W., Vogelstein B. & Nakamura Y. (1992) Germ-line mutations of the APC gene in 53 familial adenomatous polyposis patients. *Proceedings of the National Academy of Sciences of the United States of America*, **89**, 4452–6.

Mulligan L.M., Kwok J.B., Healey C.S., Elsdon M.J., Eng C., Gardner E., Love D.R., Mole S.E., Moore J.K., Papi L., Ponder M.A., Telenius H., Tunnacliffe A. & Ponder B.A.J. (1993) Germ-line mutations of the RET proto-oncogene in multiple endocrine neoplasia type 2A. *Nature*, **363**, 458–60.

Nishisho I., Nakamura Y., Miyoshi Y., Miki Y., Ando H., Horii A., Koyama K., Utsunomiya J., Baba S., Hedge P., Markham A., Krush A.J., Petersen G., Hamilton S.R., Nilbert M.C., Levy D.B., Bryan T.M., Preisinger A.C., Smith K.J., Su L.-K., Kinzler K.W. & Vogelstein B. (1991) Mutations of chromosome 5q21 genes in FAP and colorectal cancer patients. *Science*, **253**, 665–9.

Ogawa O., Eccles M.R., Szeto J., McNoe L.A., Yun K., Maw M.A., Smith P.J. & Reeve A.E. (1993) Relaxation of insulin-like growth factor II gene imprinting implicated in Wilms' tumour. *Nature*, **362**, 749–51.

Oliner J.D., Pietenpol J.A., Thiagalingam S., Gyuris J., Kinzler K.W. & Vogelstein B. (1993) Oncoprotein MDM2 conceals the activation domain of tumour suppressor p53. *Nature*, **362**, 857–60.

Papadopoulos N., Nicolaides N.C., Wei Y.-F., Ruben S.M., Carter K.C., Rosen C.A., Haseltine W.A., Fleischmann R.D., Fraser C.M., Adams M.D., Venter J.C., Hamilton S.R., Petersen G.M., Watson P., Lynch H.T., Peltomäki P., Mecklin J.-P., de la Chapelle A., Kinzler K.W. & Vogelstein B. (1994) Mutation of mutL homolog in hereditary colon cancer. *Science*, **263**, 1625–9.

Pelletier J., Bruening W., Kashtan C.E., Mauer S.M., Manivel J.C., Striegel J.E., Houghton D.C., Junien C., Habib R., Fouser L., Fine R.N., Silverman B.L., Haber D.A. & Housman D. (1991) Germline mutations in the Wilms' tumor suppressor gene are associated with abnormal urogenital development in Denys-Drash syndrome. *Cell*, **67**, 437–47.

Peltomaki P., Aaltonen L.A., Sistonen P., Pylkkanen L., Mecklin J.P., Jarvinen H., Green J.S., Jass J.R., Weber J.L., Leach F.S., Petersen G.M., Hamilton S.R., de la Chapelle A. & Vogelstein B. (1993) Genetic mapping of a locus predisposing to human colorectal cancer. *Science*, **260**, 810–2.

Ping A.J., Reeve A.E., Law D.J., Young M.R., Boehnke M. & Feinberg A.P. (1989) Genetic linkage of Beckwith-Weidemann syndrome to 11p15. *American Journal of Human Genetics*, **44**, 720–3.

Ponder B. (1990) Neurofibromatosis gene cloned. *Nature*, **346**, 703–4.

Powell S.M., Zilz N., Beazer B.Y., Bryan T.M., Hamilton S.R., Thibodeau S.N., Vogelstein B. & Kinzler K.W. (1992) APC mutations occur early during colorectal tumorigenesis. *Nature*, **359**, 235–7.

Pritchard-Jones K., Fleming S., Davidson D., Bickmore W., Porteous D., Gosden C., Bard J., Buckler A., Pelletier J., Housman D., van Heyningen V. & Hastie N. (1990) The candidate Wilms' tumour gene is involved in genitourinary development. *Nature*, **346**, 194–7.

Qian Y.W., Wang Y.C.J., Hollingsworth R.E., Jones D., Ling N. & Lee E.Y.H. (1993) A retinoblastoma-binding protein realted to a negative regulator of Ras in yeast. *Nature*, **364**, 648–52.

Rainier S., Johnson L.A., Dobry C.J., Ping A.J., Grundy P.E. & Feinberg A.P. (1993) Relaxation of imprinted genes in human cancer. *Nature*, **362**, 747–9.

Rauscher F., Morris J.F., Tournay O.E., Cook D.M. & Curran T. (1990) Binding of the Wilms' tumor locus zinc finger protein to the EGR-1 consensus sequence. *Science*, **250**, 1259–62.

Rees M., Leigh S.E.A., Delhanty J.D.A. & Jass J.R. (1989) Chromosome 5 allele loss in familial and sporadic colorectal adenomas. *British Journal of Cancer*, **59**, 361–5.

Reeve A.E., Sih S.A., Raizis A.M. & Feinberg A.P. (1989) Loss of allelic heterozygosity at a second locus on chromosome 11 in sporadic Wilms' tumor cells. *Molecular and Cellular Biology*, **9**, 1799–803.

Reifenberger G., Liu L., Ichimura K., Schmidt E.E. & Collins V.P. (1993) Amplification and overexpression of the *MDM2* gene in a subset of human malignant gliomas with out *p53* mutations. *Cancer Research*, **53**, 2736–9.

Riccardi V.M., Sujansky E., Smith A.C. & Franke U. (1978) Chromosomal imbalance in the aniridia-Wilms' tumor association: 11p interstitial deletion. *Pediatrics*, **61**, 604–10.

Rouleau G.A., Merel P., Lutchman M., Sanson M., Zucman J., Marineau C., Hoang X.K., Demczuk S., Desmaze C., Plougastel B., Pulst S., Lenoir G., Bijlsma E., Fashold R., Dumanski J., de Jong P., Parry D., Eldrige R., Aurias A., Delattre O. & Thomas G. (1993) Alteration in a new gene encoding a putative membrane-organizing protein causes neuro-fibromatosis type 2. *Nature*, **363**, 515–21.

Rubinfeld B., Souza B., Albert I., Muller O., Chamberlain S.C., Mariarz F., Munemitsu S. & Polakis P. (1993) Association of the APC gene product with β-catenin. *Science*, **262**, 1731–4.

Rustgi A.K., Dyson N. & Bernards R. (1991) Amino-terminal domains of c-*myc* and N-*myc* proteins mediate binding to the retinoblastoma gene product. *Nature*, **352**, 541–4.

Sarnow P., Ho Y.S., Williams J. & Levine A.J. (1982) Adenovirus E1B-58kd tumor antigen and SV40 large tumor antigen are physically associated with the same 54kd cellular protein in transformed cells. *Cell*, **28**, 387–94.

Sato T., Tanigami A., Yamakawa K., Akiyama F., Kasumi F., Sakamoto G. & Nakamura Y. (1990) Allelotype of breast cancer: cumulative allele losses promote tumor progression in primary breast cancer. *Cancer Research*, **50**, 7184–9.

Schildkraut J.M., Risch N. & Thompson W.D. (1989) Evaluating genetic association among ovarian, breast and endometrial cancer: evidence for a breast-ovarian relationship. *American Journal of Human Genetics*, **45**, 521–9.

Schneider R. (1992) The human protooncogene *ret*: a communicative cadherin? *Trends in Biochemical Sciences*, **17**, 468–9.

Shan B., Zhu X., Chen P.L., Durfee T., Yang Y., Sharp D. & Lee W.H. (1992) Molecular cloning of cellular genes encoding retinoblastoma-associated proteins: identification of a gene with properties of the transcription factor E2F. *Molecular and Cell Biology*, **12**, 5620–31.

Shattuck-Eidens D., McClure M., Simond J., Labrie F., Narod S., Webber B., Collins F., Freidman L., Ostermeyer E., Szabo C., King M.C., Jhanwar S., Offit K., Norton L., Gilewski T., Lubin M., Osborne M., Black D.M., Boyd M., Steel M., Ingles S., Haile R., Lindblom A., Olsson H., Borg A., Bishop D.T., Solomon E., Radice P., Spatti G., Gayther S., Ponder B., Warren W., Stratton M., Liu Q., Fujimura F., Lewis C., Skolnick M.H. & Goldgar D.E. (1995) A collaborative survey of 80 mutations in the BRCA1 breast and ovarian cancer susceptibility gene. *JAMA*, **273**, 535–41.

Simard J., Feunteun J., Lenoir G., Tonin P., Normand T., The V.L., Vivier A., Lasko D., Morgan K., Rouleau G.A., Lynch H., Labrie F. & Narod S. (1993) Genetic mapping of the breast-ovarian cancer syndrome to a small interval on chromosome 17q12–21: exclusion of candidate genes EDH17B2 and RARA. *Human Molecular Genetics*, **2**, 1193–9.

Smith K.J., Johnson K.A., Bryan T.M., Hill D.E., Markowitz S., Willson J.K., Paraskeva C., Petersen G.M., Hamilton S.R., Vogelstein B. & Kinzler K.W. (1993) The *APC* gene product in normal and tumor cells. *Proceedings of the National Academy of Sciences of the United States of America*, **90**, 2846–50.

Smith S.A., Easton D.F., Evans D.G.R. & Ponder B.A.J. (1992) Chromosome 17 allele loss in familial ovarian cancer. *Nature Genetics*, **2**, 128–31.

Sotelo-Avila C. & Gooch W.M. (1976) Neoplasms associated with the Beckwith-Weidemann syndrome. *Perspectives in Pediatric Pathology*, **3**, 255–72.

Srivastava S., Tong Y.A., Devadas K., Zou Z.-Q., Sykes V.W., Y. C., Blattner W., Pirollo K. & Chang E.H. (1992) Detection of both mutant and wild-type p53 in normal skin fibroblasts and demonstration of a shared 'second hit' on p53 in diverse tumors from a cancer-prone family with Li-Fraumeni syndrome. *Oncogene*, **7**, 987–91.

Srivastava S., Zou Z., Pirollo K., Blattner W. & Chang E.H. (1990a) Germ-line transmission of a mutated p53 gene in a cancer-prone family with Li-Fraumeni syndrome. *Nature*, **348**, 747–749.

Srivastava S., Zou Z., Pirollo K., Blattner W. & Chang E.H. (1990b) Germ-line transmission of a mutated p53 gene in a cancer-prone family with Li-Fraumeni syndrome. *Nature*, **348**, 747–9.

Su L.K., Johnson K.A., Smith K.J., Hill D.E., Vogelstein B. & Kinzler K.W. (1993) Association between wild type and mutant *APC* gene products. *Cancer Research*, **53**, 2728–31.

Su L.K., Vogelstein B. & Kinzler K.W. (1993) Association of the APC tumor suppressor protein with catenins. *Science*, **262**, 1734–7.

Takahashi R., Hashimoto T., Xu H.J., Hu S.X., Matsui T., Miki T., Bigo-Marshall H., Aaronson S.A. & Benedict W.F. (1991) The retinoblastoma gene functions as a growth and tumor suppressor in human bladder carcinoma cells. *Proceedings of the National Academy of Sciences of the United States of America*, **88**, 5257–61.

Thibodeau S.N., Bren G. & Schaid D. (1993) Microsatellite instability in cancer of the proximal colon. *Science*, **260**, 816–19.

Trahey M. & McCormick F. (1987) A cytoplasmic protein stimulates normal N-*ras* p21 GTPase, but does not affect oncogenic mutants. *Science*, **238**, 542–5.

Trofatter J.A., MacCollin M.M., Rutter J.L., Murrell J.R., Duyao M.P., Parry D.M., Eldridge R., Kley N., Menon A.G., Pulaski K., Haase V.H., Ambrose C.M., Munroe D., Bove C., Haines J.L., Martuza R., MacDonald M., Seizinger B., Short P., Buckler A. & Gusella J.F. (1993) A novel moesin-, ezrin-, radixin-like gene is a candidate for the neurofibromatosis 2 tumor suppressor. *Cell*, **72**, 791–800.

Tulinius H., Egilsson V., Olafsdottir G. & Sigvaldson H. (1992) Risk of prostate, ovarian, and endometrial cancer among relatives of women with breast cancer. *British Medical Journal*, **305**, 855–7.

van Heyningen V., Bickmore W.A., Seawright A., Fletcher J.M., Maule J., Fekete G., Gessler M., Bruns G.A.P., Huerre-Jeanpierre C., Junien C., Williams B.R.G. & Hastie N.D. (1990) Role for the Wilms tumor gene in genital development? *Proceedings of the National Academy of Sciences of the United States of America*, **87**, 5383–6.

Viskochil D., Buchberg A.M., Xu G., Cawthon R.M., Stevens J., Wolff R.K., Culver M., Carey J.C., Copeland N.G., Jenkins N.A., White R. & O'Connell P. (1990) Deletions and a translocation interrupt a cloned gene at the neurofibromatosis type 1 locus. *Cell*, **62**, 187–92.

Vogelstein B., Fearon E.R., Hamilton S.R., Kern S.E., Preisinger A.C., Leppert M., Nakamura Y., White R., Smits A.M.M. & Bos J.L. (1988) Genetic alterations during colorectal tumour development. *New England Journal of Medicine*, **319**, 525–32.

Vogelstein B., Fearon E.R., Kern S.E., Hamilton S.R., Preisinger A.C., Nakamura Y. & White R. (1989) Allelotypes of colorectal carcinomas. *Science*, **244**, 207–11.

Wallace M.R., Marchuk D.A., Andersen L.B., Letcher R., Odeh H.M., Saulino A.M., Fountain J.W., Brereton A., Nicholson J., Mitchell A.L., Brownstein B.H. & Collins F.S. (1990) Type 1 neurofibromatosis gene: identification of a large transcript disrupted in three NF1 patients. *Science*, **249**, 181–6.

Weksberg R., Shen D.R., Fei Y.L., Song Q.L. & Squire J. (1993) Disruption of insulin-like growth factor 2 imprinting in Beckwith-Wiedemann syndrome. *Nature Genetics*, **5**, 143–50.

Whyte P., Buchkovich K.J., Horowitz J.M., Friend S.H., Raybuck M., Weinberg R.A. & Harlow E. (1988) Association between an oncogene and an antioncogene: the adenovirus E1A proteins bind to the retinoblastoma gene product. *Nature*, **334**, 124–9.

Wooster R., Neuhausen S.L., Mangior J., Quirk Y., Ford D., Collins N., Nguyen K., Seal S., Tran T., Averill D., Fields P., Marshall G., Narod S., Lenoir G.M., Lynch H., Feunteun J., Derrlee P., Cornelisse C.J., Menko F.H., Daly P.A., Ormiston W., McManus R., Pye C., Lewis C.M., Cannon-Albright L.A., Peto P., Ponder B.A.J., Skolnick M.H., Easton D.F., Goldgar D.E. & Stratton M.R. (1995) Localization of a breast cancer susceptibi!'ity gene, BRCA2, to chromosome 13q12-13. *Science*, **265**, 2088–90.

Xu G.F., Lin B., Tanaka K., Dunn D., Wood D., Gesteland R., White R., Weiss R. & Tamanoi F. (1990a) The catalytic domain of the neurofibromatosis type 1 gene product stimulates *ras* GTPase and complements *ira* mutants of *S. cerevisiae*. *Cell*, **63**, 835–41.

Xu G.F., O'Connell P., Viskochil D., Cawthon R., Robertson M., Culver M., Dunn D., Stevens J., Gesteland R., White R. & Weiss R. (1990b) The neurofibromatosis type 1 gene encodes a protein related to GAP. *Cell*, **62**, 599–608.

Xu W., Mulligan L.M., Ponder M.A., Liu L., Smith B.A., Mathew C.G.P. & Ponder B.A.J. (1992) Loss of NF1 alleles in phaeochromocytomas from patients with type 1 neurofibromatosis. *Genes, Chromosomes and Cancer*, **4**, 1–6.

Yatani A., Okabe K., Polakis P., Halenback R., McCormick F. & Brown A.M. (1991) *ras* p21 and GAP inhibit coupling of muscarinic receptors to atrial K^+ channels. *Cell*, **61**, 769–76.

Yunis E., Zuniga R. & Ramirez E. (1981) Retinoblastoma, gross internal malformations, and deletion 13q14-q31. *Human Genetics*, **56**, 283–6.

8 Diet

PETER BOYLE AND PATRICK MAISONNEUVE

INTRODUCTION

Diet and nutritional factors commenced to be the focus of serious attention in the aetiology of cancer from the 1940s onwards (Tannenbaum, 1940). After initially dealing with the effect of feeding specific diets to animals receiving chemical carcinogens, research turned to the potential of associations with human cancer risk. At first, this was conducted through international comparisons of estimated national per capita food intake data with cancer mortality rates. It was consistently found that there were very strong correlations in these data, particularly with dietary fat intake and a number of types of cancer thought to be hormonally related, including cancer of the breast, prostate, ovary and endometrium (Armstrong & Doll, 1975). Of course, there are other forms of cancer associated with diet and nutritional factors including colorectal cancer; pancreas cancer; and lung, mouth, larynx and oesophageal cancer. The focus of this chapter will be the hormonally related cancers, and the epidemiological evidence of their association with diet will be reviewed.

A major problem in conducting aetiological studies in humans had always been the difficulty of assessing the contents of the diet. Much work was done on this topic during the late 1960s but particularly from the 1970s onwards. As dietary assessment methods became better, and certain methodological difficulties were identified and overcome, the science of 'Nutritional Epidemiology' emerged (Willett, 1989).

Early studies in this field were characterized by the great variability in the results obtained and in the quality of the study methodology employed. Consequently, it was difficult to reach any serious conclusion from the early publications regarding causative associations between dietary intake patterns and cancer risk. The quality of the information available from many studies during the 1980s onwards improved quite dramatically and many insights have been obtained into the dietary aetiology of a variety of cancers.

The focus of attention in human studies has largely been centred around associations with fat intake and vitamins. A summary of the epidemiological situation is likely to be quite contentious, particularly in a subject area that appears to attract more reviews than original articles. In our opinion, and we stress that it is just that, present evidence indicates that an increased intake of fat in the diet is associated with an increased risk of colorectal cancer and, probably, prostate cancer. High consumption of fruits and vegetables is associated with a reduced risk of a number of forms of cancer including lung cancer, oral cancer, pancreas cancer, larynx cancer, oesophageal cancer, bladder cancer and gastric cancer (Steinmetz & Potter, 1991). The relationship appears to be a general effect and is consistently found with many different groups of fruits and vegetables. Although many candidate mechanisms, and molecules, have been put forward to explain the relationship, there is little real evidence to suggest that it is one particular component of diet as opposed to another that is responsible.

Perhaps the most disputed relationship between dietary intake and cancer risk at the present time is that postulated to exist between adult dietary fat intake patterns and breast cancer risk. There have been nearly 30 epidemiological studies published on this topic, some *retrospective* and others *prospective.* Read and interpreted as individual studies, the reader is forced to make subjective assessments of the quality of studies and then to somehow synthesize all this information in his head, again in a subjective manner, before coming to some conclusion. The introduction of meta-analysis in the overview of randomized clinical trials has been a great boon to many areas of research. However, its use in epidemiological studies may not be entirely as straightforward as in the assessment of randomized clinical trials.

BREAST CANCER

Descriptive Epidemiology

Breast cancer is the most frequent malignancy among women, with an estimated 422,000 new cases annually in developed countries. In developing parts of the world, mammary cancer, with an estimated

298,000 new cases, lies behind the cervix uteri (344,000) in frequency (Parkin, Pisani & Ferlay, 1993). The disease is rare in males.

The highest incidence rates of breast cancer in women are exclusively from the United States (Table 8.1). Incidence rates exceeding 100 per 100,000 are reported from the white population of the San Francisco Bay Area (104.2) and the Hawaiian population of Hawaii (100.2). Rates in western Europe are considerably lower, with the highest recorded incidence rate from Geneva, Switzerland (73.5 per 100,000). The highest incidence rate in central and eastern Europe was reported from the former German Democratic Republic (46.3). Low rates are reported from other central and eastern European countries, Asia and Africa (Parkin et al., 1992).

In contrast to the situation in women, breast cancer in men is a rare disease (Table 8.1) with rates generally below 1 per 100,000 per annum.

In Singapore, the incidence of breast cancer in Hokkien and Cantonese females is some 30% greater than in Teochew, Hainanese and Hakka. An urban-rural gradient is generally found, with the incidence higher in urban compared to rural areas (Boyle et al., 1990). Although in a large number of Muslim countries – Egypt, Tunisia, Sudan, Iran, Kuwait and Pakistan – the breast, rather than the cervix uteri, is the most common female cancer site, the high relative frequencies in these countries do not necessarily mean that incidence will be high. For example, although the relative frequency in Kuwaiti females is 22%, the incidence is 15.9, whereas in Maoris a relative frequency of 20% is associated with an incidence of 59.9 per 100,000.

The continued rise in the age-specific incidence of female breast cancer, following Clemmesen's hook, is particularly marked in the highest incidence areas, whereas in several Asian countries a plateau or even a slight decline is observed after menopause. Intermediate age-incidence curves are seen for eastern European countries.

Muir et al. (1980) drew attention to similarities of cross-sectional age-incidence curves for breast cancer at various times in the past in Iceland, with current cross-sectional curves in regions of contrasting incidence, namely, Connecticut, Finland and Miyagi Prefecture, suggesting that these represented birth cohort effects reflecting differing times of entry of risk factors into the environment. Thus risk in Iceland in 1911–1929, 1930–1949 and 1950–1972 was the same as in Japan in 1959–1960, Finland in 1959–1961 and Connecticut in 1960–1962 respectively.

The change in risk of breast cancer in migrants from low incidence to high-incidence areas, and in their descendants, argues strongly for environmental influences. Incidence in Hawaii and San

Table 8.1. Current (Circa 1985) Highest and Lowest Incidence Rates for Breast Cancer Recorded Worldwide Among 166 Populations

Breast, Male ICD9 175 Registry	Cases	Rate	Breast, Female ICD9 174 Registry	Cases	Rate
Kuwait: non-Kuwaitis	10	2.2	U.S., Bay Area: white	9,736	104.20
France, Tarn	21	1.5	U.S., Hawaii: Hawaiian	351	100.2
Italy, Trieste	7	1.4	U.S., Hawaii: white	735	99.3
Bermuda: black	1	1.3	U.S., Alameda: white	2,864	99.2
Switzerland, Neuchatel	7	1.1	U.S., Seattle	8,976	94.2
Israel: born Eur. Amer.	59	1.1	U.S., Detroit: white	9,779	91.4
U.S., New York City	237	1.0	U.S., Atlanta: white	3,748	91.0
Philippines, Manila	42	1.0	U.S., Connecticut: white	10,155	88.9
France, Calvados	17	1.0	U.S., Los Angeles: O. white	16,057	88.5
Portugal, V N de Gaia	5	1.0	U.S., Alameda: black	541	83.8
U.S., Los Angeles: Chinese	0	–	Japan, Yamagata	647	17.6
Singapore: Malay	0	–	Kuwait: Kuwaitis	141	17.2
Bermuda: white & other	0	–	Israel: non-Jews	172	17.0
The Gambia	0	–	U.S., Los Angeles: Korean	48	16.9
U.S., Los Angeles: Filipino	0	–	Thailand, Chiang Mai	308	13.7
Peru, Trujillo	0	–	Mali, Bamako	44	10.2
Kuwait: Kuwaitis	0	–	Thailand, Khon Kaen	111	9.9
Canada, N. W. T. & Yukon	0	–	China, Qidong	265	9.5
U.S., Hawaii: Chinese	0	–	Algeria, Setif	85	6.4
U.S., Los Angeles: Korean	0	–	The Gambia	22	3.4

Source: From Parkin et al., 1982.

Francisco Bay Area Japanese is now double that in Japan, although the difference is less in Los Angeles (1.4-fold). A comparable phenomenon is observable for Chinese: the incidence in Singapore and Hong Kong Chinese is about 50% higher than that in Shanghai and Tianjin, but well below that in United States Chinese. In Singapore, the incidence in the Singapore-born Chinese in 1968–1982 was 29.5, while that for those born elsewhere, mainly in China, was 18.2, a difference significant for all dialect groups (Lee et al., 1988).

The incidence of breast cancer is increasing slowly in most countries, the rate of increase tending to be greatest where rates were the lowest (e.g., 3.2% per annum in Singapore Chinese, an increase most noticeable in the 0 to 49 age group). Mortality rates have also been increasing in the developing world (e.g., Japan and Hong Kong), having a tendency to remain stationary in Western countries. In the United States, mortality in white women less than 50 years of age has fallen, overall mortality being remarkably stable between 1950 and 1982 (Devesa et al., 1987).

Temporal Trends in Breast Cancer

It appears that the incidence of breast cancer in women is increasing overall in international populations (Table 8.2) and that the increases in incidence are present in all populations irrespective of the rates at the beginning of the time period.

Temporal trends in mortality from female breast cancer are interesting to examine, since incidence rates can be subject to 'artificial' influences such as the introduction and widespread uptake of screening programs. While these may affect mortality also, this is the aim of such programs and mortality is an important end point. Nine countries with long-time series of mortality data were chosen to be representative of different international scenarios (Boyle et al., 1995). Unfortunately, there are few epidemiological data available from Asia and Africa.

In Canada, the all-ages mortality rate from breast cancer has remained very stable since 1950. The truncated rate rose to a peak in 1970 and has subsequently declined slightly. There is some evidence of a downward cohort effect in mortality affecting women born since around 1920–1930 (who have been observed at premenopausal ages up to 50).

In Japan, the all-ages mortality rate and the truncated rate (35–64) both stayed constant until around 1970. Subsequently, both have risen, although the increase in the truncated rate has been more noticeable. Examination of the mortality data by birth cohort indicates that increases have been taking place consistently among birth co-

Table 8.2. Incidence of Breast Cancer in Selected Registries

Cancer Incidence in Five Continents	Volume I[a]	Volume II[b]	Volume III[c]	Volume IV[d]	Volume V[e]	Volume VI[f]
Canada, Manitoba	58.04	60.58	64.15	64.15	74.62	75.42
Canada, Saskatchewan	57.41	59.12	62.76	62.64	65.60	70.10
U.S., Alameda: white	*	62.36	76.07	78.19	78.38	99.18
U.S., Alameda: black	*	38.59	56.54	67.20	68.37	83.80
U.S., Connecticut	58.95	62.29	71.42	77.87	*	*
U.S., Connecticut: white	*	*	*	*	77.83	88.89
U.S., Connecticut: black	*	*	*	*	61.27	64.73
India, Bombay	*	20.36	20.07	21.19	24.10	24.60
Japan, Miyagi	13.16	10.96	13.04	17.40	22.00	27.75
Denmark	43.76	44.88	49.15	54.35 58.83[g]	63.07	68.62
Finland	26.07	29.35	32.93	40.07	44.72	52.50
Norway	38.80	40.97	44.38	49.64	51.81	54.78
Sweden	45.22	48.59	52.37	55.20	60.74	62.46
U.K., Birmingham	46.74	51.05	53.01	56.42	55.04	63.37
New Zealand: non-Maori	47.18[h]	50.20	52.51	62.60	57.68	64.33

[a]From Doll R., Payne P. & Waterhouse J. (Eds.) (1966) *Cancer incidence in five continents,* Vol. I. International Agency for Research on Cancer, Lyon.
[b]From Doll R., Muir C.S. & Waterhouse, J. (Eds.) (1970) *Cancer incidence in five continents,* Vol. II. International Agency for Research on Cancer, Lyon.
[c]From Waterhouse J., Muir C.S., Correa P. & Powell J. (Eds.) (1976) *Cancer incidence in five continents,* Vol. III (IARC Scientific Publication No. 15). International Agency for Research on Cancer, Lyon.
[d]From Waterhouse J., Muir C.S., Shanmugaratnam K. & Powell J. (Eds.) (1982) *Cancer incidence in five continents,* Vol. IV (IARC Scientific Publication No. 42). International Agency for Research on Cancer, Lyon.
[e]From Muir C.S., Waterhouse J.A.H., Mack T., Powell J. & Whelan S. (Eds.) (1987) *Cancer incidence in five continents,* Vol. V (IARC Scientific Publication No. 88). International Agency for Research on Cancer, Lyon.
[f]From Parkin D.M., Muir C.S., Whelan S., Gao Y.T., Ferlay J. & Powell J. (Eds.) (1992) *Cancer incidence in five continents,* Vol. VI (IARC Scientific Publication No. 120). International Agency for Research on Cancer, Lyon.
[g]Two time periods are available for this country.
[h]New Zealand: whole population.
*Data unavailable.

horts, although there does not appear to be any 'acceleration' in younger cohorts who are more likely to have been exposed to a Western-style diet (Boyle et al., 1993).

In the former Czechoslovakia, both the all-ages and the truncated mortality rates increased throughout the period of observation. This increase was also apparent when the data were examined by birth cohort, although there is a suggestion that the increasing risk may be slowing down in younger birth cohorts. If so, this should begin to influence the pattern of overall mortality rates in the coming decades. In Poland, there have been substantial increases taking place in the mortality rates of breast cancer. It appears that the mortality is still increasing slowly in younger birth cohorts. In Germany, both the all-ages and the truncated rates have increased since 1950. The risk still appears to be increasing among younger birth cohorts. In Denmark, the all-ages mortality rate increased very slightly between 1950 and 1990: after an initial increase, the truncated mortality rate has remained fairly constant since around 1970. There is some evidence of a levelling off in risk evident among the more recent born cohorts.

In the United Kingdom, all-ages mortality rates have remained virtually constant since about 1970 as have the truncated rates since about the same time. There is evidence that the cohort effect is slowing down, with very little indication of increase in younger cohorts born since approximately 1930. In Italy, there have been steep increases taking place in both the all-ages and the truncated mortality rates from breast cancer since 1950. However, when examined by birth cohort there are indications that there has been a levelling off in the age-specific rates in cohorts born since approximately 1930. In Australia, the all-ages and the truncated mortality rates from breast cancer have remained fairly stable since 1950. Cohort patterns indicate that the risk has remained virtually constant for several decades.

Aetiology of Breast Cancer

It is particularly important when considering the aetiology of breast cancer to bear in mind that other factors have been identified that influence the risk of developing the disease. Age at first birth, age at menopause, oral contraceptive usage, ionizing irradiation and a number of other risk factors have been identified and are reviewed elsewhere (Boyle, 1988)

Anthropometric Variables De Waard and his colleagues in the Netherlands first described the association between obesity and increased breast cancer risk in 1964 (de Waard et al., 1964) and has subsequently refined and championed his original hypothesis (de Waard et al., 1974; de Waard et al., 1977; de Waard et al., 1982). Weight has since been shown to be an independent risk factor for breast cancer in a wide variety of population settings: in women over 50 in Taiwan (Lin, Chen & MacMahon, 1971); in Athens (Valaoras et al., 1969); in women over 49 in Brazil (Mirra et al., 1971); in Japan (Hirayama, 1978); in Canada (Choi et al., 1978); in postmenopausal women in Israel (Lubin et al., 1985); and in others, all of which have recently been reviewed by Rose (Rose, 1986). However, the author of this latter review (Rose, 1986) admits that not all studies have been confirmatory (e.g., Wynder et al., 1978; Stavraky & Emmons, 1974; Adami et al., 1977; Soini, 1977), although the body of evidence available points to an increased risk of breast cancer at least in postmenopausal obese women.

The role of obesity in the premenopause, as well as the potential influence of other anthropometric variables on breast carcinogenesis, is currently largely ill defined (Choi et al., 1978; Helmrich et al., 1983; Talamini et al., 1984; Lubin et al., 1985; Willett et al., 1985; La Vecchia et al., 1987; Le Marchand et al., 1988). Various studies have shown an inverse relation between measures of body weight and minimal or early breast cancer in the premenopause, but the potential problem of selection bias requires careful addressing, since small breast lumps are obviously easier to detect in thinner women (Brinton et al., 1983; Willett et al., 1985; Swanson et al., 1988).

De Waard and Trichopoulos (1988) established a breast cancer hypothesis that related adolescent height and weight to subsequent breast cancer risk, the basic hypothesis being that overnutrition in early life may increase breast cellularity (Albanes & Wilnick, 1988). Based on the hypothesis that the onset of menses is linked to the attainment of a certain body mass (and the suggestion that early menarche is a risk factor for breast cancer), it was suggested that increased height and increased weight could be independent risk factors.

Direct evidence from epidemiological studies in support of this hypothesis is not strong. Studies of migrants (Locke & King, 1980), cohorts of young athletes (Frisch et al., 1987) and ballet dancers (Warren, 1980) have suggested that lower weight during adolescent and young adult life may reduce subsequent breast cancer risk. However the U.S. Nurses Health Study (Willett et al., 1985) and a prospective study of Hawaiian women (Le Marchand, 1988) reported an inverse association between adolescent body mass and premenopausal breast cancer but no relation with earlier age at menarche, height or weight.

De Waard and Baanders-van Halewign (1974) found an independent effect of height on breast cancer risk and an approximately multiplicative effect of height and weight: the relative risk rose to 3.6 for tallest/heaviest women compared to the lowest height/weight category. Subsequently, most studies have produced inconsistent results in premenopausal women (Willett et al., 1985; Kolonel et al., 1986; La Vecchia et al., 1987; Le Marchand, 1988; Swanson et al., 1988).

Parazzini and his colleagues (1989) examined the independent effects of height, weight and body mass index on breast cancer risk on a combined dataset from Italy involving 3,247 case and 3,263 controls. They found no association between height, weight, body mass index (W/H^2; $W/H^{1.5}$) or surface area and premenopausal breast cancer risk (Parazzini et al., 1989). In postmenopausal women, the risk of breast cancer was inversely related to height being (compared to women <155 cm) 0.8 in tall (>165 cm) women: the trend in risk was significant (p=.03) but not monotonic. A direct, statistically significant association emerged with weight and indices of body mass and breast cancer risk in postmenopausal women. Considering two indices of body mass (W/H^2, $W/H^{1.5}$) and relative to leaner women, the respective estimated risks of postmenopausal breast cancer increased to 1.4 and 1.3 for grossly obese women with significant trend.

Parazzini et al. (1989) found that the role of overweight was more evident in women with early age at menopause, suggesting a duration–risk effect. These observations have important theoretical implications in order to understand the role of overweight, and its biological consequences, in breast carcinogenesis. The issue can only be resolved by the collection and analysis of more data.

Physical Activity Obesity and energy intake cannot be considered independently of energy expenditure. Frisch and her colleagues (1985) investigated the prevalence of breast cancer, as measured by lifetime occurrence, among former college athletes and nonathletes. Former athletes were taller but had a lower fat/body weight ratio and had a later menarche than nonathletes. The reported relative risk for breast cancer in nonathletes as compared with athletes was 1.86 (95% C.I. 1.00, 3.47) indicating that physical activity or some related consequence was protective against breast cancer, risk being calculated after adjustment for potential confounding factors. Confirmatory findings from ballet dancers (Warren, 1980) add to this evidence, but it may be premature to ascribe the effect to physical activity, ignoring the possible related decreased body weight.

Dietary Factors Dietary practices have increasingly become the focus of attention in studies of human cancer epidemiology (Graham, 1980; American Academy of Sciences, 1982). The concept is not new;

Tannenbaum clearly demonstrated the effects of dietary deficiency and excess on carcinogenesis in 1940. Since then, there has been a search for preformed carcinogens in food items and, more recently, it has been postulated that metabolic effects of diet may influence the occurrence of cancer by indirect means and that carcinogens may be produced from dietary substrates (Armstrong, McMichael & MacLennan, 1982).

Much of the evidence linking breast cancer risk to dietary parameters has been derived from correlation studies between breast cancer incidence and mortality, with per capita intake of total fat and other nutrients in a variety of countries discussed earlier. This was implicitly related to the concept that fat intake correlated with cholesterol intake and that cholesterol, as the parent molecule of steroids, might be the source of increased oestrogens (Boyle & Leake, 1988). A direct correlation has been reported between breast cancer mortality and intake of milk, table fats, beef, calories and protein as well as fat (Gaskill et al., 1979), although the same study reported an inverse correlation with intake of eggs. Even after controlling for age at first marriage, the association between breast cancer risk and milk consumption (direct) and consumption of eggs (indirect) remained.

The incidence of breast cancer among premenopausal Japanese-American women in California is now almost as high as that for Caucasian women (Dunn, 1977). The low Japanese rates are thought to be associated with dietary practices and this has been investigated by comparison of the diet of Japanese men whose wives had developed breast cancer with that of other Japanese men (Nomura, Henderson & Leg, 1978). It was reported that husbands of the cases consumed more beef and other meat, butter/margarine/cheese, corn and wieners than the controls and that they ate less Japanese foods. If the diets of husbands and wives are similar, this would suggest that the "Western diet" poses a risk of breast cancer to women exposed to it.

Data are available from both prospective studies and several case-control studies to shed some light on the dietary hypotheses. These studies have concentrated, directly or indirectly, on dietary fat intake and include the implication that increased fat intake leads to increased fat content and size of breasts. Fat cells can provide the enzyme aromatase, which converts adrenal androgens to oestrogens – the principal source of oestrogens in postmenopausal women (Boyle & Leake, 1988).

Relative risks of between 1.6 and 2.6 were reported from a case-control study involving 77 cases for five categories of food: fried foods, fried potatoes, hard fat used for frying, dairy products (except milk) and white bread (Phillips, 1975). This study was limited by the small sample size and interpretation hampered by the failure to calculate indices of nutrient intake.

A larger study of 400 cases found total fat consumption to have the strongest association with breast cancer risk in premenopausal women, although there were weaker associations found for saturated fat and cholesterol (Miller et al., 1978). Controlling for the effect of each nutrient merely increased the risk associated with total fat consumption whereas the effects of saturated fat and cholesterol diminished. The association of total fat consumption, with breast cancer risk was the only consistent finding in the postmenopausal group.

Another large study of 577 cases found that the relative risk increased significantly with increasing frequency of consumption of beef and other red meat, pork and sweet desserts (Lubin et al., 1981) and supported a link between breast cancer and the consumption of animal fat and protein. This study did not, however, calculate nutrient densities, and interpretation may be hindered by the collection of information on cases and controls being made under different circumstances.

A case-control study based on 2,024 cases found no difference in risk between cases and controls produced by differences in ingestion of fat. Similarly, there was no difference in risk of breast cancer associated with diets containing vitamin C or cruciferous vegetables. Risk for breast cancer in women over 55 years of age increased with a lower reported intake of vitamin A in the diet (Graham et al., 1982).

A smaller case-control study from Greece found no association with fat but a significant protective effect associated with increasing consumption of salad-type vegetables (Katsouyani et al., 1986). Recent case-control studies have been providing only marginal evidence in favour of the association between dietary fat intake and breast cancer risk.

Lubin and her coworkers (1986) reported that women in the highest quartiles of fat and animal protein intake and in the lowest quartiles of fiber intake had about twice the risk of women in the lowest quartiles of fat and protein and in the highest quartile of fiber intake (Lubin, Wax & Modan, 1986). A case-control study from Hawaii reported only a suggestion that cases consumed more saturated fat and oleic acid than neighborhood controls, although the authors stated that the differences were not impressive (Hirohata et al., 1987). A similar study from France found risk increased with increasing consumption of cheese and decreased with increasing consumption of yoghurt (Le et al., 1986).

The most important study to date on breast cancer and dietary intakes was from the prospective United States Nurses' Health Study (Willett et al., 1987). In 1980, a total of 89,538 United States registered nurses who were 34 to 59 years of age and had no history of cancer completed a previously validated dietary questionnaire designed to measure individual consumption of total fat, saturated fat, linoleic acid and cholesterol as well as other nutrients. During four years of follow-up, 601 cases of breast cancer were diagnosed among the 89,538 nurses in the study. After adjustment for known determinants in multivariate analysis, the relative risk of breast cancer among women in the highest quintile of caloric-adjusted total fat intake, as compared with women in the lowest quintile, was 0.82 (95% C.I., 0.64 to 1.05). The corresponding relative risks were 0.84 (0.66, 1.08) for saturated fat, 0.88 (0.69, 1.12) for linoleic acid and 0.91 (0.70, 1.18) for cholesterol intake. Similar results were found for both postmenopausal and premenopausal women. These results suggested to the authors that a moderate reduction in fat intake by adult women is unlikely to result in a substantial reduction in the incidence of breast cancer (Willett et al., 1987). The conclusions were substantially unchanged when the follow-up was later extended (Willett et al., 1992).

This was confirmed by a follow-up study constructed from the National Health and Nutrition Examination Survey 1 (NHANES 1). This cohort is based on adults, over 25, examined in the NHANES 1 (1970–1975) cross-sectional survey of the United States population and provides a mean follow-up time of ten years. A sample of 5,485 women that included 99 breast cancer cases (34 premenopausal and 65 postmenopausal at NHANES baseline) was examined for associations with dietary intake and breast cancer risk. Dietary intake was assessed by a 24-hour recall method. For total fat and saturated fat, a significant inverse association was indicated in proportional hazards analyses. Adjustment of fat for total energy intake resulted in a smaller effect that was no longer statistically significant. Adjustment for accepted breast cancer risk factors did not change these findings (Jones et al., 1987).

A case-control study from the province of Vercelli in northern Italy reported relative risks of breast cancer for women in the highest quintile of consumption of saturated fat of 3.0 (95% C.I. 1.9, 4.7) and for the highest quintile of consumption of animal protein of 2.9 (1.8, 4.6) (Tonioli et al., 1989). They also reported a reduced risk for women who derived less than 28% of calories from fat compared to those women who derived more than 35%. These findings, based on 250 cases and 499 controls, represent the most striking association yet reported between dietary intakes and breast cancer risk.

Breast cancer incidence was monitored in a cohort of 20,341 Californian Seventh Day Adventist women followed-up for six years (Mills et al., 1989) using a limited dietary questionnaire: 215 histologically confirmed breast cancers were found among approximately

115,000 person-years of followup. Increasing consumption of high-fat animal products was not associated with an increased risk of breast cancer in any consistent fashion (nor was percent of calories from fat) after adjustment for other breast cancer risk factors. With the risk in the lowest quartile of calories from fat set to 1.0, subsequent quartiles had risks of 0.95 (95% C.I. 0.64 to 1.42), 1.19 (0.79, 1.80) and 1.21 (0.81, 1.81). The overall trend (chi-square 1.78) was not significant. Most interestingly, this study was able to address, in a limited way, associations with childhood diet by asking about vegetarian status at different periods of life: no association was found with childhood or early teenage dietary habits (vegetarian versus nonvegetarian) and adult breast cancer risk.

Several other important prospective studies have all concluded that there was no association between dietary fat intake and breast cancer risk. Such studies involving follow-up of initially disease-free women have employed hundreds of thousands of subjects followed for periods up to ten years and have been conducted in a variety of population settings: Finland (Knekt et al., 1990), Canada (Howe et al., 1991), Iowa (Kushi et al., 1992), the Netherlands (van den Brandt, 1993), New York State (Graham et al., 1992) and New York City (Tonioli et al., 1994).

Howe et al. (1990) presented the results of a combined analysis of 12 case-control studies of breast cancer and diet that estimated intake of energy and major nutrients. This analysis showed a consistent, statistically significant, positive association between breast cancer risk and saturated fat intake in postmenopausal women: the relative risk for the highest to lowest quintile was 1.46 ($p<.0001$). Howe et al. (1990) calculated that the log relative risk per 45 gm of saturated fat intake was 0.38 ± 0.085 (i.e., the relative risk will increase by 1.46 for every increase of 45 gm of saturated fat intake per day). Since the majority of women consume less that 30 gm/day in total, such a change in intake (of 45 gm/day) is entirely unrealistic. Thus, the calculated relative risk from this study gives the impression of being larger than is realistically within a preventable range. Willett and Stampfer (1990) note that quoting a relative risk like this is like calculating a change of risk (associated with weight change) as per 300 pounds. Within this study, Howe et al. (1990) compared the distribution of dietary intakes in Canada and China and calculated, based on the odds ratios calculated from the overview analysis, a relative risk of 1.3 between the two populations (which compares to the fourfold variation between incidence rates in the two populations).

Howe et al. (1990) also demonstrated a consistent protective effect for a number of markers of fruit and vegetable intake. Vitamin C had the most consistent and statistically significant inverse association with breast cancer risk: the relative risk for the highest versus lowest quintile was 0.69 (p<.0001). The authors calculated that if the dietary associations represent causality, the percentage of breast cancers that might be prevented by dietary modification in the North American population is estimated to be 24% for postmenopausal women and 16% for premenopausal women (Howe et al., 1990).

Prentice and Sheppard (1990) examined the data on dietary fat and cancer and found a strong relationship for both cross-sectional and temporal changes. This involved comparing national mortality data with national per capita food disappearance data. However, the quality and validity of these latter data were disputed in the same issue (Willett & Stampfer, 1990). Of many points raised, perhaps the most telling is that related to time trends. According to national statistics, fat disappearance increased from 39% of energy in 1961–1963 in the United States to 42% in 1975–1977. According to large, detailed national surveys, fat actually consumed has fallen from 42.1% in 1965, 36 to 40.8% in 1976–1980, 36.8% in 1985 to 36.4% in 1986. Furthermore, estimated energy intake rose from 3,191 to 3,539 kcal/day during the same period: if correct, this should have led to an average yearly weight gain of 17 kg per person. Thus, a very skeptical attitude to food disappearance data seems prudent following these observations (Willett & Stampfer, 1990).

The epidemiological literature on the relationship between vegetable and fruit consumption and breast cancer risk has recently been reviewed (Steinmetz & Potter, 1991). Six case-control studies, conducted in five different countries, have examined the association with vegetable and fruit consumption. Three of these found a significantly lower risk in association with higher intake of at least one vegetable (Katsouyanni et al., 1986; La Vecchia et al., 1987; Hislop et al., 1988; Trichopolou et al., 1995), while two found a lower risk specifically in association with high intake of carrots (Katsouyanni et al., 1986, Hislop et al., 1988). Earlier studies found no association (Graham et al., 1982; Zemla, 1986).

An index of vitamin C was calculated and analyzed by Howe et al. (1990) in his recent meta-analysis: 'vitamin C intake had the most consistent and statistically significant inverse association with breast cancer risk' (Howe et al., 1990). When beta-carotene, fibre and vitamin C were examined simultaneously, only vitamin C remained significant, which led the authors to use vitamin C intake as the marker for fruit and vegetable intake. The significant findings for vitamin C remained after fat intake was introduced into the model. The authors calculated that if all postmenopausal women in the population were to modify their saturated fat intake (to that of the lower one fifth of the population), the breast cancer rate in postmenopausal women in North America would drop by 10%. If, however, all postmenopausal women were to increase their consumption of fruit and vegetables to reach the average daily consumption of vitamin C, the breast cancer rate would fall by 16% (Howe et al., 1990). Thus for breast cancer, the protective effect of vitamin C appeared to be at least equal to the effect of saturated fat.

In reviewing the epidemiological evidence available regarding vitamin C, vitamin A, vitamin E and selenium with breast cancer risk, Garland et al. (1993) concluded that the available data supported a modest protective effect of vitamin A on breast cancer risk. Data on the relationship of vitamin C and vitamin E and breast cancer risk were limited and inconsistent. A substantial body of evidence indicated a lack of an appreciable influence of selenium intake within the range of intakes of human diets.

Boyd and his colleagues in Toronto have made a great effort to help the scientific community make up its mind about the strength of evidence published regarding the association between dietary fat intake and the risk of breast cancer (Boyd et al., 1993). Using state-of-the-art meta-analysis techniques developed in the setting of randomized clinical trials, Boyd et al. have conducted a meta-analysis of 23 studies of diet and breast cancer that were published at that time. These studies were not selected and satisfied a short list of several a priori conditions. The study is notable for both its results and the methodology employed.

Through performance of a quantitative meta-analysis, Boyd et al. (1993) assessed the epidemiological evidence from case-control and cohort studies linking dietary fat intake with breast cancer risk. All eligible studies were identified using a MEDLINE search of the years 1966 to 1993 and a secondary search of all cited references. Data were abstracted from 23 studies that examined fat as a nutrient and 19 studies that examined intakes of foodstuffs. Summary relative risks for total fat intake were examined after adjustment for potential modifying factors. The studies included in the meta-analysis were conducted in countries throughout Europe, North America, Asia and Australasia.

Among the studies that examined fat as a nutrient, the summary odds ratio comparing women in the highest fifth of daily intakes with women in the lowest fifth was 1.12 (95% C.I. 1.04–1.21). Those studies of the cohort type had a summary odds ratio of 1.01 (95% C.I. 0.90–1.13) whereas case-control studies demonstrated a relative risk of 1.21 (95% C.I. 1.10–1.34). Summary odds ratios were increased slightly among those studies which performed adjustment for energy intake: both in cohort studies (Odds Ratio = 1.03, 95% C.I. 0.92–1.16) and case-control studies (Odds Ratio = 1.42, 95% C.I. 1.17–1.72). Summary odds ratios for saturated fat were 1.36 (95% C.I. 1.17–1.58) for case-control studies and 0.95 (95% C.I. 0.84–1.08) for cohort studies. A further analysis indicated that studies conducted in Europe were more likely to demonstrate increased risks of breast cancer associated with high fat consumption. However, two studies published subsequent to Boyd et al. (1993) from populations of Europe with wide ranges of dietary fat intake both failed to demonstrate any association between fat intake and an increased risk of breast cancer (Martin-Moreno et al., 1994; Trichopoulos et al., 1994).

The findings suggest that a high dietary fat intake is associated with an increased risk of breast cancer over those women who have a lower intake. These overall findings are being driven by the results from case-control studies but particularly those conducted in European populations where the authors observe that the diet may be more varied than in North American populations. Two large subsequent studies from Europe have both gone against this observation. The large North American studies of dietary fat intake and breast cancer risk have been criticized as having too limited a range of intakes available in the population to detect the magnitude of risk being investigated.

Studies in the whole area of diet and cancer are difficult from the methodological point of view. 'Diet' is difficult to measure and a great deal of effort has gone into this over the last decade with large improvements being made in the methodology for such studies. Case-control studies have also been open to criticism for bias in the sense that cases may report eating more food overall and particularly more fat-rich foods than normal healthy women. Thus, unless great care is taken in the design and methodology of such studies, the possibility of bias exists. Cohort studies are less subject to this sort of bias and are generally considered to have advantages in this area. That is a situation that does not help interpretation of these findings: the stronger design showing no association and the weaker design demonstrating the association.

There also should be a greater attempt made to consider the role of meta-analysis in observational studies and, in particular, the problems of performing meta-analysis of epidemiological studies. Boyd et al. (1993) have endeavoured to do this but there are certain fundamental problems that still must be addressed. The technique of meta-analysis is very appropriate for the grouping together of the results from randomized trials. However, epidemiological studies of the type considered in this analysis are observational studies and there are additional considerations necessary when performing meta-analysis of such studies (Spitzer, 1991). Among the important points raised are whether such analyses can be performed without having the original material available: unless this is so it may be difficult to have adequate control of confounding. Should hospital control series be combined with studies where population controls have been obtained? How should odds ratios and confidence intervals obtained from meta-analysis be interpreted when there is obvious heterogeneity in the effects observed between studies?

This latter point is particularly relevant to the situation described here by the authors. An additional point in this study is that the authors have concentrated on comparison of the highest and lowest fifths of the distribution of intakes. These are the groups where all the outliers will tend to be found and may be somewhat heterogenous in the quality of the data themselves. Furthermore, fat intake is a continuous variable and one to which everyone is exposed: there is no truly unexposed group in nutritional epidemiology and the epidemiologist is looking for different effects associated with different levels of exposure. Limiting attention to the extreme groups ignores the continuous nature of the exposure data and will tend to give an exaggerated impression of the odds ratio associated with modest differences in levels of consumption. Of course, in the individual studies the median values of these fifths will vary for reasons of different distributions of intake between the populations considered as well as some variation due to differences in the success of the questionnaire in assessing the exposure of interest.

Another important piece of information that became available recently has been the publication of the results of the United States Nurses Health Study regarding intake of vitamins and breast cancer risk (Hunter et al., 1993). Basically, there was no association found with dietary intake of vitamin C, vitamin E or beta-carotene and breast cancer risk. However, there was a significant protective effect of vitamin A intake found. While there was a statistically significant test for linear trend, it could be argued that with the risk set to 1.0 in the lowest quintile of intake, the risk in the other quintiles was reduced to approximately 80% of this value. When the effects of vitamin supplementation were examined, it was found that the protective effect of vitamin A supplementation was confined to those women in the lowest fifth of the range of intakes (Hunter et al., 1993).

There is strong and consistent evidence that intakes of fruits and vegetables protect against a variety of forms of cancer, although breast cancer appears to be an exception (Steinmetz & Potter, 1991). The finding of a protective effect against breast cancer for a diet high in vitamin A is of considerable interest. The finding of a protective effect of vitamin A supplementation is important, although it must be interpreted as cautiously as the authors have done. There are a number of significant issues to bear in mind. Chiefly, the effect was confined to women in the lowest fifth of the entire range of dietary intakes and the data were obtained from an observational study. The authors stress the necessity for randomized trials to be conducted before advice can be given to women to take vitamin A supplements to reduce breast cancer risk.

Dietary Factors and Breast Cancer Prognosis It has been shown that survival rates from breast cancer are higher among women in areas where breast cancer rates are low (Wynder, Kajatani & Kuno, 1963; Morrison et al., 1973) and 20 years ago Haenszel (1964) suggested that factors which determine tumour development may also affect the course of the disease. This in turn suggests that different risk factors may put different cell populations at risk of transformation.

A study of the possible influence of dietary fat intake on survival was stimulated following a comparison of survival rates among breast cancer cases in Boston and Tokyo. The higher survival rates in Tokyo could not be explained by differences in age, stage, histology, parity or age at first full-term pregnancy (Morrison et al., 1976). The major distinguishing variable between Japanese and American women that is also thought to be a breast cancer risk factor is dietary fat intake. As suggested earlier, the role of fat, particularly cholesterol, has been related to possible stimulation of tumour growth by oestrogens (Boyle & Leake, 1986).

Abe et al. (1976) reported a five-year survival rate of 56% in obese women as compared to 80% in nonobese women, and Boyd et al. (1981) examined the relationship between breast cancer risk factors and subsequent prognosis and found that body weight was the only risk factor associated with survival.

A review of the relationship between obesity and breast cancer recurrence after mastectomy found that nine studies were supportive and two others nonsupportive (Rose & Boyer, 1986). The evidence of association appears strong.

Alcohol Intake Several studies have shown that alcohol consumption increases the risk of female breast cancer and few published studies contradict these findings. The evidence of an association is becoming firmer, although the risks reported are generally small (odds ratios of between 1.0 and 2.0) (see, for example, Willett et al., 1987;

Shatzkin et al., 1987; Lê, Hill & Kramer, 1984; O'Connell et al., 1987). However, the alcohol habit is so widespread that the possibility remains that it is an important determinant of breast cancer risk.

To help clarify this possible association, Longnecker et al., (1988) produced a combined analysis of published data on this subject (Hiatt & Bawol, 1984; Hiatt, Klatsky & Armstrong, 1988; Willett et al., 1987; Schatzkin et al., 1987; Harvey et al., 1987; Rosenberg et al., 1982; Webster et al., 1983; Paganini-Hill & Ross, 1983; Byers & Funch, 1982; Rohan & McMichael, 1988; Talamini et al., 1984; O'Connell et al., 1987; Harris & Wynder, 1988; Lê et al., 1984; La Vecchia et al., 1985; Begg et al., 1983; Monson & Lyon, 1975; Klatsky, Armstrong & Friedman, 1987; Williams & Horm, 1977; Katsouyanni et al., 1986; Miller et al., 1987). They found strong evidence to support a dose–response relationship from both retrospective and prospective studies. Using their calculated dose–response curves, the risk of breast cancer for an alcohol intake of 24 gm of absolute alcohol per day (roughly two drinks per day) relative to reported nondrinkers was 1.4 (95% C.I., 1.0–1.8). It would appear that at intakes of 24 gm/day or more the data are strongly supportive of an association between alcohol consumption and an increased risk of breast cancer and at lower levels of intake, weaker or modest associations are found. The evidence in favour of a dose–response relationship is strong, and the pooled relative risk of 1.1 for ever versus never drinkers does not alter these conclusions, since most women are light or moderate drinkers.

Longnecker and his co-workers (1988) do not interpret their findings as proof of causality but as being strongly supportive of an association between alcohol consumption and breast cancer risk. They calculate that, based on their results, 13% of all cases of breast cancer in the United States may be attributable to alcohol consumption.

The literature has been summarized as suggesting a need for women to be recommended to moderate their alcohol consumption until the situation is clarified (Graham, 1987). If such an association is real it may not be direct. It could arise from the direct action of alcohol on endocrine function or through an association between alcohol consumption and unmeasured causative agents. For low levels of alcohol intake the latter option could be a possible but speculative explanation of these results. However, it has recently been shown that women between 21 and 40 years who drink 30 gm of alcohol per day demonstrated increases in total oestrogen levels and amount of bioavailable oestrogens (Reichman et al., 1993). This is consistent with several epidemiological studies where the effect of alcohol consumption has been restricted to premenopausal women (Freidenreich et al., 1993)

Summary: Diet and Breast Cancer

In summary, diet, but especially a diet high in fat, particularly saturated fat, is thought from the results of animal studies and on biologic principles to influence the risk of breast cancer. Results of direct studies on humans provide conflicting and weak evidence of an association, although results from some studies are so clear and internally consistent that they cannot yet be ignored. The association has been described as being "weak in individuals as opposed to populations" (American Academy of Science, 1982). While biologically plausible, there seems to be no consistent evidence available at present from direct studies of breast cancer cases to support the association of current fat intake with breast cancer risk or total energy intake or protein (see Rohan & Bain, 1987 for a detailed review). The most powerful study to date, the prospective Nurses Health Study, reported no evidence of any increased risk for total fat, saturated fat, linoleic acid nor cholesterol in neither premenopausal or postmenopausal women (Willett et al., 1987). It may well be that the dietary influences in early life, especially at puberty, are important determinants of breast cancer risk, influencing risk by affecting endocrine function (Miller & Bulbrook, 1981) or some other mechanism (de Waard & Trichopoulos, 1988). It is an avenue that still requires attention from epidemiologists and other scientists, particularly with respect to the possible protective effects of vitamins. It may also be timely to accept that there may well be no influence of adult dietary patterns of fat consumption on the risk of developing breast cancer. The data regarding an increased risk of breast cancer with alcohol consumption are remaining firm with successive studies. Biological explanations are also beginning to emerge and it seems wise advice, based on the present evidence, that women should limit their intake of alcohol to reduce their risk of breast cancer.

PROSTATE CANCER

Prostate cancer is also an important public health problem, with over a quarter of a million new cases diagnosed worldwide in the single year 1985 (Parkin et al., 1993). The incidence of the disease is increasing rapidly in most regions of the world (Boyle, 1994; Alexander & Boyle, 1994), although the mortality rate has remained constant in generations of men born since the early years of this century (Boyle et al., 1994). The evidence that prostate cancer risk has important environmental determinants is compelling. Briefly, different populations around the world experience different levels of prostate cancer and these levels change with time usually in an orderly and predictable manner: international variation in incidence is around two orders of magnitude (Boyle et al., 1994). However, when migration takes place, groups of migrants tend to acquire the prostate cancer pattern of their new home (Haenszel, 1961). Furthermore, groups within a community whose lifestyle habits differentiate themselves from other members of the same community generally have notably different prostate cancer rates; for example, Seventh Day Adventists and Mormons (Boyle & Zaridze, 1987).

For reasons such as these it is widely thought that prostate cancer has environmental determinants, defining 'environment' in its broadest sense to include a wide range of lifestyle factors including dietary, social and cultural factors. Although these are theoretically avoidable, for prostate cancer no avoidable causes have been clearly identified, although a large number of factors have been investigated.

The presence of latent prostate cancer in a substantial proportion of middle-age and elderly men (Breslow et al., 1977), the relative lack of geographical variation in this phenomenon and the present impossibility of distinguishing true latent disease from early progressive disease presents the epidemiologists with a set of intriguing problems. In particular, these causative factors that are most relevant to the prevention of clinically relevant disease are likely to be promotional agents or late-stage carcinogens. It is not clear whether it is desirable for latent disease to be excluded in control series or ascertained in cohort studies but, in any event, few studies have attempted to do so.

Descriptive Epidemiology

Prostate cancer is a frequent cancer in old men, increasing with age through the most advanced years. The disease exhibits large ethnic and international differences, being particularly common in American blacks, among whom it ranks second after lung cancer. In 1985 it was estimated that prostatic cancer was the fourth most frequent cancer in men, with an estimated 291,000 cases occurring annually worldwide (Parkin et al., 1993). Registered incidence and mortality are increasing (Zaridze et al., 1984) and incidence and mortality rates of cancer of the prostate demonstrate wide international variation with, for example, a 120-fold difference present between areas of highest and lowest incidence, according to the most recently available statistics (Parkin et al., 1992). In areas where adequate data are available over long time periods, such as in Scotland, Connecticut (Zaridze & Boyle, 1987) and the Scandinavian countries (Hakulinen et al., 1986), the incidence has been increasing for over 30 years.

The leading 23 rates of prostate cancer are reported from North America and the black population of Bermuda. The highest incidence rates are reported from black population groups in Atlanta (102.0 per 100,000), San Francisco Bay Area (95.6), Detroit (94.2), Alameda County (93.5) and Los Angeles (82.7) (Table 8.3). The overall incidence rate among blacks in the SEER system in the United States is 82.0 per 100,000, which is considerably higher than the corresponding incidence rate in whites (61.8). The lowest incidence rates are recorded from populations in Asia and northern Africa.

In contrast to the distribution pattern of overt prostatic cancers, the frequency of the smaller noninvasive lesions denoted 'latent' carcinoma does not appear to show much international variation (Breslow et al., 1977).

Table 8.3. Current (Circa 1985) Highest and Lowest Incidence Rates of Prostate Cancer Recorded Worldwide Among 166 Populations

Prostate, Male
ICD9 185

Registry	Cases	Rate
U.S., Atlanta: black	832	102.0
U.S., Bay Area: black	944	95.6
U.S., Detroit: black	2210	94.2
U.S., Alameda: black	497	93.5
U.S., Los Angeles: black	1734	82.7
U.S., Seattle	7712	82.4
U.S., Utah	3019	77.9
U.S., New Orleans: black	582	72.9
U.S., Connecticut: black	296	65.0
Bermuda, black	45	64.0
Kuwait: Kuwaitis	27	4.4
India, Ahmedabad	143	4.1
Thailand, Chiang Mai	59	4.0
Thailand, Khon Kaen	19	2.7
India, Madras	100	2.1
Algeria, Setif	21	2.0
China, Shanghai	323	1.7
The Gambia	6	1.2
China, Tianjin	84	1.2
China, Qidong	20	0.8

Source: From Parkin et al. 1992.

The incidence of prostate cancer in blacks is much higher and often double that among whites in the same locality. Rates are intermediate, in the 30 to 50 per 100,000 range, in Canada, South America, Scandinavia, Switzerland and Oceania, whereas more moderate rates, around 20, are seen in most European countries. Very low rates, below 10, are seen in China, Japan, India and other Asian countries, as well as in the Middle East, but not in Israel, where rates are around 20, with the exception, however, of the non-Jewish population, where rates are lower.

Japanese migrants to the United States have experienced a marked increase in prostatic cancer, although the rates of the Japanese in the San Francisco Bay Area and in Los Angeles are still less than half of those of whites. Contrasts between United States Chinese and those elsewhere are even greater. In Singapore, the risk in foreign-born Chinese was 70% of that in the Singapore-born over 1968–1982. Polish migrants to the United States also acquired higher mortality rates on migration (Staszewski & Haenszel, 1965), again emphasizing the influence of the environment, probably dietary changes that modify hormone metabolism.

The incidence and mortality of prostatic cancer have been rising over time in many areas. While an average annual increase of 4.9% has been observed in Singapore Chinese and of 1.7% in the United States black population, respectively, a decrease in mortality in American blacks is, however, anticipated in the future on the basis of the decline in risk observed in the younger cohorts (Ernster et al., 1978). Similar observations have been made in Australia and in England and Wales (Holman et al., 1981). The interpretation of time trends and incidence levels is, however, not easy, depending to a degree on local practice concerning 'latent' cancer of the prostate discovered incidentally at prostatic resection or autopsy. In Malmo, Sweden, the incidence of prostate cancer was 50% higher than elsewhere: at the national level, 7.6% of 298 cases were discovered at autopsy compared to 36.4% of 177 in Malmo (National Board of Health and Welfare, 1984).

Temporal Trends in Prostate Cancer

There are substantial increases in the reported incidence of prostate cancer around the world (Table 8.4). However, in view of potential problems with 'latent carcinoma' of the prostate varying between countries for a variety of reasons compounded recently by the increasing use of transurethral prostatectomy (TURP) as a treatment for benign prostatic hyperplasia (BPH), which is associated with a 14%

Table 8.4. Incidence of Prostatic Cancer in Selected Registries

Cancer Incidence in Five Continents	Volume I[a]	Volume II[b]	Volume III[c]	Volume IV[d]	Volume V[e]	Volume VI[f]
Canada, Manitoba	30.59	31.06	37.62	43.22	44.36	54.71
Canada, Saskatchewan	33.43	39.04	39.01	46.13	57.58	52.99
U.S., Alameda: White	*	38.03	40.38	44.46	49.56	55.24
U.S., Alameda: Black	*	65.26	75.02	100.20	87.85	93.47
U.S., Connecticut	33.84	33.03	37.73	42.66	*	*
U.S., Connecticut: White	*	*	*	*	46.76	47.22
U.S., Connecticut: Black	*	*	*	*	72.28	65.00
India, Bombay	*	6.54	7.97	6.85	8.20	6.90
Japan, Miyagi	3.83	3.23	2.74	4.88	6.28	7.81
Denmark	17.71	19.45	21.76	23.02 23.64[g]	27.74	29.88
Finland	17.56	17.43	22.67	27.17	34.23	36.11
Norway	25.04	29.80	33.07	38.89	42.04	43.83
Sweden	26.51	33.47	38.80	44.36	45.89	50.20
U.K., Birmingham	17.30	18.39	17.70	18.57	18.90	24.97
New Zealand: non-Maori	34.38[h]	39.95	25.91	30.66	33.32	35.38

[a]From Doll R., Payne P. & Waterhouse J. (Eds.) (1966) *Cancer incidence in five continents,* Vol. I. International Agency for Research on Cancer, Lyon.
[b]From Doll R., Muir C.S. & Waterhouse, J. (Eds.) (1970) *Cancer incidence in five continents,* Vol. II. International Agency for Research on Cancer, Lyon.
[c]From Waterhouse J., Muir C.S., Correa P. & Powell, J. (Eds.) (1976) *Cancer incidence in five continents,* Vol. III (IARC Scientific Publication No. 15). International Agency for Research on Cancer, Lyon.
[d]From Waterhouse J., Muir C.S., Shanmugaratnam K. & Powell J. (Eds.) (1982) *Cancer incidence in five continents,* Vol. IV (IARC Scientific Publication No. 42). International Agency for Research on Cancer, Lyon.
[e]From Muir C.S., Waterhouse J.A.H., Mack T., Powell J. & Whelan S. (Eds.) (1987) *Cancer incidence in five continents,* Vol. V (IARC Scientific Publication No. 88). International Agency for Research on Cancer, Lyon.
[f]From Parkin D.M., Muir C.S., Whelan S., Gao Y.T., Ferlay J. & Powell J. (Eds.) (1992) *Cancer incidence in five continents,* Vol. VI (IARC Scientific Publication No. 120). International Agency for Research on Cancer, Lyon.
[g]Two time periods are available for this country.
[h]New Zealand: whole population.
*Data unavailable.

yield of unexpected focal carcinoma upon microscopic inspection (Murphy, 1991), and the increasing use of the prostate specific antigen test for prostate cancer (Boyle et al., 1993), examination of mortality data may give a clearer picture of changes in life-threatening prostate cancer through time, particularly since there has been little change in survival after treatment.

There are two interesting features to trends in mortality from prostate cancer. Firstly, the overall age-adjusted mortality rate is higher than the truncated rates (calculated on ages 35 to 64) and, secondly, the overall age-adjusted mortality rate increases much faster than the truncated rates if both are increasing.

In Canada, although the truncated rates have remained relatively stable since 1955, the overall age-adjusted mortality rate has been increasing since 1965. Birth cohort examination shows a slight increase in rates in successive birth cohorts for age groups over 55. In Japan, both the truncated and overall age-adjusted mortality rates have been increasing since 1955. However, the increases from overall age-adjusted mortality rates are more substantial. Examination of rates by birth cohorts suggests an increase in rates in successive birth cohorts for almost all age groups, particularly from those with ages over 65. There has not been any evidence of an acceleration in younger cohorts who are more likely to have been exposed to the modern Western diet introduced gradually to Japan following the Second World War (Boyle et al., 1993).

In the former Czechoslovakia, the overall age-adjusted mortality rates of prostate cancer have been increasing since 1955, but the truncated rates remained stable until 1968, and then were followed by a basically increasing trend. Birth cohort examination shows a continuing increase in rates in successive birth cohorts for almost all age groups examined with substantial increase from those with ages over 65. In Poland, both the truncated and overall age-adjusted mortality rates experienced a rapid increase between 1959 and 1970, and this has been followed by a relatively slower but steady increase ever since. Birth cohort examination shows an increase in rates in successive birth cohorts for almost all the age groups examined.

In Germany, both the truncated and overall age-adjusted mortality rates increased between 1955 and 1975. The rates, however, stabilized thereafter. Birth cohort examination shows an increase in rates in subsequent birth cohorts for cohorts born before 1915. For cohorts born after, the rates are quite similar. In the United Kingdom, both the truncated and overall age-adjusted mortality rates remained relatively stable between 1955 and 1975, and subsequently an increase occurred in both rates. Birth cohort examination shows similar rates for cohorts born before 1905, and a slight increase in rates in successive birth cohorts for those born after that, particularly for age groups between 50 and 74.

In Denmark, both the truncated and overall age-adjusted mortality rates showed no clear time trend until 1975, and subsequently an increase in rates occurred. Birth cohort examination did not show any systematic cohort pattern in mortality rates. However, in each age group examined, the rates experienced a slight fall in the first three cohorts and a subsequent increase in the following ones. This mortality pattern seems to exhibit a period effect rather than a birth cohort phenomenon. In Italy, the overall age-adjusted mortality has been increasing, although the truncated rates remained relatively stable between 1955 and 1987. Examination by birth cohort indicates an increase in rates in successive birth cohorts for those born before about 1910. For cohorts born after that, the mortality rates are quite similar in successive birth cohorts. In Australia, there has been no substantial change in both truncated and overall age-adjusted mortality rates between 1955 and 1988. Consequently, birth cohort examination shows the rates are quite stable in successive birth cohorts for all age groups examined.

In an attempt to investigate the nature of any changes in risk pattern for prostate cancer and to quantify any effect found, all available data in the World Health Organization Mortality Database were employed in an exercise of mathematical modelling using age-period-cohort models (Boyle et al., 1995). There was little increase noted in the cohort-specific risks in many countries subsequent to those men born around 1910. In those countries where there was an increase noted, it was small and did not exceed 1.5. Thus it was concluded that while prostate cancer incidence was rising (e.g., in Caucasians in the United States it rose by 30% between 1980 and 1988 (WHO, 1992)) the risk of fatal carcinomas was fairly stable worldwide (Boyle et al., 1994).

Aetiology of Prostate Cancer

The prostate is a primarily androgen-dependent gland controlled essentially by levels of plasma testosterone, of which 90 to 95% of the body's daily production is synthesized and secreted by the testis. However, despite this basic knowledge, in research directed to the search for endocrine or biochemical factors that could be implicated in prostatic carcinogenesis, determination of steroid or peptide hormone concentrations in plasma of patients with the disease has failed to consistently identify any endocrine disturbance, or any difference from the distribution in normal asymptomatic male, which could lead to a greater understanding of prostate cancer aetiology (Griffiths et al., 1990).

Body Mass Index Body mass index (WT/HT/HT generally expressed as kg/m^2) is determined by a complex interaction of genetic factors, total caloric intake, basal metabolic rate and total exercise.

In the American Cancer Society cohort, overweight males were shown to have a 30% increased risk of prostate cancer when compared to men within 10% of their ideal body weight (Lew & Garfinkel, 1979). Among Seventh Day Adventists the risk of fatal prostate cancer was 2.5 times elevated in overweight men (Snowden et al., 1984). However, the evidence from case-control studies has not been conclusive (Wynder et al., 1971; Graham et al., 1983), although a similar study from northern Italy found a substantial dose–response gradient (Talamini et al., 1986). Setting the risk to be 1.0 in the lowest tertile of body mass index (the *referent category*) the risk rose to 2.3 (95% CI, 2.1, 4.8) through 4.4 (1.9, 9.9) in the highest group: the test for linear trend was highly significant ($p<.0001$).

In view of this potential association, and the possible link to caloric intake, careful adjustment for body mass index in analysis of all nutritional datasets in prostate cancer epidemiology is essential (Boyle & Zaridze, 1993).

Dietary Fat Intake Hypotheses relating prostatic cancer risk to a high-fat diet are attractive on theoretical grounds (through the possible influence of fat on hormone metabolism in men; Hill et al., 1980) and arose initially from observations on the international distribution of prostatic cancer mortality (Wynder et al., 1971). Several correlation studies have reported a positive correlation between prostatic cancer occurrence, generally mortality, and national per capita fat disappearance statistics as well as strong correlations between prostate cancer mortality rates and those of other forms of cancer suspected as being associated with a high fat intake such as breast and ovarian cancer (Boyle & Zaridze, 1993). In recent times, focus has fallen on four aspects of this association:

Until the very recent past, the nutritional epidemiology of prostatic cancer could be characterized as a series of studies that have produced tantalizing results but have suffered from limitations in their design and methodology. These generally have supported the hypothesis that prostate cancer risk is increased by a diet with an increasing content of fat (Boyle & Zaridze, 1993); of at least 13 case-control studies, 10 have shown some positive evidence, but early cohort studies were less consistent.

The United States Health Professionals Follow-up Study was used to examine this association among 47,855 men aged 40 to 75 at recruitment and initially free from cancer, and who had been followed-up for four years. This is one of the first studies to include the methodologically essential adjustment for total caloric intake. In these men there was a total of 300 prostate cancers diagnosed, including 126 advanced cases. Total fat consumption was directly related to the risk of advanced cancer: the risk, after adjustment for age and total energy intake, in the highest fifth of the intake range compared to the lowest fifth was 1.79 (95% C.I., 1.04–3.07) with the test for linear trend just falling short of the usually accepted level of statistical significance (being $p = .06$). The association observed was due mainly to saturated fat (relative risk = 1.63) but was not found with vegetable fat. Among the food groups considered, red meat represented the group with the strongest association with prostate cancer risk in the highest fifth being 2.64 (95% C.I., 1.21–5.77) ($p = .02$). Fat from fish or dairy products was unrelated to risk apart from a positive association with butter. Saturated fat, monounsaturated fat and alpha-linoleic acid were associated with advanced prostate cancer, although only the association with alpha-linoleic acid remained after simultaneous adjustment for saturated fat, monounsaturated fat and linoleic acid (Giovannucci et al., 1993).

Further positive associations without adjustment for total caloric intake have been reported for animal fat in a prospective study of United States Seventh Day Adventists (Mills et al., 1989) and, more recently, a random population-based study in Hawaii (Le Marchand et al., 1994). It is interesting that the relative risk estimates in the Hawaiian and U.S. Health Professionals studies are very similar despite the differences in methodology and study population.

Discrepancies in the effects reported between case-control and cohort studies may be attributed in part to the time at which exposure was classified; if dietary fat intake has its effect at a late stage in disease development, then positive results would be anticipated in case-control studies and cohort studies with relatively short follow-up periods. In contrast, negative results should come from prospective studies with long follow-up periods as has been observed for the Lutheran Brotherhood Cohort Study (Hsing et al., 1990).

Thus, it would appear that there is an association between dietary intake of fat and the risk of prostate cancer. The recommendation to men to lower their intake of meat to reduce their risk of prostate cancer is appropriate (Giovannucci et al., 1993), although the exact mechanism of carcinogenesis remains unknown. It is often suggested that fat exerts its effect through modification of the endogenous hormonal milieu (Hill et al., 1980).

Vitamin A, Beta-carotene and Retinoids It is difficult to escape the impression given from a number of studies that the risk of prostate cancer is increased by increasing reported intake of vitamin A, particularly retinol. This may be explained at least partially by the retinol content of meat, but there is still a residual to the association that leaves the reviewer uncomfortable (Boyle & Zaridze, 1993).

The recent results from an intervention trial in smokers provide some limited reassurance on this matter. Among 23,000 Finnish male smokers entered into a randomized trial of beta-carotene versus placebo there were 138 cases of prostate cancer reported in the beta-carotene group (a rate of 16.3 per 10,000) compared to 112 (13.2 per 10,000) in the placebo group (Finnish/United States Randomised Intervention Trial of Beta-Carotene in Smokers, 1994). The age-adjusted relative risk appears to be approximately 1.24 (the confidence interval cannot be calculated from the data presented). This finding is consistent with several previous observations that the risk of prostate cancer appears to be elevated among those men who received beta-carotene but it is in a sense reassuring that if the excess is significant then it is not very large in magnitude (around 25%). However, it is clear that this putative association deserves to be a continued priority for future research, particularly in light of the increasing tendency to undertake trials of carotenoids and retinoids in the prevention of malignant disease and that the general populations of many countries are already anticipating these findings and are increasingly taking vitamins including these compounds.

Vitamin E An interesting finding, although one that was completely unexpected, from this same study (The Alpha-Tocopherol, Beta-Carotene Cancer Prevention Study Group, 1994) was a striking negative association between risk of prostate cancer and intake of vitamin E. Among men randomized to alpha-tocopherol (50 mg daily) there were 99 cases of prostate cancer observed (rate 11.7 per 10,000) compared to 151 cases among these men receiving the placebo (17.8 per 10,000). The approximate age-adjusted relative risk was 0.66.

This is the first evidence that vitamin E may be protective against prostate cancer; it is a post hoc inference and obviously requires confirmation before it can be acted upon and recommendations made to the general public. It is clearly identified, due to the magnitude of the effect, as a major priority in prostate cancer research at the present time.

Vitamin D International correlation studies suggest that vitamin D could be closely linked to the risk of prostate cancer (Schwartz & Hulka, 1990). Such a potential association was examined in the cohort of members of the Kaiser Permanente Medical Care plan in Oakland and San Francisco whose serum was collected between 1964 and 1971 (Corder et al., 1993). A total of 90 cases of prostate cancer in black men and 91 cases in white men were identified from the cohort of 250,000 men sampled: controls were selected matched for age, race and day of serum storage. In these groups of cases and controls, levels of the major metabolites of vitamin D were measured and examined in respect to prostate cancer risk. The mean serum level of 1,25-D was 1.81 pg/ml lower in cases than in matched controls: this difference was statistically significant (p = .02). The risk of prostate cancer decreased with higher levels of 1,25-D especially in men with lower levels of 25-D_3. However, the mean levels of 25-D_3 were similar in cases of prostate cancer and in controls. In men aged 57 years or older, 1,25 D was found to be an important risk for palpable and anaplastic tumours but not for tumours found incidentally at the time of surgery to treat the symptoms of benign prostatic hyperplasia or well-differentiated tumours (Corder et al., 1993).

Thus, vitamin D may be specifically relevant to the promotional events and clinically important tumours that are of public health importance. It should be considered together with the other dietary factors listed above in the aetiology of prostate cancer.

Summary: Diet and Prostate Cancer

Descriptive epidemiology has highlighted the wide geographical variation in prostate cancer occurrence and the large increases taking place in the reported incidence of the disease worldwide. Descriptive epidemiology provides compelling evidence that the large majority of prostate cancer has important environmental determinants and that a large proportion of the cases should be preventable.

However, knowledge of risk factors for prostate cancer is poor and avoidable causes have not yet been identified. Intuition tells us that the 'causes' of prostate cancer are hormonal, but at the present time neither the important hormones nor their critical levels nor their period of maximum influence have been determined. From examination of the available analytical studies, there is a dietary component to prostate cancer risk involving saturated fat intake and particularly intake of meat and (perhaps) milk: this may relate to the hormonal milieu. The role of carotenoids and retinoids remains unclear at the present time, with the suggestion of an increased risk associated with an increased intake still a cause for some concern. The possible protective roles of vitamin D and vitamin E are emerging as of potential interest and should, at least, be priorities for further research.

Although a large number of different occupations have been associated with an increased risk of prostate cancer, the only fairly consistent finding is that of the increased risk associated with occupation in agriculture. However, the increased risk is proving to be nonspecific and not related to exposure to animals, cereals or other types of farming. Recent evidence suggests that the specific factor may be exposure to herbicides and this should be followed-up as soon as possible.

There is a likelihood of important genetic effects in prostate cancer, the unravelling of which will require international cooperation. There is at the present time little evidence that having a vasectomy or benign prostatic hyperplasia leads to an increased risk of prostate cancer. There is no consistent evidence suggesting an association of prostate cancer risk with cigarette smoking (IARC, 1986), alcohol consumption (IARC, 1988), coffee consumption (IARC, 1991) or sexually transmitted diseases and prostate cancer risk (Boyle & Zaridze, 1993).

Despite this knowledge of such a litany of risk factors, there is little action that can be recommended at the present time to reduce risk of prostate cancer through alteration of lifestyle factors. The large increases in the expected numbers of cases due to the ageing of the population seem to be outwith the control of primary prevention strategies at the present time. Chemoprevention and screening appear to be priority alternatives to alteration of risk through alteration of risk factors. Screening deserves urgent evaluation through randomized trials (Boyle & Alexander, 1994), the search for prostate cancer families should be an urgent research priority and the striking protective effect involving vitamin E should be followed-up as a matter of considerable urgency.

ENDOMETRIAL CANCER

The descriptive epidemiology of endometrial cancer is in several aspects similar to that of breast cancer. High incidence rates are reported in developed countries of North America and Europe except the United Kingdom, and low rates in Japan and other cancer registration areas in Asia. Although endometrial cancer is a disease of older women, its age incidence curve shows a flattening of the slope around menopause.

Descriptive Epidemiology of Cancer of the Corpus Uteri

The highest rates of cancer of the corpus uterus are reported from the United States and Canada (Table 8.5), specifically from populations that are white or essentially white. The highest incidence rate is from the white population of the San Francisco Bay Area, where the incidence rate is 22.3 per 100,000. Low incidence rates are reported from populations of India, Southeast Asia and Africa (Table 8.5). In Israel, the incidence in Jews born in Europe or America is higher than in those born in Africa or Asia or in Israel. The Chinese and Japanese in the United States experience rates that are more than four times those in China and Japan.

Leiomyosarcoma of the uterus accounts for 6.8% of these cancers in United States black women compared to 2.2% in whites (Young et

Table 8.5. Current (Circa 1985) Highest and Lowest Incidence Rates of Endometrial Cancer Recorded Worldwide in 166 Populations

Corpus Uteri, Female ICD9 182 Registry	Cases	Rate
U.S., Bay Area: white	2186	22.3
U.S., Alameda: white	659	22.1
U.S., Seattle	2101	21.8
U.S., Detroit: white	2306	21.2
U.S., Los Angeles: O. white	3714	19.0
U.S., Hawaii: white	141	18.9
U.S., Iowa	2029	18.4
U.S., Hawaii: Hawaiian	64	18.3
Canada, Manitoba	679	18.0
U.S., Utah	720	17.7
U.S., Los Angeles: Korean	4	2.0
Bermuda: white & other	3	1.9
Brazil, Goiania	12	1.8
India, Madras	91	1.7
India, Ahmedabad	74	1.7
India, Bangalore	73	1.6
The Gambia	8	1.2
Algeria, Setif	12	1.1
Mali, Bamako	4	0.8
China, Qidong	14	0.5

Source: From Parkin et al. 1992.

al., 1981). In Singapore in 1968–1982, the proportion was 11.6% (Lee et al., 1988).

Whereas mortality rates from cancer of the corpus uteri have shown large declines, incidence trends are more variable. In the United States, a substantial increase in incidence, more marked in ages 55 to 64 and ascribed to the use of postmenopausal estrogens, occurred in the 1970s. Incidence rates have now declined to or below previous levels after the use of these drugs ceased (Austin & Roe, 1982). Increases in Europe were much smaller.

Temporal Trends in Uterine Cancer

There are modest increases in the incidence of endometrial cancer reported from European centres. In some populations the temporal trends are difficult to interpret (Table 8.6).

Mortality statistics for cervix and endometrium cancer individually are unreliable (Cuzick & Boyle, 1990) for many of the same reasons as discussed above under colorectal cancer. Thus it is necessary to consider uterus cancer as a single entity when discussing mortality data and investigating temporal trends in them. This, of course, is a major problem on account of the differences in the epidemiology of the two sites.

In Canada, both the truncated and overall age-adjusted mortality rates of uterus cancer have been decreasing rapidly since 1955. Birth cohort examination suggests a consistent decline in rates in successive birth cohorts in all age groups examined. In Japan, both the truncated and overall age-adjusted mortality rates of uterus cancer have been decreasing consistently since 1955, with a more substantial decline in truncated rates. Birth cohort examination shows a rapid decrease in rates in successive birth cohorts for those born after 1900.

In the former Czechoslovakia, a rapid decline was observed in both truncated and overall age-adjusted mortality rates of uterus cancer between 1955 and 1973. Since 1974, however, the mortality rates have been relatively stable. Birth cohort examination indicates a decrease in rates in successive birth cohorts until 1935. In Poland, both the truncated and overall age-adjusted mortality rates of uterus cancer increased between 1959 and 1964, and remained stable during the following years (1965–1969). However, the rates have declined since 1969 and more so for the truncated rates. Birth cohort examination shows a decline in rates in successive birth cohorts for those born after 1920.

In Germany, both the truncated and overall age-adjusted mortality rates of uterus cancer have been decreasing since 1955. The de-

Table 8.6. Incidence of Endometrial Cancer in Selected Registries

Cancer Incidence in Five Continents	Volume I[a]	Volume II[b]	Volume III[c]	Volume IV[d]	Volume V[e]	Volume VI[f]
Canada, Manitoba	14.28	16.52	14.21	14.21	19.76	17.96
Canada, Saskatchewan	15.45	19.06	17.34	18.75	15.75	14.64
U.S., Alameda: white	*	16.83	33.33	38.48	24.79	22.14
U.S., Alameda: black	*	18.12	13.60	10.55	10.75	10.07
U.S., Connecticut	12.73	15.31	17.78	21.32	19.34	17.56
U.S., Connecticut: white	*	*	*	*	19.34	17.56
U.S., Connecticut: black	*	*	*	*	12.47	11.12
India, Bombay	*	1.45	1.35	1.38	2.02	2.27
Japan, Miyagi	1.98	1.27	1.26	1.95	2.82	3.16
Denmark	10.68	10.96	11.43	12.58 13.02[g]	15.26	15.28
Finland	9.06	8.60	9.61	10.89	12.16	11.77
Norway	7.68	8.23	9.74	10.98	12.07	12.29
Sweden	11.14	11.99	12.10	12.97	13.24	12.66
U.K., Birmingham	7.99	8.98	8.49	9.37	9.08	10.13
New Zealand: Non-maori	10.57[h]	10.56	10.39	11.21	9.97	9.25

[a]From Doll R., Payne P. & Waterhouse J. (Eds.) (1966) *Cancer incidence in five continents,* Vol. I. International Agency for Research on Cancer, Lyon.
[b]From Doll R., Muir C.S. & Waterhouse, J. (Eds.) (1970) *Cancer incidence in five continents,* Vol. II. International Agency for Research on Cancer, Lyon.
[c]From Waterhouse J., Muir C.S., Correa P. & Powell, J. (Eds.) (1976) *Cancer incidence in five continents,* Vol. III (IARC Scientific Publication No. 15). International Agency for Research on Cancer, Lyon.
[d]From Waterhouse J., Muir C.S., Shanmugaratnam K. & Powell J. (Eds.) (1982) *Cancer incidence in five continents,* Vol. IV (IARC Scientific Publication No. 42). International Agency for Research on Cancer, Lyon.
[e]From Muir C.S., Waterhouse J.A.H., Mack T., Powell J. & Whelan S. (Eds.) (1987) *Cancer incidence in five continents,* Vol. V (IARC Scientific Publication No. 88). International Agency for Research on Cancer, Lyon.
[f]From Parkin D.M., Muir C.S., Whelan S., Gao Y.T., Ferlay J. & Powell J. (Eds.) (1992) *Cancer incidence in five continents,* Vol. VI (IARC Scientific Publication No. 120). International Agency for Research on Cancer, Lyon.
[g]Two time periods are available for this country.
[h]New Zealand: whole population.
*Data unavailable.

crease in rates has been much faster since 1968. Birth cohort examination shows a systematic decline in rates in successive birth cohorts for those born after 1920. Both truncated and overall age-adjusted mortality rates of uterus cancer in Denmark have been decreasing since 1955. Birth cohort examination suggests a consistent decline in rates in successive birth cohorts for all age groups examined.

In the United Kingdom, both the truncated and overall age-adjusted mortality rates of uterus cancer have been decreasing since 1955, with a more rapid decrease for truncated rates. Birth cohort examination shows a basically decreasing trend in rates in successive birth cohorts for those born before 1935. For cohorts born after that, the rates seem to be increasing in successive birth cohorts. In Italy, both the truncated and overall age-adjusted mortality of uterus cancer showed a consistent decrease in rates during the past decades. Birth cohort examination indicates a rapid decline in rates in successive birth cohorts for almost all the age groups examined. In Australia, both the truncated and overall age-adjusted mortality rates of uterine cancer have been decreasing since 1955. Birth cohort examination shows a decrease in rates in successive birth cohorts for those born before 1935, although the rates may be increasing in more recent cohorts.

Aetiology of Endometrial Cancer

Endometrial cancer is, in terms of hormonal correlates, the best understood gynaecological malignancy. It is strongly related to elevated levels or availability of exogenous or endogenous oestrogens, and correspondingly low levels of progestogens. It is thus related to anovularity in many women, oestrogen replacement treatment in the menopause and obesity, which increases endogenous oestrogen levels. The relative risks for long-term use and severe obesity are on the order of 5 to 10 in various populations investigated (Lew & Garfinkel, 1979). However, in terms of attributable risk, menopausal replacement treatment was the major determinant of the epidemic of endometrial cancer observed in the United States during the 1970s (Ziel & Feinkle, 1975), whereas obesity is the major established risk determinant of endometrial cancer in Europe (Parazzini et al., 1989) where menopausal hormonal replacement therapy has not been so widely used.

Recent analysis of incidence data from Sweden reveals patterns of cohort-specific risk that are compatible with the effect of oestrogen-only hormonal replacement therapy (as prescribed in the 1960s) increasing risk while the addition of progestins approximately ten years later was not so obviously associated with an increased risk (Persson et al., 1990): this is compatible with the results from case-control and cohort studies (Persson et al., 1989). Further simultaneous examination of mortality data reveals discrepancy with incidence and mortality data that the authors suggest is partly due to improved survival but also supports the hypothesis that endometrial cancers associated with exogenous oestrogens may be associated with a favourable clinical course (Persson et al., 1990).

Use of combined oral contraceptives, and the consequent relative progestin excess, considerably decreases the risk of the endometrial cancer (Schlesselman, 1991). The combined evidence from studies showed a very consistent, approximately 50% protection in ever users as compared to never users, and the risk is inversely related to duration of use. Endometrial cancer, however, is rare in younger women, and the ultimate evaluation of the public health impact of this protection is related to the observation of much reduced risks at older ages (La Vecchia et al., 1990).

Other determinants of endometrial cancer include nulliparity, late menopause and perhaps early menarche, diabetes and hypertension (Wynder et al., 1966), although it is not known whether these risk factors are partly mediated through a mutual association with overweight.

All these established and potential risk factors, however, explain only a fraction of endometrial cancer (i.e., approximately one half in Europe and perhaps two thirds in the United States), but cannot account for the 30-fold worldwide variation in the disease incidence. There is some suggestion that not only nutritional status but also diet composition is related to endometrial cancer. Ecological studies found positive correlations with consumption of meat, eggs, milk, proteins, fats and total calorie intake. The few analytical studies available suggest positive associations with total calorie intake, carbohydrates, fats and oils, and protection by green vegetables (La Vecchia, 1989). Methodologically sound studies, with adequate allowance for total energy intake, are even more important for endometrial cancer than for other cancers that are less strongly related to obesity (Shu et al., 1993).

CANCER OF THE OVARY

Ovarian cancer is a moderately frequent disease representing, however, the most frequent cause of death from gynecologic malignancies in the Western world. Ovarian cancer is the sixth most frequent form of cancer worldwide, with an estimated 162,000 incident cases in 1985 (Parkin, Pisani & Ferlay, 1993). Epithelial cystadenocarcinomas constitute the large majority of ovarian malignancies. The less frequent germ cell tumours have a younger age distribution. The range of geographic variation for this disease is rather small.

Descriptive Epidemiology

The highest incidence rate of cancer of the ovary is reported from St. Gall in Switzerland (17.0 per 100,000) (Table 8.7). High rates are also recorded from four scandinavian countries, Iceland (16.6 per 100,000), Denmark (14.9), Sweden (14.6) and Norway (14.6) (the other country, Finland, has the 82nd highest rate (9.9)). There is little geographical pattern to the regions with the lowest rates (Table 8.7).

Hawaiians and Pacific Polynesian Islanders have higher rates than Maoris, in whom the incidence is similar to that of non-Maoris in New Zealand. The highest rates reported from Europe are 17.3 in Ardèche in France (Olaya & Nectoux, 1987) and around 15 in Norway, Sweden and in Israel for women born in Europe or America. Most rates in Europe and North America range between 8 and 12. Rates for United States blacks are about two thirds of those for whites. While women in Asia have a relatively low incidence of ovarian tumours,

Table 8.7. Current (Circa 1985) Highest and Lowest Incidence Rates of Cancer of the Ovary Recorded Worldwide

Ovary etc., Female ICD9 183 Registry	Cases	Rate
Switzerland, St. Gall	307	17.0
Iceland	118	16.6
Israel: born Eur. Amer.	742	15.2
Denmark	3,058	14.9
Canada, N. W. T. & Yukon	15	14.7
U.K., N.E. Scotland	300	14.6
Sweden	5,097	14.6
Norway	2,300	14.6
U.K., S.E. Scotland	680	14.0
Czech., Boh. & Morav.	5,195	13.6
Italy, Latina	38	4.3
U.S., Los Angeles: Korean	10	4.1
India, Ahmedabad	190	4.0
Kuwait: Kuwaitis	28	3.7
France, Martinique	30	3.2
Israel: non-Jews	27	2.4
Algeria, Setif	22	1.6
China, Qidong	45	1.5
The Gambia	7	1.4
Mali, Bamako	7	1.0

in the 5 to 7 range, Chinese and Japanese who reside in the United States tend to have slightly higher rates, although less than in the white population. Little change has been observed for the disease in most registries. The rise has been slightly greater in Japan than elsewhere.

Temporal Trends in Ovarian Cancer

The incidence rate of ovarian cancer has increased gradually in most international populations (Table 8.8), even in populations where the incidence was initially low.

In Canada, ovary cancer mortality rates remained stable between 1955 and 1973; however, they declined thereafter, especially the truncated rates. Birth cohort examination suggests quite similar rates in successive birth cohorts born before 1925. For cohorts born after that, rates decreased in successive birth cohorts. In Japan, both the truncated and overall age-adjusted mortality rates have been increasing rapidly since 1955. Birth cohort examination shows a rapid increase in rates in successive birth cohorts for all age groups examined, particularly those aged over 50.

In the former Czechoslovakia, a consistent increasing trend was observed for both truncated and overall age-adjusted mortality rates since 1955. Birth cohort examination suggests a slow but steady increase in rates in successive birth cohorts for age groups over 40. In Poland, both the truncated and overall age-adjusted mortality rates increased rapidly after 1955 and peaked in 1978; these then followed a decline between 1977 and 1981. Since that time an increase in rates has again occurred, however. Birth cohort examination shows an increase in rates in successive birth cohorts. However, the rates in different age groups have shown inconsistent changes in the last time period.

In Germany, although the overall age-adjusted mortality rates remained relatively stable between 1968 and 1988, the truncated rates have been decreasing since the early 1970s. Birth cohort examination indicates a slight increase in rates in successive birth cohorts until 1920 and a decreasing trend for cohorts born thereafter. In Denmark, there has been a small increase in the overall age-adjusted mortality rates of ovary cancer between 1955 and 1972, and thereafter a small decrease. Although subject to greater variation, this pattern is also evident in the truncated rates. Examination of rates by median year of birth shows no systematic change by birth cohort.

In Italy, both the truncated and overall age-adjusted mortality rates have been increasing rapidly since 1955. Examination by birth

Table 8.8. Incidence of Ovarian Cancer in Selected Registries

Cancer Incidence in Five Continents	Volume I[a]	Volume II[b]	Volume III[c]	Volume IV[d]	Volume V[e]	Volume VI[f]
Canada, Manitoba	15.24	14.31	11.60	10.76	12.82	10.07
Canada, Saskatchewan	9.96	10.28	11.01	10.73	11.90	11.07
U.S., Alameda: white	*	12.56	13.47	14.05	12.08	12.93
U.S., Alameda: black	*	10.40	10.27	8.72	10.48	6.85
U.S., Connecticut	13.06	11.26	12.48	12.11	12.04	12.73
U.S., Connecticut: white	*	*	*	*	12.04	12.73
U.S., Connecticut: black	*	*	*	*	7.29	8.75
India, Bombay	*	6.06	4.76	7.23	7.24	6.50
Japan, Miyagi	2.16	1.90	2.78	3.39	4.23	5.15
Denmark	13.11	13.47	15.05	15.85 14.63[g]	14.52	14.85
Finland	8.92	10.07	10.43	10.88	9.84	9.98
Norway	11.51	11.52	14.16	14.57	15.29	14.58
Sweden	13.08	14.41	15.08	15.94	15.24	14.61
U.K., Birmingham	10.09	10.75	11.28	11.02	11.07	13.42
New Zealand: Non-maori	12.59[h]	11.93	11.41	11.28	10.50	10.30

[a]From Doll R., Payne P. & Waterhouse J. (Eds.) (1966) *Cancer incidence in five continents,* Vol. I. International Agency for Research on Cancer, Lyon.

[b]From Doll R., Muir C.S. & Waterhouse, J. (Eds.) (1970) *Cancer incidence in five continents,* Vol. II. International Agency for Research on Cancer, Lyon.

[c]From Waterhouse J., Muir C.S., Correa P. & Powell, J. (Eds.) (1976) *Cancer incidence in five continents,* Vol. III (IARC Scientific Publication No. 15). International Agency for Research on Cancer, Lyon.

[d]From Waterhouse J., Muir C.S., Shanmugaratnam K. & Powell J. (Eds.) (1982) *Cancer incidence in five continents,* Vol. IV (IARC Scientific Publication No. 42). International Agency for Research on Cancer, Lyon.

[e]From Muir C.S., Waterhouse J.A.H., Mack T., Powell J. & Whelan S. (Eds.) (1987) *Cancer incidence in five continents,* Vol. V (IARC Scientific Publication No. 88). International Agency for Research on Cancer, Lyon.

[f]From Parkin D.M., Muir C.S., Whelan S., Gao Y.T., Ferlay J. & Powell J. (Eds.) (1992) *Cancer incidence in five continents,* Vol. VI (IARC Scientific Publication No. 120). International Agency for Research on Cancer, Lyon.

[g]Two time periods are available for this country.

[h]New Zealand: whole population.

*Data unavailable.

cohorts shows an increase in rates in successive birth cohorts for almost all the age groups examined. In the United Kingdom, the truncated rates of ovary cancer remained relatively stable until 1978. Since then, a small decrease in rates has occurred. The overall age-adjusted mortality rates, however, showed a slight increase before 1970 and remained relatively stable thereafter. Consequently, examination of rates by birth cohorts suggests an increase in rates in successive birth cohorts until 1920 birth cohort, and a decrease for cohorts born thereafter.

In Australia, both the truncated and overall age-adjusted mortality rates did not show a clear time trend before 1965 but started to decline thereafter. Birth cohort examination shows a relatively stable rate in successive birth cohorts for those born before 1930, and a rapid decrease thereafter.

Aetiology of Ovarian Cancer

Epithelial ovarian cancer is the commonest type of ovarian neoplasia and the leading cause of death from gynaecological neoplasms in most Western countries. This term contains a very wide and diverse range of pathological entities (Richardson et al., 1985). As for other female-hormone-related neoplasms, its age curve tends to flatten off around menopause (Pike, 1987).

The risk of ovarian cancer is increased approximately twofold in nulliparous women compared to parous women. An increased risk has been suggested for late age at first birth, early menarche and late menopause, but the evidence is inconsistent.

Over a dozen studies have uniformly indicated that oral contraceptive use is protective against ovarian carcinogenesis, the incidence of epithelial invasive cancer being reduced by approximately 40% in ever users of oral contraceptives, and to a greater extent in long-term users (Rosenberg et al., 1982; La Vecchia et al., 1984; CASH, 1987; WHO, 1989). Thus, on a population scale, combined oral contraceptives have probably been the major determinant of the (favourable) decrease in ovarian cancer rates observed in several Western countries (Adami et al., 1990).

Just as in breast and endometrial cancer, nutrition and diet are the major open questions in ovarian cancer epidemiology. The American Cancer Society One Million Study showed an elevated risk of ovarian cancer among obese women (Lew & Garfinkel, 1979), but the evidence from case-control studies is largely negative, possibly on account of loss of weight secondary to the neoplastic process. Ecological studies found positive correlations with fats, proteins and calories, although these are less strong than for endometrial cancer. Case-control studies showed a possible association with total fat intake and some protection by green vegetables (La Vecchia, 1989), but further research is required in the area, particularly because diet may be more amenable to intervention than reproductive or menstrual history.

CONCLUSIONS

Much of the interest in nutrition and cancer has focussed on the possibility that fat intake could act as a dietary substrate for hormones. Consequently, those members of the population with increased levels of dietary fat intake would have increased levels of certain hormones that were influential in the development of certain forms of cancer. It appears at the present time that adult dietary fat intake has little if any influence on the risk of breast cancer and any association with ovarian or endometrial cancer is inconclusive. However, it appears likely that the risk of prostate cancer is influenced by dietary fat intake in adult life.

Thus, recommendations for the reduction in fat intake are unlikely to have much influence on the overall incidence of breast, ovarian and endometrial cancers. The possible influence of cholesterol is theoretically attractive but at present unknown (Boyle & Leake, 1988). In searching for other dietary means to reduce cancer risk, interest has focussed on several vitamins. At the present time, there is considerable interest in vitamin A, especially, and breast cancer risk, although the possibility of an association with vitamin C and fibre intake cannot be dismissed. It remains of great interest to investigate the effects of vitamin A, vitamin D and, especially, vitamin E intakes on prostate cancer risk. Encouragement to continue with this line of research has come recently from the results of a randomized intervention trial conducted in China (Blot et al., 1993).

An important consideration is that there had not been a randomized intervention trial that demonstrated a reduction in mortality from cancer of any form. Individuals aged 40 to 69 were recruited in 1985 from four communes in Linxian, China into a randomized trial to determine if dietary supplementation with specific vitamins and minerals could lower mortality from or incidence of cancer as well as mortality from other diseases in Linxian, China, where one of the world's highest rates of oesophageal/gastric cardia cancer is found together with persistently low dietary intake of several micronutrients. Study participants were randomly assigned to intervention groups according to a one half replicate of a 2^4 factorial experimental design.

This design enabled testing for the effects of four combinations of nutrients: (A) retinol and zinc; (B) riboflavin and niacin; (C) vitamin C and molybdenum; and (D) beta-carotene, vitamin E and selenium. Doses ranged from one to two times the United States recommended daily allowances. Mortality and cancer incidence during the period March 1986 to May 1991 were ascertained on 29,584 adults who received daily vitamin and mineral supplementation during this period.

The grouping of vitamins and minerals to combine in the intervention was well thought out. Factor A was retinol and zinc, which enhances the delivery of retinol to tissues. Factor B was the B group vitamins riboflavin and niacin. Factor C combined vitamin C and molybdenum which are thought to inhibit the formation of carcinogenic nitrosoamines. Factor D was a combination of fat-soluble antioxidants beta-carotene, vitamin E and selenium. Thus there were a total of eight intervention groups in this study receiving a combination of factors: AB, AC, AD, BC, BD, CD, ABCD or placebo. Half of the study population received each of the four factor nutrient combinations (e.g., half received factor A (AB, AC, AD, ABCD) and half did not (BC, BD, CD, placebo) and the subjects who received compared to those who did not receive factor A were balanced with respect to receipt of all other nutrients.

A total of 2,127 deaths occurred among trial participants during the intervention period. Cancer was the leading cause of death, with 32% of all deaths due to oesophageal cancer or stomach cancer, followed by cerebrovascular disease. Significantly (p=.03) lower total mortality (RR=0.91, 95% C.I. 0.84–0.99) occurred among those receiving supplementation with beta-carotene, vitamin E and selenium. The reduction was mainly due to lower cancer rates (RR=0.91, 95% C.I. 0.75–1.00) especially stomach cancer (RR=0.79, 95% C.I. 0.64–0.99) with the reduced risk beginning to rise about one to two years after the start of supplementation with these vitamins and minerals. No significant effects on mortality rates from all causes were found for supplementation with retinol and zinc, riboflavin and niacin, or vitamin C and molybdenum. Patterns of cancer incidence, on the basis of 1,298 cases, generally resembled those for cancer mortality.

The authors concluded that vitamin and mineral supplementation of the diet in Linxian adults, particularly with the combination of beta-carotene, vitamin E and selenium, may effect a reduction in cancer risk in this population. The results on their own are not definite, but the promising findings should stimulate further research to clarify the potential benefits of micronutrient supplementation.

Epidemiological studies have suggested a beneficial role for fruits and vegetables in the aetiology of several important forms of cancer.

However, this protective effect is not related to any single family of fruits and vegetables and the exact molecule(s) responsible for these effects is unknown. While eating more fruits and vegetables should reduce overall cancer risk, it is impossible to think of conducting a trial that randomizes individuals into two groups, one of which has an additional amount of fruits and vegetables added to their daily diet. It would, of course, be a tremendous achievement to identify the responsible elements in fruits and vegetables that confer this protection and to introduce them to the diet of the entire population.

This is an important finding (Blot et al., 1993) that is in its own way a landmark in epidemiology. The study demonstrates a reduction in cancer mortality among those receiving supplementation with beta-carotene, vitamin E and selenium. This is the first intervention study that has demonstrated a reduced rate of death from all causes among the group receiving supplementation and a reduced death rate of total cancer and stomach cancer in particular.

Thus, it has been shown for the first time that dietary supplementation can be used to reduce cancer rates in this study population. This is, of course, a special population with high cancer rates and a long history of low dietary intakes of several important micronutrients. The results from this population at a dietary extreme cannot be directly applied to most Western populations, where the diet is generally much richer in essential micronutrients. It is likely that in such a population as the latter it would take a much larger number of study participants to detect a significant reduction that may also be smaller in size. However, these findings do provide another important element to the role of antioxidants in cancer in general and should serve to stimulate both basic research and research in molecular epidemiology in this area.

Long-term studies are necessary if research on intervention is to make progress. Of course, if there were readily available intermediate end-points available they could be smaller and shorter. However, in the absence of such end-points, large studies lasting for many years are needed to investigate the efficacy of different intervention strategies. There are many difficulties in conducting such studies and organizing them. The logistics of following 30,000 individuals, supplying them with drugs, monitoring compliance and side effects, verifying end-points and follow-up is horrendous. Perhaps the greatest obstacle to conducting such studies lies in the ability to secure long-term financial support. Granting agencies are extremely reluctant to commit themselves to expensive and long-term support for individual research projects. This will be a limiting factor to making quick progress in this area: a reasonable level of funding and good organization can overcome the logistical hurdles. I think that it is of considerable significance that the funding for this study was from *internal* sources at the National Cancer Institute.

There is still much research needing to be done in the field of nutrition and cancer aetiology and it is now vital to have a closer collaboration between basic scientists and epidemiologists before greater progress can be made. A particularly contentious problem is the association between dietary fat intake and breast cancer. The meta-analysis of Boyd et al. (1993) makes an important contribution without solving all the problems. Despite a quantitative approach, there is still the subjective judgment to be made as to whether the reader only believes in the results from prospective studies ('no association') or case-control studies conducted outside North America ('positive association'). There is still great debate about the role of adult dietary fat intake in the aetiology of breast cancer and the issue will not be finally resolved by one analysis no matter how comprehensive or sophisticated. This study is, however, a very important contribution to the whole area. The authors take all studies published and use state-of-the-art statistical methodology to conduct a quantitative meta-analysis. The results are of great interest: however, they will not stop the debate raging among epidemiologists about the existence of the association between dietary fat intake and breast cancer risk, but the authors provide an important new data point in this great debate.

The demonstration of a protective effect of vitamin A supplementation among the lowest fifth of the range of dietary intakes stresses the need to conduct large, randomized intervention studies of this topic (Hunter et al., 1993). The demonstration of an effect of supplementation in such a randomized trial in China (Blot et al., 1993) gives great encouragement to proceed in this direction. However, there are difficulties of both a methodological nature and a financial nature to overcome before more large-scale trials of this nature can be performed in developed countries.

ACKNOWLEDGMENTS

This work was conducted within the framework of support from the *Associazione Italiana per la Ricerca sul Cancro* (Italian Association for Cancer Research).

REFERENCES

Abe R., Kumagai N. & Kimagai M. (1976) Biological characteristics of breast cancer in obesity. *Tohoku Journal of Experimental Medicine*, **120**, 351–9

Adami H.O., Bergstrom R., Persson I. & Sparen P. (1990) The incidence ovarian cancer in Sweden, 1960–1984. *American Journal of Epidemiology*, **132**, 446–52.

Albanes D., & Winick M. (1988) Are cell number and cell proliferation risk factors for cancer. *Journal of the National Cancer Institute*, **80**, 772–4.

Alexander F.E. & Boyle P. (1994) The rise in prostate cancer: myth or reality? In M.I. Garraway MJ (Ed.) *The epidemiology of prostate diseases*. Churchill Livingstone, Edinburgh.

American Academy of Sciences. (1982) *Nutrition and Cancer*. National Academy of Sciences, Washington, D.C.

Armstrong B.K. & Doll R. (1975) Environmental factors and cancer incidence and mortality in different countries, with special reference to dietary practices. *International Journal of Cancer*, **15**, 617–31.

Armstrong B.K., McMichael A.J. & McLennan R. (1982) Diet. In D. Schottenfeld & J. Fraumeni (Eds.): *Cancer epidemiology and prevention*. W.B. Saunders, Philadelphia.

Austin D.F. & Roe K.M. (1982) The decreasing incidence of endometrial cancer: public health implications. *American Journal of Public Health*, **72**, 65–8.

Begg C.B., Walker A.M., Wessen B. et al. (1983) Alcohol consumption and breast cancer. *Lancet*, **1**, 293–4.

Block G. (1991) Vitamin C and cancer prevention: the epidemiologic evidence. *American Journal of Clinical Nutrition*, **53**, 270–82.

Blot W.J., Li J.-Y., Taylor P., Guo W., Dawsey S., Wang G.-Q., Yang C.S., Zheng S.-F., Gail M., Li G.-Y., Yu Y., Liu B.-q., Tangrea J., Sun Y.-h., Liu F., Fraumeni J.F., Zhang Y.-H. & Li B. (1993) Nutrition Intervention Trials in Linxian, China: supplementation with specific vitamin/mineral combinations, cancer incidence, and disease-specific mortality in the general population. *Journal of the National Cancer Institute*, **85**, 1483–92.

Boyd N.F., Martin L.J., Noffel M., Lockwood G.A. & Tritchler D.L. (1993) A meta-analysis of studies of dietary fat and breast cancer risk. *British Journal of Cancer*, **68**, 627–36.

Boyd N.E., Campbell J.E., Germanson T., Thomson D.B., Sutherland D.J., & Meakin J.W. (1981) Body weight and prognosis in breast cancer. *Journal of the National Cancer Institute*, **67**, 785–9.

Boyle, P. (1988) The epidemiology of breast cancer. In U. Veronesi (Ed.) *Bailliere's Clinical Oncology*, **2**, 1–58.

Boyle P. & Leake R. (1988) Progress in understanding breast cancer: epidemiological and biological interactions. *Breast Cancer Research and Treatment*, **11**, 91–112.

Boyle P., Hsieh C.C. & Maisonneuve P. (1989) Descriptive epidemiology of breast cancer. In W. Zatonski & P. Boyle (Eds.) *100 years of vital statistics in Poland*. Inter-presse, Warsaw.

Boyle P. & Zaridze D.G. (1993) Risk factors for prostate and testicular cancer. *European Journal of Cancer*, **29A-7**, 1048–55.

Boyle P. (1994) Prostate cancer 2000: evolution of an epidemic of unknown origin. In L. Denis (Ed.) *Prostate cancer 2000*. Springer-Verlag, Heidelberg.

Boyle P., Evstifeeva T., Maisonneuve P., Macfarlane G.J. & Pagano F. Temporal trends in prostate cancer mortality: is the risk rising? *Journal of Urology* (submitted).

Boyle P. & Alexander F.E. (1994) Screening for prostate cancer: principles, methods and evaluation. *European Institute of Oncology Technical Report*, 94/03.

Boyle P., LaVecchia C., Maisonneuve P., MacFarlane G.J. & Zheng T. (1995) Cancer epidemiology and prevention. In M.J. Peckham, U. Veronesi & H. Pinedo (Eds.) *Oxford textbook of oncology*. Oxford University Press, Oxford.

Boyle P., Levi F., Lucchini F. & La Vecchia. (1993) Trends in diet-related cancers in Japan: a conundrum. *Lancet*, **342**, 752.

Byers T. & Funch D.P. (1982) Alcohol and breast cancer. *Lancet*, **1**, 799–800.

Van den Brandt P.A., van't Veer P., Goldbohm R.A., Dorant E., Volovics A., Hermus R.I.J. & Sturmans F. (1993) A prospective study on dietary fat and the risk of postmenopausal breast cancer. *Cancer Research*, **53**, 75–82.

Breslow N., Chan C.E., Dhom G., Drury R.A.B., Franks L.M., Gellei B., Lee Y.S., Lundberg S., Sparke B., Sternby N.H. & Tulinius H. (1977) Latent carcinoma of prostate at autopsy in seven areas. *International Journal of Cancer*, **20**, 680–8.

Corder E.H., Guess H.A., Hulka B., Friedman G.D., Sadler M., Vollmer R.T., Lobaugh B., Drezner M.K., Vogelman J.H. & Orentreich N. (1993) Vitamin D and prostate cancer: a prediagnostic study with stored data. *Cancer Epidemiol, Biomarkers and Prevention*, **2**, 467–72

Cuzick J. & Boyle P. (1988) Trends in cervix cancer mortality. *Cancer Surveys*, **7**(3), 417–41.

Devesa S.S., Silverman D.T., Young J.L. et al. (1987) Cancer incidence and mortality among whites in the United States, 1974–1984. *Journal of the National Cancer Institute*, **79**, 701–70.

de Waard F., Baanders-van Halewijn E.A., & Huizinga J. (1964) The bimodal age distribution of patients with mammary carcinoma. *Cancer*, **17**, 141–51.

de Waard F. & Baanders-van Halewijn E.A. (1974) A prospective study in general practice on breast cancer risk in post menopausal women. *International Journal of Cancer*, **14**, 153–60.

de Waard F., Cornelis J.P., Aoki K., & Yoshida M. (1977) Breast cancer incidence according to weight and height in two cities of the Netherlands and in Aichi prefecture, Japan. *Cancer*, **40**, 1269–75.

de Waard F. (1982) Nutritional etiology of breast cancer: where are we now, and where are we going? *Nutrition and Cancer*, **4**, 85–9.

de Waard F. & Trichopoulos D. (1988) A unifying theory of breast cancer aetiology. *International Journal of Cancer*, **41**, 666–9.

Enstrom J.E. (1980) Health and dietary practices and cancer mortality among California Mormons. In J. Cairns, L.J. Lyon, M. Skolnick (Eds.) *Cancer incidence in defined populations, Banbury report no. 4*. Cold Spring Harbor Laboratory, New York.

Friedenreich C.M., Howe G.R., Miller A.B. & Jain M.G. (1993) A cohort study of alcohol consumption and risk of breast cancer. American Journal of Epidemiology, **137**, 512–20.

Frisch R.E., Wyshak G., Albright N.L., Albright T.E., Schiff I., Jones K.P., Witschi J., Shiang E., Kuff E., Marguglio M. (1985) Lower prevalence of breast cancer and cancers of the reproductive system among former college athletes compared to nonathletes. *British Journal of Cancer*, **52**, 885–91.

Garland M., Willett W.C., Manson J.E. & Hunter D.J. (1993) Antioxidant micronutrients and breast cancer. *Journal of the American College of Nutrition*, **12**, 400–11.

Gaskill S.P., McGuire W.L., Osborn C.K. & Stern M.P. (1979) Breast cancer mortality and diet in the United States. *Cancer Research*, **39**, 3628–37.

Giovannucci E., Rimm E.B., Colditz G.A., Stampfer M.J., Ascherio A., Chute C.C. & Willett W.C. (1993) A prospective study of dietary fat and risk of prostate cancer. *Journal of the National Cancer Institute,* **85**, 1571–9.

Graham S. (1980) Diet and cancer. *American Journal of Epidemiology,* **112**, 247–52.

Graham S., Marshall J., Mettlin C., Rzepka T., Nemoto T. & Byers T. (1982) Diet in the epidemiology of breast cancer. *American Journal of Epidemiology,* **116**, 68–75.

Graham S. (1987) Alcohol and breast cancer. *New England Journal of Medicine,* **78**, 1211–13.

Graham S., Haughey B., Marshall J., Priore R., Byers T., Rzepka T., Mettlin C. & Pontes J.E. (1983) Diet in the epidemiology of carcinoma of the prostate gland. *Journal of the National Cancer Institute,* **70**, 687–92.

Graham S., Zielezny M., Marshall J., Priore R., Freudenheim J., Brasure J., Haughey B., Nasca P. & Zded M. (1992) Diet in the epidemiology of postmenopausal breast cancer in the New York State cohort. *American Journal of Epidemiology,* **136**, 1327–37.

Greenwald P., Damon A., Kirmss V. & Polan A.K. (1974) Physical and demographic features of men before developing cancer of the prostate. *Journal of the National Cancer Institute,* **53**, 341–6.

Griffiths K. et al. (1990) Endocrine factors in the initiation, diagnosis and treatment of prostatic cancer. In K. Voight & C. Knabbe (Eds.) *Endocrine dependent tumours,* Raven Press, New York.

Haenszel W. (1961) Cancer mortality among the foreign-born in the United States. *Journal of the National Cancer Institute,* **26**, 37–132.

Haenszel W.M. (1964) Contributions of end results data to cancer epidemiology. In S.J. Cutler (Ed.) *International symposium on end results of cancer therapy.* NCI Monograph 15, pp. 21–33.

Hakulinen T., Andersen A.A., Malker B. et al. (1987) Trends in cancer incidence in Nordic countries. *Acta Pathologica, Microbiologica et Immunologica Scandinavica (A), Supplement 288,* **94**, 1–269.

Harris R.E. & Wyner E.L. (1988) Breast cancer and alcohol consumption: a study in weak associations. *Journal of the American Medical Association* **259**, 2867–71.

Harvey E.B., Schairer M.S., Brinton L.A. et al. (1987) Alcohol consumption and breast cancer. *Journal of the National Cancer Institute,* **78**, 657–61.

Helmrich S.P., Shapiro S., Rosenberg L. et al. (1983) Risk factors for breast cancer. *American Journal of Epidemiology,* **117**, 35–45.

Hiatt R.A. & Bawol R.D. (1984) Alcoholic beverage consumption and breast cancer incidence. *American Journal of Epidemiology,* **120**, 676–83.

Hiatt R.A., Klatsky A.L. & Armstrong M.A. (1988) Alcohol consumption and the risk of breast cancer in a pre-paid health plan. *Cancer Research,* **48**, 2284–87.

Hill P., Wynder E.L., Garnes H. & Walker A.R.P. (1980) Environmental factors, hormone status and prostatic cancer. *Preventive Medicine,* **9**, 657–66.

Hirayama T. (1978) Epidemiology of breast cancer with special reference to the role of diet. *Preventive Medicine,* **7**, 173–95.

Hirohata T., Nomura A.M.Y., Hankin J.H., Kolonel K.N. & Lee J. (1987) An epidemiologic study on the association between diet and breast cancer. *Journal of the National Cancer Institute,* **78** 595–600.

Hislop T.G., Kan L., Coldman A.J. et al. (1988) Influence of oestrogen receptor status on dietary risk factors for breast cancer. *Canadian Medical Association Journal,* **138**, 424–30.

Howe G.R., Hirohata T., Hislop T.G. et al. (1990) Dietary fat and risk of breast cancer: combined analysis of 12 case-control studies. *Journal of the National Cancer Institute*, **82**, 561–69.

Howe G.R., Friedenreich C.M., Jain M. & Miller A.B. (1991) A cohort study of fat intake and risk of breast cancer. *Journal of the National Cancer Institute*, **83**, 336–40.

Hsing A., McLaughlin J., Schuman L., Bjelke E., Gridley G., Wacholder S., Co Chien H. et al. (1990) Diet, tobacco use and fatal prostate cancer: results of the Lutheran Brotherhood cohort study. *Cancer Research*, **50**, 6836–40.

Hunter D.J., Manson J., Colditz G.A., Stampfer M.J., Rosner B., Hennekens C.H., Speizer F.E. & Willett W.C. (1993) A prospective study of the intake of vitamins C, E, and A and the risk of breast cancer. *New England Journal of Medicine*, **329**, 234–40.

IARC (International Agency for Research on Cancer) Monographs on the Evaluation of the Carconogenic Risk of Chemicals to Man. (1986) *Volume 38. Tobacco smoking*. IARC,Lyon.

IARC (International Agency for Research on Cancer) Monographs on the Evaluation of Carcinogenic Risk to Humans. (1988) *Volume 44. Alcohol drinking*. IARC, Lyon.

IARC (International Agency for Research on Cancer) Monographs on the Evaluation of Carcinogenic Risk to Humans. (1991) *Volume 51. Coffee, tea, mate, methylxanthines (caffeine, theophylline, theobromine) and methylglyoxal*. IARC, Lyon.

Jones D.Y., Schatzkin A., Green S.B. et al. (1987) Dietary fat and breast cancer in the National Health and Nutrition Examination Survey I Epidemiologic Follow-up Study. *Journal of the National Cancer Institute*, **79**, 465–71.

Katsouyanni K., Trichopoulos D., Boyle P., Xirouchaki E., Trichopoulou A., Lisseos B., Vasilaros S. & MacMahon B. (1986) Diet and breast cancer: a case-control study in Greece. *International Journal of Cancer*, **38**, 815–20.

Kinlen L.J. (1980) Mortality in relation to abstinence from meat in certain orders of religious sisters in Britain. In J. Cairns, L.J. Lyon, M. Skolnick (Eds.) *Cancer incidence in defined populations*, pp 135–43, Banbury Report No. 4. Cold Spring Harbor Laboratory, New York.

Kinlen L.J., Hermon C. & Smith P.G. (1983) A proportional study of cancer mortality among members of a vegetarian society. *British Journal of Cancer*, **48**, 355–61.

Klatsky A.L., Armstrong M.A. & Friedman G.D. (1987) Alcohol consumption an 17-year cancer mortality. *American Journal of Epidemiology*, **126**, 770.

Knekt P., Albanes D., Seppanen R., Aromaa A., Jarvinen R., Hyvonen L., Teppo L. & Pukkala E. (1990) Dietary fat and risk of breast cancer. *Journal of the National Cancer Institute*, **83**, 336–40.

Kolonel L.N., Nomura A.M.Y., Lee J. & Hirohata T. (1986) Anthropomeric indicators of breast cancer risk in postmenopausal women in Hawaii. *Nutrition and Cancer*, **8**, 247–56.

Kushi L.H., Sellers T.A., Potter J.D., Nelson C.L., Munger R.G., Kaye S.A. & Folsom A.R. (1992) Dietary fat and postmenopausal breast cancer. *Journal of the National Cancer Institute*, **84**, 1092–9.

La Vecchia C., Franceschi S. & Decarli A. (1984) Oral contraceptive use and the risk of epithelial ovarian cancer. *British Journal of Cancer*, **50**, 31–4.

La Vecchia C., Decarli A., Franceschi S. et al. (1985) Alcohol consumption and the risk of breast cancer in women. *Journal of the National Cancer Institute*, **75**, 61–5.

La Vecchia C., Decarli A., Franceschi S. et al. (1987) Dietary factors and the risk of breast cancer. *Nutrition and Cancer*, **10**, 205–14.

La Vecchia C. (1989) Nutritional factors and cancers of the breast, endometrium and ovary. *European Journal of Cancer and Clinical Oncology*, **25**, 1945–51.

Lê M.G., Hill C. & Kramer A. (1984) Alcoholic beverage consumption and breast cancer in a French case-control study. *American Journal of Epidemiology*, **120**, 350–7.

Lê M.G., Moulton L.H., Hill C. & Kramer A. (1986) Consumption of dairy produce and alcohol in a case-control study of breast cancer. *Journal of the National Cancer Institute*, **77**, 633–6.

Lee H.P., Day N.E. & Shanmugaratnam K. (Eds.) (1988) *Trends in cancer incidence in Singapore 1968–1982*. IARC Scientific Publications No. 91, Lyon, IARC.

Le Marchand L., Kolonel L.N., Earle M.E. & Mi M.P. (1988) Body size at different periods of life and breast cancer risk. *American Journal of Epidemiology*, **128**, 137–52.

LeMarchand L., Kolonel L., Wilkens L.R., Myers B.C. & Hirohata T. (1994) Animal fat consumption and prostate cancer: a prospective study in Hawaii. *Epidemiology*, **5**, 276–82.

Lew E.A. & Garfinkel L. (1979) Variations in mortality by weight among 750,000 men and women. *Journal of Chronic Diseases*, **32**, 163–76.

Lin T.M., Chen K.P. & MacMahon B. (1971) Epidemiologic characteristics of cancer of the breast in Taiwan. *Cancer*, **27**, 1497–1504.

Locke F.B. & King H. Cancer mortality risk among Japanese in the United States. *Journal of the National Cancer Institute*, **65**, 1149–56.

Lubin J.H., Blot W.J. & Burns P.E. (1981) Breast cancer following high dietary fat and protein consumption. *American Journal of Epidemiology*, **114**, 422–37.

Lubin F., Wax Y., and Modan B. (1986) Role of fat, animal protein and dietary fiber in breast cancer aetiology: a case-control study. *Journal of the National Cancer Institute*, **77**, 605–12.

Lyon J.L., Gardner J.W. & West D.W. (1980) Cancer risk and lifestyle: Cancer among mormons from 1967–1975. In J. Cairns, J.L. Lyon, & M. Skolnick (Eds.) *Cancer incidence in defined populations. Banbury report no. 4.* Cold Spring Harbor, New York.

Miller A.B., Kelly A., Choi N.W., Mathews V., Morgan R.W., Munan L., Burch J.C., Feather J., Howe G.R. & Jain M. (1978) A study of diet and breast cancer. *American Journal of Epidemiology*, **107**, 499–509.

Miller A.B. & Bulbrook R.D. (1981) The epidemiology and etiology of breast cancer. *New England Journal of Medicine*, **305**, 1246–8.

Miller D.R., Rosenberg L., Clarke A.E. et al. (1987) Breast cancer risk and alcoholic beverage drinking. *American Journal of Epidemiology*, **126**, 736.

Mills P., Beeson L., Philips R. & Fraser G. (1989) Dietary habits and breast cancer incidence among Seventh Day Adventists. *Cancer*, **64**, 582–90.

Mirra A.P., Cole P. & MacMahon B. (1971) Breast cancer in an area of high parity: Sao Paulo, Brazil. *Cancer Research*, **31**, 77–83.

Monson R.R. & Lyon J.L. (1975) Proportional mortality among alcoholics. *Cancer*, **36**, 1077–9.

Morrison A.S., Black M.M., Lowe C.R., MacMahon B. & Yuasa S. (1973) Some international differences in histology and survival in breast cancer. *International Journal of Cancer*, **11**, 261–7.

Morrison A.S., Lowe C.R., MacMahon B., Ravnihar B. & Yuasa S. (1976) Some international differences in treatment and survival in breast cancer. *International Journal of Cancer*, **18**, 269–73.

Muir C.S., Choi N.W. & Schifflers E. (1980) Time trends in cancer mortality in some countries – their possible causes and significance. In *Proceedings of the Skandia International Symposium, Stockholm*, pp. 269–309.

Murphy W.M., Dean P.J., Brasfield J.A. & Tatum L. (1986) Incidental carcinoma of the prostate. *American Journal of Surgical Pathology*, **10**, 170–4.

National Board of Health and Welfare (of Sweden), The Cancer Registry. (1984) *Cancer Incidence in Sweden, 1981*. Stockholm socialstyrelsen.

Nomura A., Henderson B.E. & Leg J. (1978) Breast cancer and diet among Japanese in Hawaii. *American Journal of Clinical Nutrition*, **31**, 202–5.

O'Connell D.L., Hulka B.S., Chambless L.E., Wilkinson W.E. & Deubner, D.C. (1987) Cigarette smoking, alcohol consumption and breast cancer risk. *Journal of the National Cancer Institute*, **78**, 229–34.

Paganini-Hill A. & Ross R.K. (1983) Breast cancer and alcohol consumption. *Lancet*, **2**, 626–7.

Parazzini F., Negri E., La Vecchia C. et al. Population attributable risk for endometrial cancer in Northern Italy. *European Journal of Cancer and Clinical Oncology*, **25**, 1451–6.

Parazzini F., La Vecchia C., Negri E., Bruzzi P., Palli D., Brinton L. & Boyle P. (1990) Anthropometric variables and risk of breast cancer. *International Journal of Cancer*, **45**, 397–402.

Parkin D.M., Muir C.S., Whelan S., Gao Y.T., Ferlay J. & Powell J. (Eds.) *Cancer Incidence in Five Continents*, Vol. VI, IARC Scientific Publication Number 120. IARC, Lyon.

Parkin D.M., Pisani P. & Ferlay J. (1993) Estimates of the world wide incidence of eighteen major cancers in 1985. *International Journal of Cancer*, **54**, 594–606.

Persson I., Adami H.O. & Berkvist L. (1989) Risk of endometrial cancer after treatment with ostrogens alone or in conjunction with progestogens: results of a prospective study. *British Medical Journal*, **298**, 146–151.

Persson I., Schmidt M., Adami H.O., Bergstrom R., Petterson B. & Sparen P. (1990) Trends in endometrial cancer incidence and mortality in Sweden, 1960–1984. *Cancer Causes and Control*, **1**, 201–8.

Phillips R.L. (1975) Role of life-style and dietary habits in risk of cancer among Seventh Day Adventists. *Cancer Research*, **35**, 3513–22.

Phillips R.L., Kuzma J.W. & Lotz T.M. (1980) Cancer mortality among comparable members versus non-members of the Seventh Day Adventist Church. In J. Cairns, L.J. Lyon & M. Skolnick (Eds.) *Cancer incidence in defined populations, Banbury report no. 4*. Cold Spring Harbor Laboratory, New York.

Pike M.C. (1987) Age-related factors in cancers of the breast, ovary, and endometrium. *Journal of Chronic Diseases*, **40**, (Suppl. 2), 595–695.

Prentice R.L. & Sheppard L. (1990) Dietary fat and cancer: consistency of the epidemiologic data, and disease prevention that may follow from a practical reduction in fat consumption. *Cancer Causes and Control*, **1**, 81–98.

Reichman M.E., Judd J.T., Longcope C., Schatzkin A., Clevidence B.A., Nair P.P., Campbell W.S. & Taylor P.R. Effects of alcohol consumption on plasma and urinary hormone concentrations in premenopausal women. *Journal of the National Cancer Institute*, **85**, 722–7.

Richardson G.S., Scully R.E., Nikrui N. & Nelson J.H. (1985) Common epithelial cancer of the ovary. Part I. *New England Journal of Medicine,* **312**, 415–24.

Rohan T.E. & Bain C.J. (1987) Diet in the etiology of breast cancer. *Epidemiologic Reviews,* **9**, 120–145.

Rohan T.E. & McMichael A.J. (1988) Alcohol consumption and risk of breast cancer. *International Journal of Cancer,* **41**, 695–9.

Rohan T.E. & McMichael A.J. (1988) Oral contraceptive agents and breast cancer: a population-based case-control study. *Medical Journal of Australia,* **149**, 520–6.

Rose D.P. (1986) Dietary factors and breast cancer. *Cancer Surveys,* **95**, 671–88.

Rose D.P. & Boyar A.P. (1986) Dietary fat and cancer risk: the rationale for intervention. In B.S. Reddy, L.A. Cohen (Eds.) *Diet nutrition and cancer: a critical evaluation.* pp. 151–66. CRC Press, Boca Raton, FL.

Rosenberg L., Shapiro S., Slone D. et al. (1982) Epithelial ovarian cancer and combination oral contraceptives. *Journal of the American Medical Association,* **247**, 3210–12.

Shatzkin A., Jones D.Y., Hoover R.N., Taylor P.R., Brinton L.A., Ziegler R.G., Harvey E.B., Carter C.L., Licitra L.M., Dufour M.C. & Larson D.B. (1987) Alcohol consumption and breast cancer in the epidemiologic follow-up study of the first National Health and Nutrition Examination Survey. *New England Journal of Medicine,* **316**, 1169–73.

Shatzkin A., Palmer J.R., Rosenberg L., Helmrich S.P., Miller D.R., Kaufman D.W., Lesko S.M. & Shapiro S. (1987) Risk factors for breast cancer in black women. *Journal of the National Cancer Institute,* **78**, 213–17.

Schlesselman J.J. (1991) Oral contraceptives and neoplasia of the uterine corpus. *Contraception,* **43**, 557–79.

Schuman L.M., Mandel J., Blackard C., Bauer H., Scarlett J. & McHugh R. (1977) Epidemiologic study of prostatic cancer: preliminary report. *Cancer Treatment Reports,* **61**, 181–6.

Schuman L.M., Mandel J., Radke A. et al. (1982) Some selected features of the epidemiology of prostatic cancer: Minneapolis-St. Paul, Minnesota case-control study, 1976–1979. In K. Magnus (Ed.) *Trends in cancer incidence, causes and practical implications,* pp. 345–54. Hemisphere Press, Washington, D.C.

Schwartz G.G. & Hulka B.S. (1990) Is vitamin D deficiency a risk factor for prostate cancer? (Hypothesis).

Shu X.O., Brinton L.A., Gao Y.T. et al. (1989) Population-based case-control study of ovarian cancer in Shanghai. *Cancer Research,* **49**, 3670–4.

Shu X.O., Gao Y.T., Yuan J.M. et al. (1989) Dietary factors and epithelial ovarian cancer. *British Journal of Cancer,* **59**, 92–6.

Spitzer W.O. (1991) Meta-meta analysis: unanswered questions about aggregating data. *Journal of Clinical Epidemiology,* **44**, 103–7.

Steinmetz K.A. & Potter J.D. (1991) Vegetables, fruits and cancer. *Cancer Causes and Control,* **2**, 325–57.

Swanson C.A., Jones D.Y., Schatzkin A., Brinton L.A. & Ziegler R.G. (1988) Breast cancer risk assessed by anthropometry in NHANES 1 epidemiological followup study. *Cancer Research,* **48**, 5363–7.

Talamini R., La Vecchia C., DeCarli A. et al. (1986) Nutrition, social factors and prostatic cancer in a Northern Italian population. *British Journal of Cancer,* **53**, 817–21.

Tannenbaum A. (1940) Relationship of body weight to cancer incidence. *Archives of Pathology,* **30**, 508–17.

The Alpha-Tocopherol, Beta-Carotene Cancer Prevention Study Group. (1994) The effect of vitamin E and beta carotene on the incidence of lung cancer and other cancers in male smokers. *New England Journal of Medicine,* **330**, 1029–35.

Toniolo P., Riboli E., Protta F., Charrel M. & Cappa A.P.M. (1989) Calorie-providing nutrients and risk of breast cancer. *Journal of the National Cancer Institute,* **81**, 278–86.

Tonioli P., Riboli E., Shore R.E. & Pasternack B. (1994) Consumption of meat, animal products, protein, and fat and risk of breast cancer: a prospective study. *Epidemiology,* **5**, 391–7.

Trichopoulou A., Katsouyani K., Stuver S., Tzala L., Gnardellis C., Rimm E. & Trichopoulos D. (1995) Consumption of olive oil and specific food groups in relation to breast cancer risk in Greece. *Journal National Cancer Institute,* **87**, 110–7.

Valaoras V.G., MacMahon B., Trichopoulos D. & Polychronopoulou A. (1969) Lactation and reproductive histories of breast cancer patients in Greater Athens, 1965–1967. *International Journal of Cancer,* **4**, 350–61.

Warren M.P. (1980) The effects of exercise on pubertal progression and reproduction function in girls. *Journal of Clinical Endocrinology and Metabolism,* **51**,1150–7.

Webster L.A., Layde P.M., Wingo P.A. et al. (1983) Alcohol consumption and risk of breast cancer. *Lancet,* **2**, 724–6.

Willett W.C., Browne M.L., Bain C. et al. (1985) Relative weight and risk of breast cancer among premenopausal women. *American Journal of Epidemiology,* **122**, 731–40.

Willett W.C., Stampfer M.J., Colditz G.A., Rosner B.A., Hennekens C.H. & Speizer F.E. (1987) Dietary fat and the risk of breast cancer. *New England Journal of Medicine,* **316**, 22–8.

Willett W.C., Stampfer M.J., Colditz G.A., Rosner B.A., Hennekens C.H. & Speizer, F.E. (1987) Moderate alcohol consumption and risk of breast cancer. *New England Journal of Medicine,* **316**, 1174–80.

Willett W.C. (1989) *Nutritional epidemiology.* Oxford University Press, Oxford.

Willett W.C. & Stampfer M.J. (1990) Dietary fat and cancer: another view. *Cancer Causes Control,* **1**, 103–10.

Willett W.C., Hunter D.J., Stampfer M.J., Colditz G., Manson J.A.E., Spiegelman D., Rosner B.A., Hennekens C.H. & Speizer F.E. (1992) Dietary fat and fibre in relation to risk of breast cancer. *Journal of the American Medical Association,* **268**, 2037–44.

Williams R.R. & Horm J.W. (1977) Association of cancer sites with tobacco and alcohol consumption and socioeconomic status of patients: interview study from the Third National Cancer Survey. *Journal of the National Cancer Institute,* **58**, 525–47.

World Health Organisation. (1992) Trends in prostate cancer 1980–1988. *WHO Weekly Epidemiological Record,* **67**, 281–8.

Wynder E.L., Kajatani T. & Kuno J. (1963) Comparison of survival rates between American and Japanese patients with breast cancer. *Surgery, Gynecology and Obstetrics,* **117**, 196–200.

Wynder E.L., Escher G.C. & Mantel N. (1966) An epidemiological investigation of cancer of the endometrium. *Cancer,* **19**, 489–520.

Wynder E.L., Mabuchi K. & Whitmore W.F. (1971) Epidemiology of cancer of the prostate. *Cancer*, **28**, 344–60.

Zaridze D.G. & Boyle P. (1987) Cancer of the prostate: epidemiology and aetiology *British Journal of Urology*, **59**, 493–502.

Zemla B. (1984) The role of selected dietary elements in breast cancer risk among native and migrant populations in Poland. *Nutrition and Cancer*, **6**, 187–95.

Ziel H.K. & Finkle W.D. (1975) Increased risk of endometrial carcinoma among users of conjugated estrogens. *New England Journal of Medicine*, **293**, 1167–70.

PART 3

The Biological Basis for Treatment of Endocrine-Dependent Tumours

9

Breast Cancer: New Biological Approaches to Treatment

ROBERT B. DICKSON AND ROBERT CLARKE

INTRODUCTION

Normal breast development, breast carcinogenesis, and progression of breast cancer are all regulated by hormonal factors. The best defined of these factors are the steroids and peptides produced by the glandular epithelium of the ovaries, pituitary, endocrine pancreas, thyroid and adrenal cortex. These hormones act following initial interaction with either nuclear or cell surface receptors. In addition, normal and malignant mammary tissues are able to synthesize locally acting hormone-like substances acting as autocrine or juxtacrine regulators of cell growth. The polypeptide growth factors are the most widely studied of these local factors, which include prostaglandins and fatty acids. Polypeptide growth factors appear to act primarily through cell surface receptors, many of which function as protein kinases. In the mammary gland, a significant body of evidence suggests that the three main differentiated cell types communicate through paracrine mechanisms, but additional autocrine mechanisms may also exist, particularly for epithelial cells.

The mammary gland initially develops from an epithelial rudiment at the nipple. There is an initial stage of ductal penetration into the fat which seems to depend upon poorly defined, local factors. During the process of puberty, ductal elongation and branching occurs. This process is under positive regulation by ovarian oestrogenic steroids and pituitary growth hormone (or its local mediator, insulin-like growth factor I, IGF-I). The final stage in differentiation, known as lobuloalveolar development, occurs during pregnancy. Lobuloalveolar development is under the influence of many endocrine hormones and these include prolactin, growth hormone, insulin, glucocorticoids, estrogen and progesterone. When lobuloalveolar growth is completed, lactational differentiation takes over, and during this stage there may be direct, inhibitory effects of lactogenic hormones, such as prolactin, on local growth factor pathways as milk is produced (Fenton & Sheffield, 1993). Terminal epithelial differentiation results in secretory cells, which are characterized by their ability to produce milk proteins, such as casein, and lipids. Milk is also known to be a very rich source of growth factors, which may be important in mammary growth and differentiation as well as in neonatal development. Following weaning, withdrawal of the hormones of pregnancy is characterized by apoptosis of the differentiated luminal cells (Strange et al., 1992). The epithelial cells degrade their own DNA and the tissue undergoes autoproteolytic destruction as differentiated function is lost. A similar cyclicity occurs in the proliferation and development of the gland in the normal woman during the menstrual cycle (Anderson, Battersby & Macintyre, 1988). Proliferation of the epithelium is maximal in the luteal phase of the cycle, as progesterone in the presence of estrogen, peaks (Anderson, Battersby & Macintyre, 1988). Apoptosis then closely follows the cessation of proliferation. It is of special interest that proliferation in the mammary gland is out of phase with proliferation in the endometrium. Thus, the concept of progesterone as a hormone that opposes the actions of oestrogen on proliferation appears to be restricted to the endometrium.

It is probable that different types of ovarian-controlled, hormonally dependent proliferative processes occur in the mammary gland, according to developmental stage. During puberty, oestrogen-dependent growth may occur by expansion of a stem cell population within the invading, terminal ramifications of the ductal network. During normal cyclic proliferation and the cyclic proliferation of pregnancy-lactation, an oestrogen- and progesterone-dependent growth process may lead to expansion of a separate, or more differentiated 'stem cell' population within the ducts and their terminal alveoli (Daniel & Silberstein, 1987). It is likely that each of these distinct, hormone-dependent proliferative processes also depends upon poorly defined local influences from stromal cells. Historically, most studies of breast development, proliferation, differentiation and carcinogenesis have focussed on the epithelium. Recently, studies have focussed on the characterization of different mammary stromal cell types and their role in proliferation and differentiation (Haslam, 1990). An important feature of mammary differentiation is the organizing influence exerted by the basement membrane (Streuli, Bailey & Bissell, 1991). The basement membrane is a complex tissue lattice-like scaffold that is synthesized and assembled at the interface of epithelium and its underlying stroma. Its primary constituents include type IV collagen, laminin, fibronectin and heparin sulfate proteoglycans. Current research focusses on the processes of the regulatory influences governing synthesis, assembly and degradation. The basally located, scattered myoepithelial cells possess high levels of collagenase IV (Monteagudo et al., 1990) and may be critical in basement membrane turnover and gland remodelling.

Hormonal Control of Breast Cancer

Breast cancer is characterized by progressively disregulated proliferation, loss of certain epithelial characteristics, genomic instability and the development of metastases. Beatson, in the 1890s, established that ovarian endocrine influences are of primary importance in the control of metastatic breast cancer in premenopausal women. In rodent models of carcinogen-induced and spontaneous mammary cancer, it has been shown that both progesterone and oestrogens are able to support initial tumour formation and early tumour growth (Robinson & Jordan, 1987). It has also been shown that early stages in neoplasia are quite sensitive to growth factor stimulation (Medina et al., 1993), while the most malignant metastatic stages overproduce significant levels of growth factors and are refractory to their exogenous supplementation.

The prolonged administration of sustained high doses of oestrogens, and progestin can lead to the development of malignant mammary tumors in specific rodent strains. It is likely that the mechanism of action of oestrogens and progestins in both normal and malignant rodent and human breast is complex and involves oestrogen, acting through its receptor to induce expression of progesterone receptors. However, other mechanisms may also exist. For example, it may be that the oestrogenic and progestational components of the oral contraceptives are risk factors for breast cancer (Anderson, Battersby & Macintyre, 1988; McCarty, 1989; Committee on the relationship between oral contraceptives and breast cancer, 1991), but it now appears that the majority of women taking oral contraceptives do not have a significantly increased risk of breast cancer (Committee on the relationship between oral contraceptives and breast cancer, 1991). Established risk factors in breast cancer include family history, prior patient history and late pregnancy. An early pregnancy is protective (Committee on the relationship between oral contraceptives and breast cancer, 1991). Controversy surrounds the possibility that a high-fat diet places women at increased risk of the disease (Willett et al., 1992).

Oestrogen receptors (ERs) and progesterone receptors (PRs) have been localized by immunohistochemistry to a luminal subpopulation of ductal and lobular epithelial cells in women and rodents. Paradoxically, these receptors appear to be absent from terminal end-bud epithelial cells, the most proliferative regions of the gland. It is not yet clear whether steroid receptor positive cells serve a precursor role in breast cancer, although circumstantial evidence would appear to suggest the possibility (Dulbecco, 1990). About one third of breast cancers are hormonally responsive at the time they become metastatic. It is a paradox that in the treatment of human breast cancer, a variety of antihormonal therapies such as ovariectomy, hypophysectomy, GnRH agonists, aromatase inhibitors, antioestrogens and antiprogestogens, as well as oestrogen or progestogens have been used successfully to control metastatic disease (Early Breast Cancer Trialists' Collaborative Group, 1992).

As a general class, hormone unresponsive, ER- and PR-negative breast cancers seem to differ in many respects from their steroid receptor positive counterparts. These differences include higher proliferative and invasive rates, expression of certain growth factor receptors (high EGF and *erb*B_2 but low IGF-I receptors), elevated expression of drug metabolizing enzymes, more aberrant nuclear morphology, and loss of epithelial differentiation markers. These differences appear to indicate at least two distinct stages of differentiation of breast cancer (Vickers, Dickson & Cowan, 1988). It is not yet clear whether this arises because of the existence of multiple different cell types of tumour origin or because they represent different stages in the malignant progression from a single cancer precursor cell type. It is of interest that virtually all breast cancers are characterized by expression of ductal luminal keratins (Taylor-Papadimitriou & Lane, 1987). In addition, ER-positive cell lines have been observed in vitro to acquire the characteristics of ER-negative lines during the acquisition of resistance to adriamycin or the withdrawal of oestrogen (Vickers, Dickson & Cowan, 1988). These observations could be construed as an argument that breast cancers may be derived from a luminal, ER- and PR-positive stage of differentiation and that malignant progression could encompass wholesale phenotypic differentiation from this luminal lineage.

Oestrogen and progesterone and receptors

Measurements of ER predicate which patients are of good prognosis and may benefit from hormonal therapy. Although qualitative and quantitative measurements of the ER are employed to predict clinical responsivity of a tumour to hormonal therapy, this correlation is not absolute. Although more than 60% of human breast cancers are ER-positive, at best, only two thirds of these ER-positive tumors are expected to respond to endocrine therapy (Allegra & Lippman, 1980). In addition, 5 to 10% of the patients designated ER-negative respond to endocrine therapy. The progesterone receptor status has been used to increase the precision with which ER predicts prognosis. In normal endometrial tissue as well as in breast cancer cell lines, PR expression is regulated by oestrogen (Eckert & Katzenellenbogen, 1981). However, it is not known if ER regulates PR in normal human mammary epithelium or if ER and PR coexist in the same luminal cells. Although the presence of PR increases the likelihood of hormone dependency of a tumour, this relationship is not absolute. Retrospective studies have demonstrated that only 70% of PR-positive and 25 to 30% of PR-negative tumours respond to hormone therapy.

Reasons for this discrepancy between measured levels of receptors and their predictive values may include laboratory error, differential metabolism of tamoxifen, the ability of defective ER to regulate gene expression in the absence of ligand, the ability of defective or phosphorylated ER to bind ligand but not regulate gene expression, or their ability to induce constitutive synthesis of oestrogen-regulated proteins. In this context recent studies that established that alternatively spliced or mutant ERs with the potential to be constitutively activated may be common in breast cancer are of special interest (Dotzlaw, Alkhalaf & Murphy, 1992). Additional, more informative ER assays, such as binding of the ER to an oestrogen-responsive DNA element (ERE) or mutational analysis of ER by the polymerase chain reaction (PCR) or other techniques, may be necessary to more accurately predict tumour response to endocrine therapy.

Some uncertainty underlies the different function of ER as expressed endogenously in ER-positive lines versus heterotypically by expression vector in formerly ER-negative breast cancer cell lines. Several studies have shown that in contrast to its function in ER-positive cell lines, ER expressed in ER-negative cell lines functions to suppress cell growth while functioning normally in other respects (Jiang & Jordan, 1992). It is not yet established whether this is due to dominant or recessive genes. However, a recent study with an antioestrogen resistant, ER-positive but PR-negative subline of MCF-7 suggests that loss of PR expression is a recessive phenotype (Paik, Blair & Lippman, 1992). The cellular enzyme protein kinase C has been recently implicated in down-modulation of ER mRNA, inactivation of ER function, and in independently inducing some oestrogen-responsive genes with AP-1 sites in their promoters during malignant progression. Protein kinase C consists of cytoplasmic-nuclear enzymes with serine-threionine specificity for phosphate addition to other cellular proteins. It has been shown that protein kinase C is more highly expressed in ER-negative and drug resistant breast cancer as compared with ER-positive breast cancer. Stimulation of ER-positive breast cancer with an activator of protein kinase C, such as the phorbol ester 12-0-tetradeconyl phorbol-13-acetic (TPA or PMA) leads to down-regulation of ER and destabilization of its mRNA and phosphorylation of residual ER coincident with loss of its function (Tzuckerman, Zhang & Pfahl, 1991; Saceda et al., 1991). Other current investigations suggest that other sites of phosphorylation of ER and PR induced by growth factors, cAMP, dopamine agonists, and other hormones may constitutively activate the steroid receptors (Aronica & Katzenellenbogen, 1993).

MECHANISMS OF ACTION OF ANTIHORMONES AND CYTOTOXIC DRUGS

Common Interactions and Effects

The majority of breast tumours are initially responsive to both cytotoxic drugs and to various endocrine therapies. There are compelling theoretical reasons to combine chemotherapy and hormonal treatment. However, there have been few studies that have rigorously used in vivo experimental models to determine the nature of chemohormonal interactions and resistance, and to obtain data that would establish a scientific rather than a theoretical basis for designing chemohormonal regimens. Early studies were based on the simplistic rationale that cytotoxic drugs would preferentially kill the proliferating, generally hormone-unresponsive cells, while endocrine treatments would kill the more slowly proliferating hormone-dependent cells. Although this remains a valid concept, it is now apparent that there is considerable complexity in the interactions among cytotoxic drugs and hormones. For example, both agents can produce effects on cell cycle distribution. Endocrine agents can reverse multidrug resistance (Leonessa et al., 1994) and cytotoxic drugs can reduce response to antioestrogens (Clarke et al., 1986). We will discuss the relevance of some of the more recently described interactions in the following sections.

Antioestrogens – Mechanism of Action

It is widely accepted that the inhibitory effects of antioestrogens are primarily mediated through interactions with the ER.

The ability of tamoxifen to compete with oestrogen for binding to ER in vitro has been extensively described. This interaction appears complex, rather than reflecting a simple competitive inhibition of oestrogen binding. Many antioestrogens are inhibitory in the absence of oestrogen (Clarke et al., 1989). It has therefore been suggested that the antioestrogen/ER complex may have intrinsic inhibitory properties (Clarke et al., 1989). This implies that the antioestrogen/ER complex may itself have the ability to directly influence the expression of specific genes.

The ligand-occupied ER is a nuclear protein with gene regulatory functions mediated through binding to specific ERE. The affinity of the tamoxifen/ER complex for double-stranded DNA is significantly less than that of oestrogen/ER complex (Evans, Baskevitch & Rochefort, 1982). The ability of the antioestrogen/ER/ERE structures to subsequently influence gene expression appears to be significantly less than that of the oestrogen ER/ERE complexes. The partial agonist properties of tamoxifen and its metabolites may be the result of the antioestrogen/ER complex binding to ERE. The steroidal antioestrogen ICI 182,780 is a pure antagonist. The ICI 182,780/ER complex appears to alter receptor dimerization and turnover (Dauvois et al., 1992). The genes that are specifically influenced by these antioestrogen/ER interactions are unknown, but probably include those responsible for influencing TGF-β production, secretion and activation (Knabbe et al., 1987). PR expression also is induced by tamoxifen. Information is not available that allows us to fully evaluate the biological effects of antioestrogen binding to calmodulin, protein kinase C, or to membrane calcium channels, or neurotransmitter receptors of antioestrogen-induced perturbations in membrane function (Knabbe et al., 1987). These interactions occur at high doses of antioestrogens and in tumour cells regardless of their ER content and their biological relevance is unclear. Antioestrogens have systemic effects on immunological function that may also be important in the context of lymphoreticular cell infiltration in some breast tumours where the major desmoplastic components include mediators of cellular immunity.

Antioestrogens – Cell Cycle Effects

The withdrawal of hormones from hormone-dependent tissues is often accompanied by a decrease in growth fraction, which may be the result of an induction of apoptosis. Inhibition of human breast cancer cells growing in vitro by tamoxifen is also associated with a reduced rate of incorporation of [^{3}H]-DNA precursors into DNA (Clarke et al., 1986).

Cell populations rescued from tamoxifen inhibition by oestrogen treatment enter S phase in a synchronous manner. Oestrogen leads to a 50% reduction in G_0/G_1 and a 175% increase in S phase cells. Various studies have shown that tamoxifen induces a blockade in early G_1 in MCF-7 cells growing in vitro (Benz et al., 1983) which results in reduced recruitment of cells into S phase.

Results obtained with MCF-7 and T61 tumor xenografts growing in athymic nude mice have been contradictory. While tamoxifen inhibits the T61 human breast cancer xenograft, there is no clear blockade in $G_0\backslash G_1$ (Brunner et al., 1985). The tamoxifen-induced inhibition of MCF-7 cell growth has not been confirmed by in vivo studies which have shown tamoxifen increased cell loss without significant alterations in cell cycle profile (Brunner et al., 1989; Osborne, Coronado & Robinson, 1987). Clearly, a final resolution of the mechanisms of in vivo $G_0\backslash G_1$ tumour blockade by tamoxifen is required.

Cytotoxic Drugs – Cell Cycle Effects

The majority of cytotoxic drugs used in the treatment of breast cancer exhibit marked cell cycle specificity. Agents such as methotrexate and 5-fluorouracil (5-FU) act close to the G_1/S boundary; Others such as the vinca alkaloids act in M phase. Cells that are not killed by these agents may ultimately progress through the cell cycle. However, these cells have frequently acquired considerable genetic damage, and they or their subsequent generations may fail to complete further cell cycles. In some cases, the degree of genetic damage is sufficient to trigger apoptosis, a process often associated with G_0/G_1 arrest.

Since the targets for many cytotoxic drugs are closely associated with specific cell cycle related events, most of these agents are primarily effective in rapidly cycling cell populations. Tumours with high growth fractions and/or growth rates are generally most sensitive to the effects of cytotoxic drugs. The most effective sequential combination chemotherapy regimens are often those where the drugs are administered coincident with the cell kinetic recovery from response to a prior agent. For example, recovery from S-phase specific agent is accompanied by an increase in the number of cells in S/G_2, thereby producing a cell population more sensitive to the cytotoxic effects of an agent acting in a later phase of the cell cycle. Combination chemotherapy using drugs acting in different phases of the cell cycle has been used to effect in the treatment of testicular cancer and many other tumours.

Effects of Endocrine Therapies on ER Expression

Various cytotoxic drugs used in the treatment of breast cancer can transiently reduce ER expression in breast cancer cells in vitro, and these agents include Adriamycin, methotrexate, 5-FU, vincristine and melphalan (Clarke et al., 1986; Muller et al., 1980). ER levels can recover rapidly following only one cycle of cytotoxic treatment (Clarke et al., 1986; Yang & Samaan, 1983). However, prolonged exposure to Adriamycin, sufficient to induce stable resistance, results in a permanent loss of both ER and PGR expression (Vickers et al., 1988). Both the transient and constitutive down-regulation of steroid hormone receptors are sufficient to markedly reduce or completely ablate sensitivity to antioestrogens (Vickers et al., 1988).

Clinical studies reporting cytotoxic drug-induced alterations in ER levels in breast cancer patients have led to contradictory reports. While changes from ER positivity to negativity have been reported after relapse from tamoxifen therapy (Encarnacion et al., 1993), the majority of tumours do not appear to change their ER status following chemotherapy (Allegra & Lippman, 1980). Whether remaining ERs are fully functional is unclear. However, the ability of cells in vitro to recover ER expression rapidly following one course of cytotoxic drug treatment (Clarke et al., 1986) is more suggestive of a transient rather than constitutive loss of ER expression/function.

The mechanisms responsible for the drug-induced inhibition of ER expression remain unknown. It is possible that cytotoxic agents that can alter protein function (e.g., alkylating agents that induce protein cross-linkage) could interact directly with the ER protein and inhibit its ability to bind ligand or antibodies. We and others have observed that cytotoxic drugs do not alter the affinity of ER for ligand (Clarke et al., 1986; Muller et al., 1980; Yang & Samaan, 1983; Morris & Stephen, 1983). Thus, significant allosteric inhibition seems unlikely. Since ER ligands exhibit considerable stereospecificity, competitive inhibition also seems unlikely. 5-FU is often misincorporated into RNA and so may inhibit ER expression by reducing receptor synthesis (Clarke et al., 1986). Adriamycin, melphalan and vincristine all inhibit ER synthesis, but this occurs at concentrations where these agents do not significantly alter the rate of total protein synthesis (Clarke et al., 1986). Drugs such as Adriamycin that intercalate within DNA and those such as melphelan that can crosslink DNA strands could alter the rate of ER gene transcription. Alterations in mRNA stability and rates of transcription or translation may also contribute to cytotoxic drug-induced reductions in ER levels.

DRUG AND ENDOCRINE RESISTANCE

The Antioestrogen Resistant Phenotype

The acquisition of antioestrogen resistance by antioestrogen-responsive tumours occurs with a very high frequency. However, rather than attempt to reverse or delay the acquisition of resistance, most therapeutic strategies involve the cessation of hormone treatment and subsequent cytotoxic chemotherapies. The lack of resistance-modifying regimens reflects the paucity of information concerning the primary mechanism of resistance. The most widely accepted mechanism of action for antioestrogens relate to the events resulting from the association of antioestrogen with ER as described above. Consequently, the agents currently identified that appear capable of perturbing sensitivity to antioestrogens appear to function through increasing the level of expression of ER. It remains unclear whether a loss of ER expression and/or function is the primary mechanism for antioestrogen resistance. Tumor heterogeneity for ER expression metabolism of triphenylethylenes to oestrogenic metabolites and reduced cellular drug accumulation have all been implicated as potential resistance mechanisms.

Agents that Increase ER Expression – Interferons

Interferons have demonstrated little significant clinical activity when administered as single agents or in combination with other drugs. However, interferons potentiate the inhibitory effects of antioestrogens in ER-positive human breast cancer cells in vitro. For example, interferon-α2 increases the antiproliferative effects of tamoxifen in ZR-75-1 cells (Van Den Berg et al., 1987). Combinations of interferon-β (Goldstein et al., 1989; Kangas, Nieminen & Cantell, 1985) and/or interferon-γ and antioestrogens can interact synergistically in some experimental models (Van Den Berg et al., 1987; Porzsolt et al., 1989; Goldstein et al., 1989; Kangas, Niemann & Cantell, 1985).

The effects of antioestrogens are primarily mediated through ER, and those of interferon through interactions with their own specific receptors. Specific receptors for interferons have been demonstrated on ZR-75-1 (Kangas, Niemann & Cantell, 1985), MCF-7 and Hs578T human breast cancer cell lines (Goldstein et al., 1989). Tamoxifen upregulates expression of interferon receptors in ZR-75-1 cells (Kangas, Niemann & Cantell, 1985). ER expression in ZR-75-1 (Van Den Berg et al., 1987) and MCF-7 cells (Martin et al., 1991) is increased following exposure to human interferon-α. Interferon-β increases ER levels in CG-5 human breast cancer cells (Bezwoda & Meyer, 1990). Fibroblast interferon increases ER levels in the skin metastases of breast cancer patients. While some investigators have not observed interferon-induced effects on ER, the ability of interferons to modulate antioestrogen responsiveness/resistance appears to be established.

The effects of interferon/antioestrogen combinations in vitro are generally observed at noninhibitory concentrations (Bezwoda & Meyer, 1990). Thus, comparable clinical regimens could utilize doses of interferons that are not associated with significant dose-limiting toxicity. Preliminary clinical data are emerging in support of the data obtained from the in vitro and in vivo experimental models. The results are encouraging (Porzsolt et al., 1989; Recchia et al., 1990) and indicate that further studies clearly are warranted.

Agents That Increase ER Expression – Retinoids

Retinoids can lead to a prolongation of the secretory status of normal mammary glandular epithelium growing in vitro (Strum & Reseau, 1986). The majority of ER-positive human breast cancer cell lines express retinoic acid receptors (Marth, Mayer & Daxenbichler, 1984). Retinoic acid increases ER expression in MCF-7 cells (Batra & Bengstonn, 1978). Retinoic acid also inhibits the expression of FGF-2 (bFGF), FGF-4 (kFGF) and TGF-α in a human teratocarcinoma cell line (Miller et al., 1990). Since these growth factors are implicated in breast cancer cell growth and mediating the effects of oestrogens, it may be that they have a regulatory role in their makeup. Retinoids affect cell-mediated immunity and have been implicated in mediating antioestrogen inhibition through an immunomodulatory effect.

Noncross-Resistance Between Triphenylethylene and Steroidal Antioestrogens

Responses to second-line endocrine therapy may follow an initial response or a failure to respond to a prior endocrine treatment. Since the steroidal and nonsteroidal antioestrogens may use different post-receptor binding mechanisms to inhibit cells, we wished to address the issue of cross-resistance between these two agents. We have selected hormone-independent MCF-7 variants (Brunner et al., 1993). Cells resistant to 4-hydroxytamoxifen in vitro and in vivo (MCF-7/LCC-2) retain ER expression, hormone-independent growth both in vivo and in vitro, and some degree of oestradiol responsivity (Brunner et al., 1993). Furthermore, MCF-7/LCC-2 cells are not cross-resistant to the steroidal antioestrogens ICI 182,780 (Brunner et al., 1993) and ICI 164,384 (Coopman et al., 1994). These data suggest that patients failing tamoxifen might respond to a steroidal antioestrogen. Preliminary data clearly demonstrate responses to ICI 182,780 in patients that have failed tamoxifen (Nicholson et al., 1993). Thus, the endocrine responsiveness of the MCF-7/LCC-2 cells accurately predicted a pattern of endocrine responsiveness not previously reported in breast cancer patients.

Antihormone Effects on *MDR1*-mediated Drug Resistance

A multidrug-resistant phenotype is characterized by the expression of a plasma-membrane-associated 170-kDa glycoprotein (gp170), the product of the human *MDR1* gene. This protein acts as a chemotherapy drug efflux pump. Many of the more widely used drugs in breast cancer treatment, including the vinca alkaloids and the anthracycline antibiotics, are substrates for gp170. Expression of *MDR1* mRNA and/or gp170 has been widely reported in breast tumours (Sanfilippo et al., 1991; Verrelle et al., 1991). In some studies, detectable levels of its expression in breast tumours correlate with failure of cytotoxic chemotherapy (Sanfilippo et al., 1991), poor prognosis (Verrelle et al., 1991) and/or in vitro resistance to cytotoxic drugs (Sanfilippo et al., 1991). However, other groups have failed to demonstrate *MDR1*/gp170 expression in breast tumours (Merkel et al., 1989). The precise functional and biological relevance of gp170-mediated multidrug resistance in breast cancer is undetermined.

The level of gp170/*MDR1* expression in breast tumours is generally much lower than that observed in the other solid tumours that can acquire this form of multidrug resistance (Merkel et al., 1989). The level of expression required to induce a clinically resistant tumour has not been established. However, the narrow therapeutic window associated with these drugs implies that a low level of expression may be sufficient at least in some tissues.

While several hormonal agents have been demonstrated to either partly reverse gp170-mediated multidrug resistance in vitro or bind to gp170 (Brunner et al., 1989; Osborne, Coronado & Robinson, 1987; Chatterjee & Harris, 1990), many studies used MCF-7–derived MCF-7^{ADR} cells that express multiple drug resistance mechanisms considerably greater than that achievable in patients we have transfected

MCF-7 cells with a retroviral vector encoding for the constitutive expression of the *MDR1* gene (Clarke et al., 1992). These cells retain sensitivity to the ER-mediated inhibitory effects of tamoxifen.

Since tamoxifen alone has inhibitory effects in these cells, it was necessary to utilize an experimental design that would enable us to determine the nature of its interaction with gp170 substrates in *MDR1*-resistant cells. We performed extensive isobologram analyses of cytotoxicity data, and observed that tamoxifen interacts synergistically with both vinblastine and Adriamycin in MCF-7^{MDR1} cells (Leonessa et al., 1994). These data have clear implications for the design of clinical trials to investigate the gp170-reversing abilities of tamoxifen in cancer patients.

GROWTH FACTORS, RECEPTORS AND ONCOGENES IN TUMOUR GROWTH AND PROGRESSION

Identification of Relevant Growth Factors

Recent studies have begun to address the local tissue effects of oestrogen and progesterone in the promotion and growth of malignancy. Tissue regulation by these hormones is modulated in a complex fashion by growth factors, cellular adhesion molecules and diverse serum actions. There has been great interest in locally acting peptide hormones as mediators and modulators of steroid action. Early studies pointed to the importance of the transforming growth factors (TGFs) in breast cancer. This group of growth factors is now known to represent several families of polypeptides that are synthesized and secreted by a wide variety of normal and retroviral, chemical or oncogene-transformed human and rodent cell lines.

Two major classes of structurally and functionally distinct transforming growth factor families have been defined: TGFα and TGFβ. TGFα and TGFα–like peptides are members of a large family ranging from apparent molecular masses of 6 kDa to at least 44 kDa. Most members of this family compete with the EGF for binding to the same receptor, activate receptor tyrosine-specific kinase activity and have growth stimulatory properties. The TGFα–related growth factors are all single-chain polypeptides with a consensus pattern of three intrachain disulfide bonds. The most well-characterized family members bind to a common receptor (EGF receptor) and include TGFα, epidermal growth factor (EGF), vaccinia growth factor (VGF), amphiregulin, heparin-binding EGF (Hb EGF) and a factor termed cripto-1. More recently, another family member, termed betacellulin (Eckert et al., 1991) has been cloned. Finally, a separate heparin-binding subfamily which includes heregulin and *neu*-differentiating factor (NDF) has been identified and cloned. Rat and human homologues are identical in sequence, and do not appear to bind to the EGF receptor (Falls et al., 1991). NDF and heregulin bind to *erb*B_2. EGF receptor, c-*erb*B, c-*erb*B_3, and c-*erb*B_4 make up a very closely related family of tyrosine kinase–linked receptors. Contrary to initial reports, recent work has suggested that heregulin/NDF binds directly to the *erb*B_4 receptor and may associate only indirectly to *erb*B_2 (Plowman et al., 1993). No ligands for the *erb*B_3 receptor are known. All four of these receptors and all of the EGF-related growth factors except VGF and betacellulin have been detected in breast cancer.

The TGF-β family of growth factors consists of at least three related gene products, each forming 25-kDa homodimeric species, all of which are found in breast cancer. There is a complex pattern of interaction of these species with two separate soluble-binding proteins and with the three molecular weight classes of TGF-β receptors. Members of each class of these receptors have now been cloned and sequenced. While one of these receptors appears to be a nonsignalling, binding protein, the others appear to deliver signals via a serine-threonine specific kinase activity. TGF-β and TGF-α have been found in the urine, as well as pleural and peritoneal effusions of cancer patients (Butzou et al., 1993) and in some normal tissues (Basilico & Moscatelli, 1992). In addition, TGF-β overexpression is associated with progression of breast cancer (Gorsch, 1992). Treatment of normal and malignant epithelial tissue with TGF-β of all subtypes generally has a growth inhibitory and sometimes differentiating effect. Three other inhibitory factors may be relevant to breast cancer: mammary-derived growth inhibitor (MDGI) (Grosse et al., 1992), mammostatin (Ervin et al., 1989) and α-lactalbumin (Thompson et al., 1992). The existence of receptors for these three factors have not been established at present.

At least five other classes of growth factors are also relevant to breast cancer. Insulin-like growth factors, multiple binding proteins, platelet-derived growth factors A and B and fibroblast growth factors have been under intense study for several years. Each of these growth factors binds to its own multimember class of tyrosine-kinase-encoding receptors. A recently described growth factor, mammary-derived growth factor 1 (MDGF-1), has been found in human milk and in conditioned medium from human breast cancer cell lines (Bano, Solomon & Kidwell, 1985). This glycosylated, monomeric, non–disulfide-linked 62-kDa growth factor stimulates stromal collagen production and may also play a role in growth regulation of normal and malignant human mammary epithelium. Its receptor is known to include a 130-kDa protein that also stimulates tyrosine phosphorylation of a 180-kDa cellular protein (Bano et al., 1990).

It has been suggested that transformation of cells from normal to malignant may be indirectly associated with or may directly result from increased production of growth stimulatory factors or decreased production of growth inhibitory substances. Other hypotheses invoke altered responsiveness to either or both of transforming groups of growth factors. To fully test these hypotheses it is important to understand pathways of growth control in neoplastic cells, and in the normal cells from which the cancer is derived. Recent developments in serum-free culture conditions have facilitated the study of growth regulation in normal human mammary epithelial cells. Though human mammary epithelial cells may now be cultured in vitro, it is not yet clear that the cultured subtype is of the lineage or differentiation type(s) that would give rise to breast cancer in a woman. For example, receptors for oestrogen and progesterone have not been demonstrated in these cells, and some populations appear to have a basal epithelial 'stem cell' character.

Studies on steroid-growth factor interactions in human mammary tissue have been restricted to the malignant epithelium. In hormone responsive human breast cancer cells, growth stimulation by oestrogen is accompanied by an increase in growth stimulatory TGF-α and IGF-II production (King et al., 1989), whereas growth inhibition of hormone responsive breast cancer cell lines in vitro and primary tumours in vivo by an antioestrogen is paralleled by augmented secretion of growth inhibitory TGF-β (Butta et al., 1992). Similar effects have been observed with progestins: TGF-α, EGF and the EGF receptor was induced, while TGF-β was inhibited (antiprogestins had the opposite effect) (Musgrove, Lee & Sutherland, 1991). Steroids and growth factors have also been observed to cooperate in the induction of certain other indicator genes such as pS2 and cathepsin D (Musgrove, Lee & Sutherland, 1991). In hormone independent breast cancer cell lines, growth factors are constitutively produced. These results are consistent with, but do not prove, a role for growth factors in the expression of a more malignant phenotype and escape from normal hormonal control.

Regulation of Growth Factors

Recent studies have begun to evaluate the mechanisms and consequences of induction of TGF-α and TGF-β family members. TGF-α, amphiregulin and TGF-β_2 are both under transcriptional control by oestrogen and antioestrogen, but the effects of progestins and antiprogestins have been less well characterized. The transcriptional regulation of TGF-α depends upon a palindromic, imperfect consensus ERE in the region of the gene 5′ to the coding region (Saeki et al., 1991). Oestrogenic regulation of the TGF-α–regulated factor amphiregulin has also been demonstrated (Normanno et al., 1993). Under typical cell culture conditions in plastic dishes oestrogen stimulates while progestins inhibit proliferation of hormone responsive breast cancer cell lines. In contrast, in anchorage independent colony formation in soft agar culture, both oestrogen and progesterone can be growth stimulatory. Under such anchorage independent conditions, it has been shown, using antigrowth factor antibodies that oestrogen and progesterone induced TGF-α and inhibited TGF-β (Manni, Wright & Buck, 1991). One study (Colletta et al., 1991) has shown that under anchorage dependent conditions the novel synthetic progestin gestodine inhibits hormone dependent breast cancer cells partly via TGF-β induction.

Growth factor and growth factor receptor genes have been transfected into hormone responsive breast cancer cell lines to study malignant progression. While transfection of TGF-α or the EGF receptor had very little effect, minor growth-enhancing effects have been reported for the IGF-II gene and for the *erb*B^2 proto-oncogene. In striking contrast, very strong enhancement of tumor growth and the development of metastases was observed after transfection of FGF-4 into MCF-7 cells. Whether this enhancement is a direct or indirect effect is not yet known.

Finally, studies in vivo in the nude mouse are providing additional perspectives on the roles of growth factors in breast cancer proliferation. Infusion of EGF or IGF-I is capable of limited stimulation of tumor growth of MCF-7 implanted in the athymic nude mouse (Dickson, McManaway & Lippman, 1986). TGF-β infusions in the nude mouse nodes were carried out in an attempt to block proliferation of the highly responsive MDA-MB-231 cell line. Unexpectedly, tumor growth was unaffected but the animals developed cachexia, multiple organ fibrosis and splenic regression (Zugmaier et al., 1991). The effects of endogenous TGF-β produced by hormone independent breast tumours have been further characterized and neutralizing anti–TGF-β antibodies have been shown to suppress tumour growth and enhance natural killer cell (NK) immune function (Arteaga et al., 1993).

Thus a new picture of growth factor function is emerging from in vivo studies. In normal breast tissue the function of growth factors may include stimulation of epithelial proliferation by TGF-α, IGF and members of the FGF family and inhibition of epithelial proliferation by TGF-β and other inhibitory factors. However, in cancer, growth factor overproduction, perturbation of signal transduction mechanisms, and loss of tissue compartmentalization may lead to aberrant function. This may contribute to tumour growth and the development of metastases and by the process of angiogenesis or blood vessel infiltration (TGF-β, FGF), desmoplasia and collagen deposition (MDGF-1, TGF-β, TGF-α) and immune suppression (TGF-β). Some of these tumour–host interactions are described in greater detail in later sections of this chapter.

EGF RECEPTOR AND *erb*B$_2$ AS TARGETS OF THERAPY

EGF Receptor (EGFR)

In comparing hormone dependent and hormone independent breast cancer cell lines and tumours the absence of ER in conjunction with expression of high levels of EGFR is often noted (Klijn et al., 1992). The EGFR is a 170,000-dalton transmembrane glycoprotein with tyrosine kinase activity. Binding of EGF to its receptor results in the intracellular internalization and down-regulation of the receptor, and also leads to autophosphorylation of EGFR in addition to phosphorylation of other substrates. Overexpression of EGFR has been shown to result in EGF-dependent transformation of rodent fibroblasts, implicating the receptor in the process of cellular transformation. The extensive homology between EGFR and the avian erythroblastosis v-*erb*B oncogene also strongly suggests that EGFR is the cellular homologue of v-*erb*B (Downward et al., 1984).

High EGFR levels in breast tumours have been shown to correlate strongly with a poor prognosis, independent of ER status (Klijn et al., 1992). In addition, high expression of EGFR seems to occur early in the natural history of such breast cancers; its overexpression is detected simultaneously in primary and metastatic biopsies of breast cancer (Lacroix et al., 1989). Most studies with clinical specimens have utilized a membrane binding assay for EGFR. There is a great need to develop a standardized immunohistochemical approach to quantify EGFR in paraffin-fixed clinical biopsy material. High expression of EGFR is often accompanied by a low-level expression of ER, suggesting a mechanistic link between up-regulation of EGFR and hormone independence (Klijn et al., 1992). This inverse correlation also holds true in many breast cancer cell lines, with EGFR expression varying by more than two orders of magnitude from ER-positive to

ER-negative cells (Davidson et al., 1990). Additionally, substances that alter EGFR and ER expression, such as oestrogen and phorbol esters (e.g., TPA), generally have opposite effects on these two receptors (Saceda et al., 1991).

The usefulness of EGFR as a prognostic indicator and its inverse relationship with ER in both tumours and cell lines point out our need to understand the mechanisms that control EGFR in breast cancer. To date, there are few data on the molecular basis of EGFR gene expression in this disease. In general, human tumour cell lines exhibit substantial variation in their level of EGFR (King et al., 1985), and the mechanisms responsible for elevated EGFR can also differ. Cell lines have been identified with EGFR gene amplification accompanied by gene rearrangements that produce altered transcripts, gene amplification without rearrangement and overexpression of EGFR in the absence of gene amplification. Human cell lines with a nonrearranged EGFR gene contain two major species of EGFR mRNA (10 kb and 5.6 kb), and the level of these transcripts generally correlates with the amount of EGFR protein. It has been shown that messenger RNA levels correlate with the amount of protein, and that these differences in expression are controlled at least in part at the transcriptional level; EGFR gene amplification appears to be uncommon, occurring in less than 5% of breast tumours (Davidson et al., 1987). EGF receptor-directed blocking antibodies inhibit proliferation in cell lines expressing TGF-α and an amplified EGF receptor gene (Ennis et al., 1989). However, this has only limited possibilities as a therapeutic approach due to the low incidence of EGF receptor gene amplification in breast cancer. It is of interest that mammary epithelial cells with an amplified c-*myc* oncogene show hypersensitivity to stimulation by the EGF receptor pathway in vitro and to rapid tumourigenesis by this pathway in vivo in transgenic mice (Valverius et al., 1990). Several research groups are now testing various EGF-receptor–directed toxin conjugates as anticancer drugs.

c-*erb*B_2

About 10 to 30% of breast, gastric, and ovarian cancer overexpress the c-*erb*B_2 gene product at a sufficiently high level that the protein can be detected by immunohistochemical staining. This characteristic has facilitated rapid development of assays of the c-*erb*B_2 gene product as a marker of prognosis. Overexpression in adenocarcinoma of the lung, ovary, stomach (Kern et al., 1990), pancreas (Hall et al., 1990) and endometrial carcinoma (Berchuck et al., 1991) have been reported. There has been some confusion in the literature because of the terminology used by different groups who independently identified the c-*erb*B_2 gene. c-*erb*B_2 and HER-2 both refer to an identical human homologue of the *neu* oncogene in rat. In this review, we use the term 'c-*erb*B_2 protein'. The normal function of the c-*erb*B_2 protein is not known; nor is the function of the structurally related c-*erb*B_3 or c-*erb*B_4 receptors. In breast cancer, amplified *erb*B_2 is associated with poor prognosis and possible resistance to chemotherapy and endocrine therapy. However, the biological explanation for these effects is not yet clear; *erb*B_2 expression seems to relate to tumour growth, but not directly to metastasis (Yu et al., 1993). *erb*B_2 amplification in association with overexpressed Ha-*ras* is of especially poor prognosis (Dati et al., 1991). It is also of interest that the c-*erb*B_2 gene product and EGF receptor seem to form heterodimers and this phenomenon is associated with an especially poor prognosis when co-expression occurs at high levels. The development of *erb*B_2-directed toxin conjugates is a very active area of current research (Carter et al., 1992).

New Therapeutic Strategies to Block Tumour Growth

A large number of tyrosine kinase-associated oncogenes, including EGF receptor and *erb*B_2, are now known to modulate growth via a complex signal transduction cascade involving phosphorylation of the *ras* oncogene, *raf* oncogene, MAP kinase kinase, MAP kinase, and finally induction of transcription regulatory factors. The development of drugs able to modulate this cascade could represent a major new theme in anticancer drugs (Sadowski et al., 1993). Current approaches involve tyrosine kinase inhibitors such as tyrophostins (Levitski, 1992) and inhibitors of *ras* farnesylation (Kohl et al., 1993).

Recent studies have also suggested that cAMP regulates the tyrosine kinase signal transduction cascade. cAMP inhibits *raf* via phosphorylation, which results in the blockade of proliferative stimuli. Thus, protein kinase A–activating drugs have potential as new anticancer agents (Wu et al., 1993).

NEW APPROACHES TO THE BLOCKADE OF ANGIOGENESIS AND METASTASIS IN BREAST CANCER

De-differentiation, Stromal-Epithelial Interactions and Metastasis

Two separate but interdependent cellular processes occur during the progression of breast cancer. These are the loss of differentiation and of tissue compartmentalization. Several molecular systems may be involved in this process. In the case of de-differentiation, it appears that loss of cell–cell attachment, altered cell substructum attachment and altered cytoskeletal organization are important. In metastases, the same three factors are thought to be significant, but in addition, cell motility, proteolysis and the ability to survive and proliferate at distant sites are considered to be essential.

E-Cadherin (uvomorulin or L-CAM) is one of the principal cell–cell adhesion molecules. E-Cadherin is a significant factor in the processes of cell motility (Strange et al., 1991). Loss of expression of E-cadherin is associated with acquisition of a more motile, fibroblastic morphology in breast cancer and with increased invasiveness (Sommers et al., 1991). A subset of E-cadherin–negative breast cancer cells exists that expresses the mesenchymal intermediate filament vimentin, along with epithelial keratins, and has a strongly motile, invasive phenotype (Sommers et al., 1991; Thompson et al., 1992). This phenotype is associated with poor histologic grade in clinical breast cancer (Gamallo et al., 1993). This progression to phenotype has been observed by other investigators in bladder cancer and melanoma, where it has been termed an 'epithelial-mesenchymal transition' (EMT) (Hendrix et al., 1992). EMT also occurs during embryogenesis.

The process of metastasis is marked initially by local invasion of the cancer across the basement membrane to the stroma. This transition is thought to involve local proteolysis and tumour migration. Several proteolytic enzymes are thought to be involved in this process and the most important are probably the two collagen IV-selective degrading enzymes termed 92-kDa (MMP-9) and 72-kDa (MMP-2) gelatinase. Also implicated in invasion are plasmin, and cathepsins D, B and L (Kane & Gottesman, 1990). Although cathepsin D is a marker of poor prognosis and is hormonally regulated in breast cancer, it is considered unlikely to be a critical mediator of metastasis. This is because its pH optimum is extremely acidic, its presence in tumor homogenates is probably a result of inflammatory cell and finally because its levels do not correlate with invasion. Urokinase, which triggers plasmin release and the matrix metalloproteinases are the most widely studied new group of enzymes currently under investigation for their antimetastatic therapy (Crowley et al., 1993; Stetler-Stevenson, Liotta & Brown, 1992). Antiurokinase directed peptides have antimetastic potential (Crowley et al., 1993). The metalloproteinases are regulated by specific inhibitors, termed 'tissue inhibitors of metalloproteinases' (TIMPs). The gelatinases are secreted with TIMP-1 and TIMP-2 (Stetler-Stevenson, Liotta & Brown, 1992). TIMP-1 and TIMP–2 are thus potential antimetastasis drugs, although their half-lives are rather short in vivo. Other broad-spectrum antimetalloproteinase peptides and drugs are also under development (Tsuchiya et al., 1993).

It appears that loss of expression of the oestrogen and progesterone receptors may be associated with an EMT process in breast cancer (Thompson et al., 1992). The exact mechanism of EMT remains unknown, but it seems to be associated with primary defects in arrangement of desmosomal and cytoskeletal proteins (Boyer et al., 1989). Since protein kinase C (PKC) expression seems to increase during malignant progression and chemotherapy resistance and since a primary substrate of PKC is an actin filament cross-linking protein thought to be involved in motility (Lee, Karaszkiewicz & Anderson, 1992), it is possible that PKC plays a role in EMT regulation. PKC is also known to mediate induction of multiple matrix-degrading proteases via AP-1 promoter interactions, cell-substrate adhesion via NF-κB promoter interactions, and breast cancer cell invasiveness (Eck et al., 1993). Since retinoids are known to antagonize AP-1 regulated genes via RAR and RXR receptors, retinoids may have antimetastatic potential (Salbert et al., 1993). In addition, bryostatin-1 appears to be a relatively nontoxic anti-PKC drug with therapeutic potential (Hornung et al., 1992).

Cell-substratum attachment also seems critical in the process of differentiation and metastasis. Expression of high levels of a nonintegrin, 67-kDa receptor for laminin have been reported to be correlated with progression of breast and colon cancer (Mortignone et al., 1993). This laminin receptor is strongly induced by oestrogen and progesterone in breast cancer cell lines (Castronova et al., 1989). Other studies have implicated the heterodimeric integrin class of attachment molecules as necessary for metastasis (McCormick & Zetter, 1992).

Growth Factors, Proteases, Angiogenesis and Metastasis

It is not yet known what cellular events trigger the cascade of processes involved in local invasion and metastasis. Increased cellular motility may be significant and several motility-promoting molecules may be implicated and this group includes the FGF family members, and a growth factor termed 'hepatocyte growth factor' (HGF, or scatter factor), which acts through the c-*met* tyrosine kinase oncogene. One of the first steps in metastasis is tumour embolus formation in the bloodstream and subsequent entrapment in capillary networks. This process is thought to depend upon platelet activation and, in an attempt at limiting this step, antimetastatic prostacyclines are under development (Schneider & Schirner, 1993). Several model systems have been established for the study of invasion, and matrigel, a re-polymerized basement membrane extract, has been of particular value. Using this system it has been observed that ER-negative cells are generally more invasive than ER-positive cells. This process is oestrogen enhanced. Interestingly, tamoxifen is sufficiently oestrogenic to induce invasion in breast cancer cell lines, whereas the pure antioestrogen ICI 164,384 suppresses invasion (Thompson et al., 1990).

Invasive breast cancer is, by definition, marked by abnormal stromal-epithelial interaction. This was noted several years ago in the context of increased motility of tumor fibroblasts (Greg et al., 1989). More recently, this type of study has been extended to include characterization of fibroblast growth factor secretions. Interestingly, the growth factor IGF-II is expressed by breast tumor–derived fibroblasts, whereas IGF-I is expressed by normal breast fibroblasts (Cullen et al., 1992). Many other growth factors including FGF-1, FGF-2 and FGF-5 are also secreted by breast fibroblasts, regardless of source (Cullen et al., 1992). A recent study has also implicated stromal production of the protease stromelysin III as an early marker of invasive breast cancer (Lamacher et al., 1900). Finally, the matrix component tenascin appears to be synthesized in areas of invasion (Sakakura, Ishihara & Yatani, 1991).

Angiogenesis is an important event leading to the dissemination of breast cancer. Angiogenesis is necessary for tumour growth beyond a few millimeters in diameter. There are many growth factors, which include FGFs, EGF-related factors, TGF-βs, HGF and VEGF (acting through the FLK oncogene) thought to be mediators of angiogenesis (Millauer et al., 1993). Some emerging antiangiogenic therapies target these growth factors with structural antagonists (Kim et al., 1991), while others (Cogy AGM 1470 (now called TNP 470)), do not have established mechanisms of action. Chemotherapy seems to interact synergistically with this type of therapy, which leads to tumour infusion (Teicher, Sotomayor & Huang, 1992). It is of great interest that recent studies have observed a close, perhaps causal relationship between breast tumour angiogenesis and the extent of metastases in patients (Widner et al., 1992).

Several recent in vivo model systems of human breast cancer metastasis have been developed. In general, hormone independent breast cancer cells are more likely to be locally invasive in the nude mouse than hormone dependent cells. One hormone independent line, MDA-MB-435, has been developed into a hematogenesis metastases model in the nude mouse. This line can be widely metastatic in six to nine months, and inoculation site and dietary fat content strongly are determinants of tumour growth and metastatic spread (Meschter, Connolly & Rose, 1992).

Studies in a variety of systems suggest that release of heparin-binding growth factors such as the members of the FGF family can significantly contribute to angiogenesis and metastases. For example, in multistep development of human fibrosarcoma, bFGF release is closely associated with angiogenesis (Kandel et al., 1991). Also, FGF-4 expression is closely associated with metastases in spontaneous mouse mammary carcinoma (Murakami, Tanaka & Matsuzawa, 1990). Amplification of the genes for FGF-3 (Int-2) and FGF-4 occur with a frequency of 15% in human breast cancer and both genes are located in 11q13. However, expression of these two genes at the mRNA and protein levels is uncommon and it is now suspected that a more important gene also exists on the amplicon. A likely candidate is the cyclin D1-a cell cycle related gene (Schuuring et al., 1992). A recent study has also shown that FGF-4 transfection into human MCF-7 breast cancer cells strongly promotes tumour growth and metastasis. In this study the gene encoding the enzyme lacZ, which renders cells easily stainable, was utilized in preparing the model. LacZ gene co-transfection with FGF-4 afforded clear indication of metastatic cells. By three weeks ipsilateral lymph nodes were 100% positive; by six weeks other more distant lymph nodes, lung and kidney were positive; and by 12 weeks multiple organs showed evidence of metastases. The nature of the most important heparin-binding growth factors in human breast cancer remains of interest, and a recent report identified the heparin-binding–growth-associated neurotropic molecule known as pleiotropin in breast cancer cell lines (Wellstein et al., 1992).

Potential Novel Therapies of Angiogenesis and Metastasis

There is now the hope that identification of molecular determinants of growth, apoptosis, angiogenesis, metastasis and drug resistance will lead to new breast cancer therapies. In particular, strategies for coupling bacterial toxins to growth factors and antibodies directed toward cell surface receptors and tumour antigens seem to be a real possibility. It is possible that programmed cell death is inducible with treatment. In this context, antagonists, chemotherapeutic drugs and differentiation agents may be of value (Henderson, Ross & Pike, 1993). It may also be possible to attach therapeutically the processes of angiogenesis leading to metastasis. The literature would suggest that prevention of endothelial invasion of the tumour with antiprotease anti–growth factor, or antiadhesion strategies might inhibit metastases. Likewise, similar strategies might also have direct effects on the invasive potential of tumour cells. There is also much current enthusiasm concerning the potential for gene therapy. Ideal candidates for this would be the attempted transfection of wild-type *Rb-1* or *p53* tumor suppressor genes in breast tumours that had either lost expression entirely or expressed mutant proteins. Theoretically, this could be achieved by a retroviral vector strategy. Obvious hurdles in such approaches, however, would be development of administrative programme routes, target cell specificities and efficient incorporation techniques for such therapy and the probability that ultimately multiple tumour suppressors might become mutated (Muncaster et al., 1992). Finally novel inhibitors for the p170 glycoprotein resistance pump are in development and could be used to increase effectiveness of current chemotherapeutic agents (Leonessa et al., 1994). However, many other mechanisms of resistance might exist for antihormonal and cytotoxic drugs.

CONCLUSIONS

Although this chapter has focussed on treatment, pharmacologic prevention of breast cancer seems to be a realistic hope. At present there are ongoing trials of tamoxifen in high-risk women. Other potentially viable prevention strategies have been proposed using retinoids, vitamin D, progestins, antiprogestins or GnRH analogues. Another approach involves the potential of the local induction of growth inhibitory TGF-β. Tamoxifen, antiprogestin and retinoids are known to have this characteristic (Dickens & Colletta, 1993). Other prevention strategies have diet as their focus. Lowered fat and increased vegetable consumption coupled with adequate exercise have been proposed (Willett et al., 1992). Finally, better application of mammography and biopsy techniques is almost certain to make a positive impact on the disease (Willett et al., 1992).

Perhaps one of the most exciting long-term hopes is a better understanding of the role of mammary differentiation. Knowledge of how to pharmacologically or dietarily interrupt proliferative processes and how to induce differentiation is likely to lead to new effective future strategies in breast cancer prevention and treatment (Henderson, Ross & Pike, 1991).

REFERENCES

Allegra J.C. & Lippman M.E. (1980) Estrogen receptor status and the disease-free interval in breast cancer. *Recent Results in Cancer Research,* **71**, 20–5.

Anderson T.J., Battersby S. & Macintyre C.C.A. (1988) Proliferative and secretory activity in human breast during natural and artificial menstrual cycles. *American Journal of Pathology*, **130**, 193–204.

Aronica S.M. & Katzenellenbogen B.S. (1993) Stimulation of estrogen receptor-mediated transcription and alteration in the phosphorylation state of the rat uterine estrogen receptor by estrogen, cyclic adenosine monophosphate, and insulin-like growth factor-1. *Molecular Endocrinology*, **7**, 743–52.

Arteaga C.L., Carty-Dugger T., Moses H.L., Hurd S.D. & Pietenpol J. (1993) Transforming growth factors β_1 can induce estrogen independent tumorigenicity of human breast cancer cells in athymic mice. *Cell Growth and Differentiation*, **4**, 3448–53.

Bano M., Kidwell W.R., Lippman M.E. & Dickson R.B. (1990) Characterization of MDGF-1 receptor in human mammary epithelial cell liver. *Journal of Biological Chemistry*, **265**, 1874–80.

Bano M., Soloman D.S. & Kidwell W.R. (1985) Purification of mammary derived growth factor 1 (MDGF 1) from human milk and mammary tumors. *Journal of Biological Chemistry*, **260**, 5745–52.

Basilico C. & Moscatelli D. (1992) The FGF family of growth factors and oncogenes. *Advances in Cancer Research*, **59**, 115–65.

Batra S. & Bengstonn B. (1978) Effects of diethylstilbestrol and ovarian steroids on the contractile movements in rat uterine smooth muscle. *Journal of Physiology*, **276**, 329–42.

Benz C., Cadman E., Gwin J., Wu T., Amara J., Eisenfeld A. & Dannies P. (1983) Tamoxifen and 5-fluorouracil in breast cancer: cytotoxic synergism in vitro. *Cancer Research*, **43**, 5298–303.

Berchuck A., Rodriguez G., Kinney R.B., Soper J.T., Dodge R.K., Clarke-Pearson D. & Bast R. (1991) Overexpression of HER-2/neu in endometrial cancer is associated with advanced stage disease. *American Journal of Obstetrics and Gynecology*, **164**, 15–21.

Bezwoda W.R. & Meyer K. (1990) Effect of α-interferon, 17β-estradiol, and tamoxifen on estrogen receptor concentration and cell cycle kinetics of MCF-7 cells. *Cancer Research*, **50**, 5387–91.

Boyer B., Tucker G.C., Valles A.M., Franke W.W. & Thiery J.P. (1989) Rearrangements of desmosomal and cytoskeletal proteins during the transition from epithelial to fibroblastoid organization in cultured rat bladder carcinoma cells. Journal of Cell Biology, **109**, 1495–509.

Brunner N., Bronzert D., Vindelov L.L., Rygaard K., Spang-Thomsen M. & Lippman M.E. (1989) Effect of growth and cell cycle kinetics of estradiol and tamoxifen on MCF-7 human breast cancer cells grown in vitro in nude mice. *Cancer Research*, **49**, 1515–20.

Brunner N., Frandsen T.L., Holst-Hansen C., Bei M., Thompson E.W., Wakeling A.E., Lippman M.E. & Clarke R. (1993) MCF7/LCC2: A 4-hydroxytamoxifen resistant human breast cancer variant which retains sensitivity to the steroidal antiestrogen ICI 182780. *Cancer Research*, **53**, 3229–32.

Brunner N., Spang-Thomsen M., Vindelov L., Wolff J. & Engelholm S.A. (1985) Effect of tamoxifen on the receptor-positive T61 and the receptor negative T60 human breast carcinomas grown in nude mice. *European Journal of Cancer and Clinical Oncology*, **21**, 1349–54.

Butta A., MacLennan K., Flanders K.C., Sacks N.P.M., Smith I., McKinna A., Dowsett M., Wakefield L.M., Sporn M.B., Baum M. & Colletta A.A. (1992)

Induction of transforming growth factor β_1 in human breast cancer *in vivo* following tamoxifen treatment. *Cancer Research,* **52**, 4261–4.

Butzow R., Fukushima D., Twardzik D.R. & Ruoslahti E. (1993) A 60-kD protein mediates the binding of transforming growth factor-β to cell surface and extracellular matrix proteoglycans. *Journal of Cell Biology,* **122**, 721–7.

Carter P., Presta L., Gorman C.M., Ridgway J.B.B., Henner D., Wong W.L.T., Rowland A.M., Kotts C., Carver M.E. & Shepard H.M. (1992) Humanization of an anti-p185 HER2 antibody for human cancer therapy. *Proceedings of the National Academy of Sciences of the United States of America,* **89**, 4285–9.

Castronova V., Taraboletti G., Liotta L.A. & Sobel M.E. (1989) Modulation of laminin receptor expression by estrogen and progestins in human breast cancer. *Journal of the National Cancer Institute,* **81**, 781–7.

Chatterjee M. & Harris A.L. (1990) Reversal of acquired resistance to adriamycin in CHO cells of tamoxifen and 4-hydroxytamoxifen: role of drug interaction with alpha 1 acid glycoprotein. *British Journal of Cancer,* **62**, 712–17.

Clarke C.L. & Sutherland R.L. (1990) Progestin regulation of cellular proliferation. *Endocrine Reviews,* **11**, 266–301.

Clarke R., Brunner N., Thompson E.W., Glanz P., Katz D., Dickson R.B. & Lippman M.E. (1989) The inter-relationships between ovarian-independent growth, antiestrogen resistance and invasiveness in the malignant progression of human breast cancer. *Journal of Endocrinology,* **122**, 331–40.

Clarke R., Currier S., Kaplan O., Lovelace E., Boulay V., Gottesman M.M. & Dickson R.B. (1992) Effect of P-glycoprotein expression on sensitivity to hormones in MCF-7 human breast cancer cells. *Journal of the National Cancer Institute,* **84**, 1506–12.

Clarke R., Morwood J., Van Den Berg H.W., Nelson J. & Murphy R.F. (1986) The effect of cytotoxic drugs on estrogen receptor expression and response to tamoxifen in MCF-7 cells. *Cancer Research,* **46**, 6116–19.

Colletta A.A., Wakefield L.M., Howell F.V., Danielpour D., Baum M. & Sporn M.B. (1991) The growth inhibition of human breast cancer cells by a novel synthetic progestin involves the induction of transforming growth factor beta. *Journal of Clinical Investigation,* **87**, 277–83.

Committee on the relationship between oral contraceptives and breast cancer, IOM, DHPDP. (1991) *Oral contraceptives and breast cancer,* pp. 1–185. National Academy Press, Washington, D.C.

Coopman P., Garcia M., Brunner N., Derocq D., Clarke R. & Rochefort H. (1994) Antiproliferative and antiestrogenic effects of ICI 164,384 in 4-OH-tamoxifen-resistant human breast cancer cells. *International Journal of Cancer,* (in press).

Crowley C.W., Cohen R.L., Lucas B.K., Liu G., Shuman M.A. & Levinson A.D. (1993) Prevention of metastasis by inhibition of the urokinase receptor. *Cell Biology,* **90**, 5021–5.

Cullen K.J., Smith H.S., Hill S., Rosan N. & Lippman M.E. (1992) Growth factor mRNA expression by human breast fibroblasts from benign and malignant lesions. *Cancer Research,* **51**, 4978–85.

Daniel C.W. & Silberstein G.B. (1987) Developmental biology of the mammary gland. In M.C. Neville & C.W. Daniel (Eds.) *The mammary gland,* pp. 3–36. Plenum Press, New York.

Dati C., Muraca R., Tazartes O., Antoniotti S., Perroteau I., Giai M., Cortese P., Sismondi P., Saglio G. & DeBortoli M. (1991) c-erbB-2 and ras expression levels in breast cancer are correlated and show a cooperative association with unfavorable clinical outcome. *International Journal of Cancer*, **47**, 833–8.

Dauvois S., Danielian P.S., White R. & Parker M.G. (1992) Antiestrogen ICI 164,384 reduces cellular estrogen receptor content by increasing its turnover. *Proceedings of the National Academy of Sciences of the United States of America*, **89**, 4037–41.

Davidson N.E., Gelmann E.P., Lippman M.E. & Dickson R.B. (1987) Epidermal growth factor receptor gene expression in estrogen receptor-positive and negative human breast cancer cell lines. *Molecular Endocrinology*, **1**, 216–23.

Dickens T.-A. & Colletta A.A. (1993) The pharmacological manipulation of members of the transforming growth factor beta family in the chemoprevention of breast cancer. *Bio Essays*, **15**: 71–4.

Dickson R.B., McManaway M. & Lippman M.E. (1986) Estrogen induced factors of breast cancer cells partially replace estrogen to promote tumor growth. *Science*, **232**, 1540–3.

Dotzlaw H., Alkhalaf M. & Murphy L.C. (1992) Characterization of estrogen receptor variant mRNA's from human breast cancers. *Molecular Endocrinology*, **5**, 773–85.

Downward J., Yarden Y., Mayes E., Scarce G., Totty N., Stockwell P., Ullrich A., Schlessinger J. & Waterfield M.D. (1984) Close similarity of epidermal growth factor receptor and v-*erb*B oncogene protein sequence. *Nature* (London), **307**, 521–7.

Dulbecco R. (1990) Experimental studies in mammary development and cancer: relevance to human cancer. *Advances in Oncology*, **5**, 3–6.

Early Breast Cancer Trialists Collaborative Group (1992) Systemic treatment of early breast cancer by hormonal, cytotoxic, and immune therapy. *Lancet*, **339**, 1–15, 71–85.

Eck S.L., Perkins N.D., Carr D.P. & Nabel G.J. (1993) Inhibition of phorbol ester-induced cellular adhesion by competitive binding of NF-kB in vivo. *Molecular and Cellular Biology*, **13**, 6530–6.

Eckert K., Granetzny A., Fischer J. & Grosse R. (1991) Relationship between 43 kDa epidermal growth factor-related activity, clonogenic activity, and clinical parameters for breast cancer. *Anticancer Research*, **11**, 2125–30.

Eckert R.L. & Katzenellenbogen B.S. (1981) Human endometrial cells in primary tissue culture: modulation of the progesterone receptor level by natural and synthetic estrogens in vitro. *Journal of Clinical Endocrinology and Metabolism*, **52**, 699–708.

Edwards D.P., Chamness G.C. & McGuire W.L. (1979) Estrogen and progesterone receptor proteins in breast cancer. *Biochimica et Biophysica Acta*, **560**, 457–86.

Encarnacion C.A., Ciocca D.R., McGuire W.L., Clarke G.M., Fuqua S.A.W. & Osborne C.K. (1993) Measurement of steroid hormone receptors in breast cancer patients on tamoxifen. *Breast Cancer Research and Treatment*, **26**, 225–336.

Ennis B.W., Valverius E.M., Lippman M.E., Bellot F., Kris R., Schlessinger J., Masui H., Goldberg A., Mendelsohn J. & Dickson R.B. (1989) Anti EGF receptor antibodies inhibit the autocrine stimulated growth of MDA-MB-468 breast cancer cells. *Molecular Endocrinology*, **3**, 1830–8.

Ervin P.R., Kaminski M., Cody R.L. & Wicha M.S. (1989) Production of mammostatin, a tissue-specific growth inhibitor, by normal human mammary cells. *Science*, **244**, 1585–7.

Evans E., Baskevitch P.P. & Rochefort H. (1982) Estrogen receptor-DNA interaction: difference between activation by estrogen and antiestrogen. *European Journal of Biochemistry*, **128**, 185–91.

Falls D.L., Rosen K.M., Corfas G., Lane W.S. & Fischbach G.D. (1993) ARIA, a protein that stimulates acetylcholine receptor synthesis, is a member of the neu ligand family. *Cell*, **72**, 801–15.

Fenton S.E. & Sheffield L.G. (1993) Prolactin inhibits epidermal growth factor (EGF)-stimulated signaling events in mouse mammary epithelial cells by altering EGF receptor function. *Molecular Biology of the Cell*, **4**, 773–80.

Gamallo C., Palacios J., Suarez A., Pizarro A., Navarro P., Quintanilla M. & Cano A. (1993) Correlation of E-cadherin expression with differentiation grade and histological type in breast carcinoma. *American Journal of Pathology*, **142**, 987–93.

Goldstein D., Bushmeyer S.M., Witt P.L., Jordan V.C. & Borden E.C. (1989) Effects of type I and II interferons on cultured human breast cells: interactions with estrogen receptors and with tamoxifen. *Cancer Research*, **49**, 2698–702.

Gorsch S.M. (1992) Immunohistochemical staining for transforming growth factor beta associates with disease progression in human breast cancer. *Cancer Research*, **52**, 6949–52.

Greg A.M., Schor A.M., Rushton G., Ellis I. & Schor S.L. (1989) Purification of the migration stimulating factor produced by fetal and breast cancer patient fibroblasts. *Proceedings of the National Academy of Sciences of the United States of America*, **86**, 2438–42.

Grosse R., Bohmer F.D., Binas B., Kurtz A., Spitzer E., Muller T. & Zschiesche W. (1992) Mammary-derived growth inhibitor. In R.B. Dickson & M.E. Lippman (Eds.) *Genes, oncogenes and hormones*, pp. 69–96. Kluwer Academic Publishers, Boston.

Hall P.A., Hughes C.M., Staddon S.L., Richman P.I. et al. The c-erb B-2 protooncogene in human pancreatic cancer. *Journal of Pathology*, **161**, 195–200.

Haslam S.Z. (1990) Stromal-epithelial interactions in normal and neoplastic mammary gland. In M.E. Lippman & R.B. Dickson (Eds.) *Regulatory mechanisms in breast cancer*, pp. 401–20. Kluwer, Boston.

Henderson B.E., Ross R.K. & Pike M.C. (1993) Hormonal chemoprevention of cancer in women. *Science*, **259**, 633–8.

Hendrix M.J.C., Seftor E.A., Chu Y.W., Seftor R.E.B., Nagle R.B., McDaniel K.M., Leong S.P.L., Yohem K.H., Leibovitz A.M., Meyskens F.L., Jr., Conaway D.H., Welch D.R., Liotta L.A. & Stetler-Stevenson W. (1992) Coexpression of vimentin and keratins by human melanoma tumor cells: correlation with invasive and metastatic potential. *Journal of the National Cancer Institute*, **84**, 165–72.

Hornung R.L., Pearson J.W., Beckwith M. & Longo D.L. (1992) Preclinical evaluation of bryostatin as an anticancer agent against several murine tumor cell lines: *in vitro versus in vivo* activity. *Cancer Research*, **52**, 101–7.

Jiang S.Y. & Jordan V.C. (1992) Growth regulation of estrogen receptor-negative breast cancer cells transfected with complementary DNAs for estrogen receptor. *Journal of the National Cancer Institute*, **84**, 580–91.

Kandel J., Bossy-Wetzel E., Radvanyi F., Klagsbrun M., Folkman J. & Hanahan D. (1991) Neovascularization is associated with a switch to the export of bFGF in the multistep development of fibrosarcoma. *Cell*, **66**, 1095–104.

Kane S.E. & Gottesman M.M. (1990) The role of cathepsin L in malignant transformation. *Seminars in Cancer Biology*, **1**, 127–36.

Kangas L., Nieminen A.-L. & Cantell K. (1985) Additive and synergistic effects of a novel antiestrogen toremifene (Fc-1157a) and human interferons on estrogen responsive MCF-7 cells in vitro. *Medical Biology*, **63**, 187–90.

Kern J.A., Schwartz D.A., Nordberg J.E., Weiner D.B., Greene M., Torney L. & Robinson R.A. (1990) p185neu expression in human lung adenocarcinomas predicts shortened survival. *Cancer Research*, **50**, 5184–7.

Kim I., Manni A., Lynch J. & Hammond J.M. (1991) Identification and regulation of insulin-like growth factor binding proteins produced by hormone-dependent and -independent human breast cancer cell lines. *Molecular and Cellular Endocrinology*, **78**, 71–8.

King C.R., Kraus M.H., Williams L.T., Merlino G.T., Pastan I.H. & Aaronson S.A. (1985) Human tumor cell lines with EGF receptor gene amplification in the absence of aberrant sized mRNAs. *Nucleic Acids Research*, **13**, 8477–86.

King R.J.B., Wang D.Y., Daley R.J. & Darbre P.D. (1989) Approaches to studying the role of growth factors in the progression of breast tumors from the steroid sensitive to insensitive state. *Journal of Steroid Biochemistry*, **34**, 133–8.

Klijn J.G.M., Berns P.M.J.J., Schmitz P.I.M. & Foekens J.A. (1992) The clinical significance of epidermal growth factor receptor (EGF-R) in human breast cancer: a review on 5232 patients. *Endocrine Reviews*, **13**, 3–15.

Knabbe C., Lippman M.E., Wakefield L.M., Flanders K.C., Derynck R. & Dickson R.B. (1987) Evidence that transforming growth factor-beta is a hormonally regulated negative growth factor in human breast cancer cells. *Cell*, **48**, 417–28.

Kohl N.E., Mosser S.D., deSolms S.J., Giuliani E.A., Pompliano D.L., Graham S.L., Smith R.L., Scolnick E.M., Oliff A. & Gibbs J.B. (1993) Selective inhibition of ras-dependent transformation by a farnesyltransferase inhibitor. *Science*, **260**, 1934.

Lacroix H., Iglehart J.D., Skinner M.A. & Kraus M.H. (1989) Overexpression of erbB-2 or EGF receptor proteins present in early stage mammary carcinoma is detected simultaneously in matched primary tumors and regional metastases. *Oncogene*, **4**, 145–51.

Lamacher J.M., Podhajcer O.L., Chenard M.P., Rio M.C. & Chambon P. (1990) A novel metalloproteinase gene specifically expressed in stromal cells of breast carcinomas. *Nature* (London), **348**, 699–704.

Lee S.A., Karaszkiewicz J.W. & Anderson W.B. (1992) Elevated level of nuclear protein kinase C in multidrug-resistant MCF-7 human breast carcinoma cells. *Cancer Research*, **52**, 3750–9.

Leonessa F., Jacobsin M., Boyle B., Lippman J., McGarvey M. & Clarke R. (1994) The effect of tamoxifen on the multidrug resistant phenotype in human breast cancer cells: isobologram, drug accumulation and gp-170 binding studies. *Cancer Research*, **54**, 441–7.

Levitzki A. (1992) Tyrophostins: tyrosine kinase blockers as novel antiproliferative agents and dissectors of signal transduction. *FASEB Journal*, **6**, 3275–82.

McCarty K.S. (1989) Proliferative stimuli in the normal breast: estrogens or progestins. *Human Pathology*, **20**, 1137–8.

McCormick B.A. & Zetter B.R. (1992) Adhesive interactions in angiogenesis and metastasis. *Pharmacology and Therapeutics*, **53**, 239–60.

Manni A., Wright C. & Buck H. (1991) Growth factor involvement in the multihormonal regulation of MCF-7 breast cancer cell growth in soft agar. *Breast Cancer Research and Treatment*, **20**, 43–52.

Marchionni M.A., Goodearl A.D.J., Chen M.S., Bermingham-McDonogh O., Kirk C., Hendricks M., Danehy F., Misumi D., Sudhalter J., Kobayashi K., Wroblewski D., Lynch C., Baldassare M., Hiles I., Davis J.B., Hsuan J.J., Totty N.F., Otsu M., McBurney R.N., Waterfield M.D., Stroobant P. & Gwynne D. (1993) Glial growth factors are alternatively spliced erbB2 ligands expressed in the nervous system. *Nature*, **362**, 312–18.

Marth C., Mayer I. & Daxenbichler G. (1984) Effect of retinoic acid and 4-hydroxytamoxifen on human breast cancer cell lines. *Biochemical Pharmacology*, **33**, 2217–21.

Martignone S., Menard S., Bufalino R., Cascinelli N., Pellegrini R., Tagliabue E., Andreola S., Rilke F. & Colnaghi M.I. (1993) Prognostic significance of the 67-kilodalton laminin receptor expression in human breast cancer carcinomas. *Journal of the National Cancer Institute*, **85**(5), 200–6.

Martin H.J., McKibben B.M., Lynch M. & Van Den Berg H.W. (1991) Modulation by oestrogen and progestin/antiprogestin of alpha interferon receptor expression in human breast cancer cells. *European Journal of Cancer*, **27**, 143–6.

Medina D., Kittrell F.S., Oborn C.J. & Schwartz M. (1993) Growth factor dependency and gene expression in preneoplastic mouse mammary epithelial cells. *Cancer Research*, **53**, 668–74.

Merkel D.E., Fuqua S.A.W., Tandon A.K., Hill S.M., Buzdar A.U. & McGuire W.L. (1989) Electrophoretic analysis of 248 clinical breast cancer specimens for P-glycoprotein overexpression of gene amplification. *Journal of Clinical Oncology*, **7**, 1129–36.

Meschter C.L., Connolly J.M. & Rose D.P. (1992) Influence of regional location of the inoculation site and dietary fat on the pathology of MDA-MB-435 human breast cancer cell-derived tumors grown in nude mice. *Clinical and Experimental Metastasis*, **10**, 167–73.

Millauer B., Wizigmann-Voos S., Schnurch H., Martinez R., Møller N.P.H., Risau W. & Ullrich A. (1993) High affinity VEGF binding and developmental expression suggest Flk-1 as a major regulator of vasculogenesis and angiogenesis. *Cell*, **72**, 835–46.

Miller W.H., Moy D., Li A., Grippo J.F. & Dmitrovsky E. (1990) Retinoic acid induces down-regulation of several growth factors and proto-oncogenes in a human embryonal cancer cell line. *Oncogene*, **5**, 511–17.

Monteagudo C., Merino M.J., San-Juan J., Liotta L.A. & Stetler-Stevenson W.G. (1990) Immunohistochemical distribution of type IV collagenase in normal, benign, and malignant breast tissue. *American Journal of Pathology*, **136**, 585–92.

Morris I.D. & Stephen T.M. (1983) In vitro and in vivo interactions of methotrexate and other antimetabolites with the oestrogen high affinity receptors of the rat uterus. *British Journal of Cancer*, **47**, 433–7.

Muller R.E., Sheard B.E., Traish A. & Wotiz H.H. (1980) Effect of chemotherapeutic agents on the formation of estrogen-receptor complex in human breast tumor cytosol. *Cancer Research*, **40**, 2941–2.

Muncaster M.M., Cohen B.L., Phillips R.A. & Gallie B.L. (1992) Failure of *RB1* to reverse the malignant phenotype of human tumor cell lines. *Cancer Research*, **52**, 654–61.

Murakami A., Tanaka H. & Matsuzawa A. (1990) Association of *hst* gene expression with metastatic phenotype in mouse mammary tumor cells. *Cell Growth and Differentiation*, **1**, 225–31.

Musgrove E.A., Lee C.S.L. & Sutherland R.L. (1991) Progestins both stimulate and inhibit breast cancer cell cycle progression while increasing expression of transforming growth factor α, epidermal growth factor receptor, c-*fos*, and c-*myc* genes. *Molecular and Cellular Biology*, **11**, 5032–43.

Nicholson R.I., Gee J.M.W., Anderson E., Dowsett M., DeFriend D., Howell A., Robertson J.F.R., Blamey R.W., Baum M., Saunders C., Walton P. & Wakeling A.E. (1993) Phase I study of a new pure antiestrogen ICI 182,780 in women with primary breast cancer: immunohistochemical analysis. *Breast Cancer Research and Treatment*, **27**, 135.

Normanno N., Qi C.-F., Gullick W.J., Persico G., Yarden Y., Wen D., Plowman G., Kenney N., Johnson G., Kim N., Brandt R., Martinez-Lacaci I., Dickson R.B. & Salomon D.S. (1993) Expression of amphiregulin, cripto-1, and heregulin α in human breast cancer cells. *International Journal of Oncology*, **2**, 903–11.

Osborne C.K., Coronado E.B. & Robinson J.P. (1987) Human breast cancer in athymic nude mice: cytostatic effects of long-term antiestrogen therapy. *European Journal of Cancer and Clinical Oncology*, **23**, 1189–96.

Paik S., Blair O. & Lippman M.E. (1992) Dominance of tamoxifen sensitive phenotype in MCF-7/LY-2 somatic cell hybrids (abstr.). *Proceedings of the American Society for Cancer Research*, **33**, 1645.

Perkins A.S. & Vande Woude G.F. (1993) Principles of molecular cell biology of cancer: oncogenes. In V.T. DeVita, S. Hellman & S.A. Rosenberg (Eds.) pp. 35–59. J.B. Lippincott, Philadelphia.

Plowman G.D., Culouscou J.-M., Whitney G.S., Green J.M., Carlton G.W., Foy L., Neubauer M.G. & Shoyab M. (1993) Ligand-specific activation of HER4/p180^{erbB4}, a fourth member of the epidermal growth factor receptor family. *Proceedings of the National Academy of Sciences of the United States of America*, **90**, 1746–50.

Porzsolt F., Otto A.M., Trauschel B., Buck C., Wawer A.W. & Schonenberger H. (1989) Rationale for combining tamoxifen and interferon in the treatment of advanced breast cancer. *Journal of Cancer Research and Clinical Oncology*, **115**, 465–9.

Pouillart P., Palangie T., Jouve M., Garcie G.E., Fridman W.H., Magdalena H., Falcoff E. & Billianus A. (1982) Administration of fibroblast interferon to patients with advanced breast cancer: possible effects on skin metastastis and on hormone receptors. *European Journal of Cancer and Clinical Oncology*, **18**, 929–35.

Quian X.L., Decker S.J. & Greene M.I. (1992) p185-c-neu and epidermal growth factor receptor associate into a structure composed of activated kinases. *Proceedings of the National Academy of Sciences of the United States of America*, **89**, 1330–4.

Recchia F., Morgante A., Ercole C., Marchionni F. & Rabitti G. (1990) Differentiation induction and tamoxifen (TMX) therapy for stage IV breast cancer (BC). Preliminary report of a phase II study (abstr.). *Proceedings of the American Society of Clinical Oncology*, **9**, 193.

Robinson S.P. & Jordan V.C. (1987) Reversal of the antitumor effects of tamoxifen by progesterone in the DMBA-induced rat mammary carcinoma model. *Cancer Research*, **47**, 5386–90.

Saceda M., Knabbe C., Dickson R.B., Lippman M.E., Bronzert D., Lindsey R.K., Gottardis M.M. & Martin M.B. (1991) Posttranslational destabilization of estrogen receptor mRNA in MCF-7 cells by 12-0-tetradecanoyl phorbol-13-acetate. *Journal of Biological Chemistry*, **266**, 17809–14.

Sadowski H.B., Shuai K., Darnell J.E., Jr. & Gilman M.Z. (1993) A common nuclear signal transduction pathway activated by growth factor and cytokine receptors. *Science*, **261**, 1739.

Saeki T., Cristiano A., Lynch M.J., Brattain M., Kim N., Normanno N., Kenney N., Ciardiello F. & Salomon D.S. (1991) Regulation by estrogen through the 5′-flanking region of the transforming growth factor α gene. *Molecular Endocrinology*, **5**, 1955–63.

Sakakura T., Ishihara A. & Yatani R. (1991) Tenascin in mammary gland development: from embryogenesis to carcinogenesis. In M.E. Lippman & R.B. Dickson (Eds.) *Regulatory mechanisms in breast cancer*, pp. 365–82. Kluwer, Boston.

Salbert G., Fanjul F., Piedrafita J., Lu X.P., Kim S., Tran P. & Pfahl M. (1993) Retinoic acid receptors and retinoid X receptor-α down-regulate the transforming growth factor-β_1 promoter by antagonizing AP-1 activity. *Molecular Endocrinology*, **7**, 1347–56.

Sanfilippo O., Ronchi E., De Marco C., Di Fronzo G. & Silvestrini R. (1991) Expression of P-glycoprotein in breast cancer tissue and in vitro resistance to doxorubicin and vincristine. *European Journal of Cancer*, **27**, 155–8.

Schneider M.R. & Schirner M. (1993) Antimetastatic prostacylin analogs. *Drugs Fut.*, **18**, 29–48.

Schuuring E., Verhoven E., Mooi W.J. & Michalides R.J.A.M. (1992) Identification and cloning of two overexpressed genes U 21B31/PRAD 1 and ems-1 within the amplified chromosome 11q13 region in human carcinomas. *Oncogene*, **7**, 355–61.

Shing Y., Christofori G., Hanahan D., Ono Y., Sasada R., Igarashi K. & Folkman J. (1993) Betacellulin: a mitogen from pancreatic β cell tumors. *Science*, **259**, 1604–7.

Sommers C.L., Thompson E.W., Torri J.A., Kemler R., Gelmann E.P. & Byers S.W. (1991) Cell adhesion molecule uvomorulin expression in human breast cancer cell lines: relationship to morphology and invasive capacities. *Cell Growth and Differentiation*, **2**, 365–72.

Stetler-Stevenson W.G., Liotta L.A. & Brown P.D. (1992) Role of type IV collagenases in human breast cancer. In R.B. Dickson & M.E. Lippman (Eds.) *Genes, oncogenes and hormones*, pp. 21–42. Kluwer, Boston.

Strange R., Li F., Friis R.R., Reichmann E., Haenni B. & Burri P.H. (1991) Mammary epithelial differentiation *in vitro*: minimum requirements for a functional response to hormonal stimulation. *Cell and Growth Differentiation*, **2**, 549–59.

Strange R., Li F., Suarer S., Burkhardt A. & Friis R.R. (1992) Apoptic cell death and tissue remodelling during mouse mammary gland involution. *Development*, **115**, 49–58.

Streuli C.H., Bailey N. & Bissell M.J. (1991) Control of mammary epithelial differentiation: basement membrane induces tissue-specific gene expression in the absence of cell-cell interaction and morphological polarity. *Journal of Cell Biology*, **115**, 1383–95.

Strum J.M. & Reseau J.H. (1986) Effects of B-retinyl acetate on human breast epithelium in explant culture. *American Journal of Anatomy*, **175**, 35–48.

Taylor-Papadimitriou J. & Lane E.B. (1987) Keratin expression in the mammary gland. In M.C. Neville & C.W. Daniel (Eds.) *The mammary gland*, pp. 181–216. Plenum Press, New York.

Teicher B.A., Sotomayor E.A. & Huang Z.D. (1992) Antiangiogenic agents potentiate cytotoxic cancer therapies against primary and metastatic disease. *Cancer Research*, **52**, 6702–4.

Thompson E.W., Katz D., Shima T.B. et al. (1990) ICI 164,384: a pure antiestrogen for basement membrane invasiveness and proliferation of MCF-7 cells. *Cancer Research*, **49**, 6929–34.

Thompson E.W., Paik S., Brunner N., Sommers C.L., Zugmaier G., Clarke R., Shima T.B., Torri J., Donahue S., Lippman M.E., Martin G.R. & Dickson R.B. (1992) Association of increased basement membrane invasiveness with absence of estrogen receptor and expression of vimentin in human breast cancer cell lines. *Journal of Cellular Physiology*, **150**, 534–44.

Thompson M.P., Farrell H.M., Mohanam S., Liu S., Kidwell W.R., Bansal M.P., Cook R.G., Kotts C.E. & Bano M. (1992) Identification of human milk α-lactalbumin as a cell growth inhibitor. *Protoplasma*, **167**, 134–44.

Tsuchiya Y., Sato H., Endo Y., Okada Y., Mai M., Sasaki T. & Seiki M. (1993) Tissue inhibitor of metalloproteinase 1 is a negative regulator of the metastatic ability of a human gastric cancer cell line, KKLS, in the chick embryo. *Cancer Research*, **53**, 1397–1402.

Tzukerman M., Zhang X.K. & Pfahl M. (1991) Inhibition of estrogen receptor activity by the tumor promoter 12-O-tetradecanylphorbol-13-acetate: a molecular analysis. *Molecular Endocrinology*, **5**, 1983–92.

Valverius E.M., Cisardiello F., Heldin N.E., Blondel B., Merlo G., Smith G., Stampfer M.R., Lippman M.E., Dickson R.B. & Salomon D.S. (1990) Stromal influences on transformation of human mammary epithelial cells overexpressing c-*myc* and SV 40T. *Journal of Cellular Physiology*, **145**, 207–16.

Van Den Berg H.W., Leahey W.J., Lynch M., Clarke R. & Nelson J. (1987) Recombinant human interferon alpha increases oestrogen receptor expression in human breast cancer cells (ZR-75-1) and sensitises them to the anti-proliferative effects of tamoxifen. *British Journal of Cancer*, **55**, 25–7.

Velu T.J., Beguinot L., Vass W.C., Willingham M.C., Merlino G.T., Pastan I. & Lowry D.R. (1987) Epidermal growth factor dependent transformation by a human EGF receptor proto-oncogene. *Science*, **238**, 1408–10.

Verrelle P., Meissonnier F., Fonck Y., Feillel V., Dionet C., Kwiatkowski F., Plagne R. & Chassagne J. (1991) Clinical relevance of immunohistochemical detection of multidrug resistance P-glycoprotein in breast carcinoma. *Journal of the National Cancer Institute*, **83**, 111–16.

Vickers P.J., Dickson R.B., & Cowan K.H. (1988) Multidrug-resistance in human breast cancer. *Trends in Pharmacological Sciences*, **9**, 443–5.

Vickers P.J., Dickson R.B., Shoemaker R. & Cowan K.H. (1988) A multidrug-resistant MCF-7 human breast cancer cell line which exhibits cross-resistance to antiestrogens and hormone independent tumor growth. *Molecular Endocrinology*, **2**, 886–92.

Wellstein A., Fang W., Khatri A., Lu Y., Swain S., Dickson R.B., Susse R., Riegel A.T. & Lippman M.E. (1992) A heparin-binding growth factor secreted from breast cancer cells is homologous to a developmentally regulated cytokine. *Journal of Biological Chemistry*, **267**, 2582–8.

Widner N., Semple J.P., Welsch W.R. & Folkman J.R. (1991) Tumor angiogenesis and metastases-correlation in invasive breast carcinoma. *New England Journal of Medicine*, **324**, 1–8.

Willett W.C., Hunter D.J., Stampfer M.J., Colditz G., Manson J.E., Spiegelman D., Rosner B., Hennekens C.H. & Speizer F.E. (1992) Dietary fat and fiber in relation to risk of breast cancer. *Journal of the American Medical Association*, **268**, 2037–44.

Wu J., Dent P., Jelinek T., Wolfman A., Weber M.J. & Sturgill T.W. (1993) Inhibition of the EGF-activated MAP kinase signaling pathway by adenosine 3′,5′-monophosphate. *Science*, **262**, 1065–9.

Yang K.-P. & Samaan N. (1983) Reduction of the estrogen receptor concentration in MCF-7 human breast carcinoma cells following exposure to chemotherapeutic drugs. *Cancer Research*, **43**, 3534–8.

Yu D., Shi D., Scanlon M. & Hung M. (1993) Reexpression of *neu*-encoded oncoprotein counteracts the tumor-suppressing but not the metastasis-suppressing function E1A. *Cancer Research*, **53**, 5784–90.

Zugmaier G., Paik S., Wilding G., Knabbe C., Bano M., Lupu R., Deschauer B., Simpson S., Dickson R.B. & Lippman M.E. (1991) Transforming growth factor beta 1 induces cachexia and systemic fibrosis without an antitumor effect in nude mice. *Cancer Research*, **51**, 3590–4.

Zyad A., Bernard J., Clarke R., Tursz T., Brockhaus M. & Chouaib S. (1994) Human breast cancer cross-resistance to TNF and adriamycin: relationship to MDR1, MnSOD and TNF gene expression. *Cancer Research*, **54**, 825–31.

10

The Biological Basis for the Treatment of Prostate Cancer

JONATHAN WAXMAN, ANDREW STUBBS AND HARDEV PANDHA

INTRODUCTION

Prostate cancer has become an epidemic. It has doubled in incidence over the last 20 years, and in the United States in 1994 became the commonest cancer of man, overtaking lung cancer in the prevalence stakes. This change has been accompanied by an increased interest in prostate cancer research, once a waif at the Cancer Research Ball, and now a dowager sitting at the top table of priority funding. This chapter seeks to explore whether any current laboratory research into this malignancy has shed light on the clinical behaviour of prostate cancer in man. The majority of laboratory work is carried out on cell lines, originating from human tumours, and any objective review might suggest that research based on these cell lines is irrelevant to the clinical situation. This is because although prostate cancer is remarkably common, only three human immortalized cell lines are freely available for study. One can only conclude that these lines are not representative of any clinical reality, and that results from laboratory studies must not reflect the situation in man. Despite this reservation, there have been remarkable findings, remarkable for their implications for our understanding of the endocrine basis of hormone-dependent malignancy. In this chapter, we will review the known biology of prostate cancer, correlating where possible science with clinical findings.

DOMINANT ONCOGENES

ras Oncogenes

The viral oncogene v-*ras* is implicated in the aetiology of sarcomas in rats. The human homologues of v-*ras* are the *ras* family of cellular oncogenes, Harvey, Kirsten and n-*ras*. The product of this oncogene is a 21,000 kDa protein p21, which is located on the inner cell membrane and functions in signal transduction in a process that initially involves the binding of a growth factor to a receptor, and results in the phosphorylation of guanidine nucleotides and protein kinase activation. *ras* mutations can result in amino acid substitutions in the p21 molecule. These substitutions result in a constitutionally activated membrane signalling process that leads to the expression of the malignant phenotype. A wide range of human tumours are found to express abnormal p21 proteins.

In an early study, expression of the *ras* oncogene product was examined in normal prostatic tissue, hypertrophic prostate and prostate cancer. p21 expression was examined by immunohistochemistry using the RAP-5 antibody, which reacts with normal human cellular Harvey, Kirsten and n-*ras* p21 as well as p21 molecules with amino acid substitutions at positions 12 and 61. The seven BPH specimens examined did not express p21 *ras*, whereas 23 of 29 carcinomas did and expression correlated with differentiation (Table 10.1).

The RAP-5 antibody has a wide range of immunoreactivity. More specific studies of the *ras* oncogene have been based on DNA hybridization techniques performed in order to assess the frequency of *ras* gene mutations in prostate cancer together with the frequency of expression of the wild-type sequence. Polymerase chain reaction (PCR) was performed for codons of interest followed by hybridization with sequence-specific oligodeoxynucleotide probes. The wild-type allele was identified in all prostate specimens but mutations were found in only 1 of 24 tumour specimens, an A to G transition at codon 61 of the Harvey *ras* gene. A further mutation was identified in one of five prostate tumour cell lines (Carter, Epstein & Isaacs, 1990). This low incidence of *ras* mutation is in contrast with the high frequency of mutations in pancreatic cancer but similar to that found in breast and renal tumours.

Table 10.1. ras p21 Expression in Benign and Malignant Prostate

	ras Positivity
Benign	0/9
Well differentiated	2/6
Moderately differentiated	4/6
Poorly differentiated	17/17

Source: From Viola et al. 1986.

Amongst the many mysteries that scientists are seeking explanations for in the Temple of Molecular Biology is the ability of a cell to metastasize within a host. There is evidence that implicates the *ras* oncogene in the process of metastasis. Transfection of the Dunning AT2.1 cell line, which has low metastatic potential with plasmids containing the Ha-*ras* oncogene, confers metastatic ability (Partin et al., 1988). Ha-*ras* expressing transfectants metastatized in over 80% of inoculated rats as compared with 10% of nontransfected controls (Treiger & Isaacs, 1988).

These observations on the highly nonrepresentive Dunning cell line are highly unlikely to have any bearing whatsoever upon the situation in human cancer. This is because of the low incidence of *ras* mutations in human prostate cancer biopsies, as described above.

myc Oncogenes

The viral oncogene v-*myc* is associated with the development of leukaemias in chickens. The human homologue of this oncogene, c-*myc*, is overexpressed in leukaemias, lymphomas and lung cancer. Those belonging to the *myc* family of oncogenes are termed housekeeping genes and are concerned with the regulation of many cellular processes. The level of c-*myc* transcription in prostatic tissue was examined by Northern blot analysis in two normal prostates, eleven patients with benign hypertrophy and seven patients with carcinoma of the prostate. Mean levels of c-*myc* transcripts were significantly high in the carcinoma specimens. c-*myc* transcript levels in a small series was, however, found to vary with tumour grade and was highest in the well-differentiated cancers (Fleming et al., 1986).

These data are of dubious significance because there is considerable overlap when the standard deviations of the mean transcript levels are compared (Table 10.2).

The series of patients described are small in number, and so no significant conclusions can really be drawn as regards the significance

Table 10.2. c-myc Transcript Levels in Prostatic Tissue

	c-*myc* Transcript Levels
Normal	2 units
BPH	26 +/− 19 units
Carcinoma	54 +/− 40 units

of c-*myc* expression in prostate cancer. Further studies are warranted but have not followed this paper, which was published over 9 years ago.

The LNCaP cell line is the only available human hormone-sensitive prostatic cancer cell line. This model has been used to examine the relationship between androgens and oncogenes. LNCaP cells were grown in culture and oncogene expression assessed in the presence and absence from the culture media of the synthetic androgen mibolerone. c-*myc* RNA levels were shown to be reduced by exposure to this synthetic androgen and this process was found to be mediated via the androgen receptor and involves a limitation of c-*myc* mRNA initiation and elongation (Wolf et al., 1992).

Other Dominant Oncogenes

Very little is known about the role of other dominant oncogenes and in particular the interaction between oncogenes and sex steroids in prostate cancer. In order to investigate this interaction, the prostate cancer cell lines PC3, PC82, PC133 and PC135 were examined for the presence of the oncogenes *fes*, *int*-1, *abl*, the *ras* family, *myb*, *fos*, *fms*, *myc*, and *sis* mRNA. High levels of Ha-*ras*, c-*myc* and *fos* expression were shown in all cell lines, but the hormone-dependent cell line PC82 expressed the highest levels of *fos* expression. The viral homologue of *fos* is implicated in animal sarcomas. Withdrawal of androgen from the culture medium led to a tenfold reduction in *fos* mRNA expression, a twofold reduction in Ha-*ras* expression and no significant changes in c-*myc* expression. These changes were seen within 3 days of withdrawal of androgen from the culture medium (Rijinders et al., 1985). PC82 differs from the other prostate cancer lines studied in that it is androgen dependent and more differentiated. It can only be grown in male nude mice, whereas the other lines will grow in both male and female nude mice. In a similar fashion to the c-*myc* story, the application of these results to the human situation is still not known and has not been investigated further 10 years from the publication of these findings.

TUMOUR SUPPRESSOR GENES

Retinoblastoma Gene

The retinoblastoma tumour suppressor gene was one of the first known members of the family of tumour suppressor genes. The retinoblastoma gene (RB) encodes a nuclear protein that is widely expressed in normal tissues. The loss of the gene or its mutation leads to an abnormal product with loss of function and it is this event that is the primary change in the development of a retinoblastoma.

RB mutations occur not only in retinoblastoma but also in breast cancer, small cell lung cancer and many other tumour groups. Bookstein and others examined the expression of the RB gene in DU145 and PC3, which are human hormone unresponsive, and LNCaP cell lines. The DU145 cell line expressed an abnormal RB product. Normal RB gene was transfected into DU145 cells and effective transfection led to the loss of ability of these cells to form tumours in nude mice (Bookstein et al., 1990). Abnormalities of RB expression have been assessed in human prostate cancer specimens and found to be infrequent (Bookstein & Allred, 1993). Once again a laboratory insight has relevance to a cell line but no importance in the human situation.

p53 Gene

The p53 gene is an essential part of the regulatory mechanisms controlling cell proliferation. p53 was first identified in 1979 as a cellular protein associated with the T antigen of the SV40 and the E1B adenovirus 5 gene product. Mutational deletion of this gene, which is associated with loss of heterozygosity at loci on chromosome 17p13, occurs in a wide variety of human tumours and in particular cancers of the colon, lung and breast. Abnormality of p53 expression is described in up to 80% of some malignancies. There have been a number of reports describing the incidence of p53 gene mutations in prostate cancer. The incidence of p53 mutations is low in prostate cancer. In one series 2 of 21 prostate tumours had p53 mutations (Uchida et al., 1993) and in another only one of 85 prostatic cancer specimens had p53 mutations (Voeller et al., 1994). This low incidence of p53 mutations suggests that this tumour suppressor gene has no relevance to prostate cancer development.

GROWTH FACTORS AND THEIR RECEPTORS

Gonadotrophin-Releasing Hormone and Its Receptor

Agonist analogues of the hyperthalamic hormone gonadotrophin-releasing hormone (GnRH) have been used as treatments for prostate cancer for the last 15 years. They are conventionally thought to act by down-regulating the pituitary gonadal axis, producing by this means castrate levels of testosterone. Clues from clinical practice suggested that this analysis of the biochemical basis for the activity of the agonists may not be correct.

We have investigated whether there is a direct effect of these agonists at the level of the tumour through specific GnRH-releasing receptors. Analysis showed the presence of a high-affinity receptor with a binding constant of approximately 10^{-9} M present in the LNCaP cell line. Nonspecific low-affinity binding of GnRH was present in the DU145 cell line. This receptor has biological significance in that addition of the agonist to culture media led to a dose-dependent short-term stimulation of growth and increase in DNA in the absence of any other added hormone (Figure 10.1). There was no stimulatory effect on the hormone-insensitive cell lines.

Assays were performed of the culture media from the prostate cancer cell lines and these were both found to contain GnRH-like radioimmunoactivity in amounts dependent on the cell numbers growing in the culture media. Positivity was found in both the hormone-unresponsive and -responsive cell lines. Prostate cancer and benign hypertrophy specimens were examined for the presence of receptors and for ligand, and 80% of both groups were receptor and ligand positive (Qayum et al., 1990). It may therefore be that this peptide receptor and its ligand have relevance to the human condition. These results suggest that GnRH is a growth factor for hormone-dependent prostate cancer and that the only difference between hormone sensitivity and insensitivity is the presence or absence of the receptor for gonadotrophin-releasing hormone. These results also provide us with information as to the possible cause of the relentless progression from a hormone-dependent to -independent phenotype in this condition. It may be that mutation of the gene encoding the cell surface receptor may be causal. It is also possible that there may be deletion of the gene encoding this receptor.

This work provides the first example of the use of a peptide therapy for cancer that acts by interfering with autocrine control mechanisms.

Epidermal Growth Factor Receptor and c-*erb*B2

The epidermal growth factor receptor is a transmembrane glycoprotein with tyrosine kinase activating activity. The receptor is distributed within a wide range of normal human tissue, and elevated levels have been reported in a variety of human tumours. There are significant similarities between the gene encoding the epidermal growth factor receptor and the oncogene c-*erb*B2 and there are homologies between epidermal growth factor receptor and the *erb*B2 product. The ligand for epidermal growth factor receptor is epidermal growth factor, which is found in saliva, urinary tract and prostatic fluid. The ligands for c-*erb*B2 include transforming growth factor alpha (TGF-α). Epidermal growth factor receptor and c-*erb*B2 oncogene product levels correlate with tumour grade, nodal status, prognosis and response to treatment in breast cancer and bladder cancer.

An RNase protection assay was used to examine mRNA levels in 38 patients with carcinoma and 35 patients with benign hypertrophy of the prostate. Significantly higher levels were found in carcinoma tissue (Morris & Green Dodd, 1990). This finding suggests that enhanced expression of the epidermal growth factor receptor gene may have a role in the regulation of prostatic tumour growth, possibly by an autocrine pathway. Immunohistochemistry was used to assess epidermal growth factor levels in ten patients with benign hypertrophy, 42 patients with benign hypertrophy adjacent to carcinoma, and 20 treated and 65 untreated carcinoma specimens. Three (6%) of the benign hypertrophy specimens stained for EGF – and these were cases in which carcinoma was adjacent to the hypertrophic prostatic tissue – and 44 (68%) of the prostate cancer specimens stained. There was no significant correlation between epidermal growth factor staining tumour differentiation or stage (Fowler et al., 1988).

Immunohistochemistry employing a polyclonal antibody was used to examine for the c-*erb*B2 protein in 13 benign hypertrophy specimens and 21 carcinomas. Twelve of the benign specimens and nine of the malignant tumours expressed the c-*erb*B2 protein (Ware et al., 1991). c-*erb*B2 expression was examined by immunohistochemistry using the *her*-2 9G6 monoclonal antibody. Overexpression was reported in 16 of 100 prostate cancers and correlated with poorly differentiated tumour grade but not with stage (Ross et al., 1993).

It would seem that c-*erb*B2 and EGFR do not provide significant information with regard to the biology of prostate cancer.

Fibroblast Growth Factor

The production of basic fibroblast growth factor and expression of the fibroblast growth factor receptor were examined in the LNCaP DU145 and PC3 cell lines. Marked differences were noted in the three cell lines. LNCaP did not produce measurable amounts of basic fibroblast growth factor, expressed small amounts of fibroblast growth factor receptor mRNA and its growth was stimulated by the addition of exogenous basic fibroblast growth factor to culture medium. The DU145 line produced measurable amounts of biologically active fibroblast growth factor and expressed large amounts of receptor mRNA. Growth of this cell line was increased by the addition of basic fibroblast growth factor to the culture medium and of FGF-like fractions extracted from DU145 cells.

In contrast, the PC3 line produced measurable amounts of basic fibroblast growth factor and expressed fibroblast growth factor receptor RNA but did not demonstrate a growth response to added basic fibroblast growth factor or to DU145 cell line extracts (Nakamoto et al., 1992). This finding is probably of little significance in that it fails to relate to any of the known biological characteristics of the different lines.

Transforming Growth Factor

The AXC/SSh rat prostate cancer cell line was examined for transforming growth factor beta (TGF-β) receptors and contained between 2,000 and 10,000 binding sites per cell. The binding capacity for TGF-β was in the range 24 to 160 pM, suggesting that this receptor might have biological significance and this was confirmed by the observation of both inhibitory and stimulatory effects of TGF-β on cellular thymidine incorporation (Shain et al., 1990).

The significance of this finding is not known. This study was carried out on an atypical animal line and not on human lines nor on human prostatic tissue. In addition no examination was performed of the synthesis of TGF-like molecules in the culture media of the prostate cancer cell line. This has been assayed in the DU145 cell line where TGF-α like activity was found (MacDonald, Chisolm & Habib, 1990). The relevance of these findings to the human situation is unknown.

THE EFFECTS OF THE STROMAL ENVIRONMENT ON PROSTATE TUMOUR GROWTH

There must be something unique about the interaction between bone stromal cells and prostate cancer cells because of the frequency with which this tumour spreads to bone and because of the distinctive pattern of that spread. In no other condition is such marked sclerosis of the bone seen in such a significant proportion of cases. This has been "explained" by the nature of the venous drainage of the prostate, which is through the lumbar sacral plexus and thence to the spine. This is, of course, somewhat implausible.

Stromal cells which include fibroblasts are the source of very many growth factors. In a series of experiments, LNCaP cells were co-

Table 10.3. LNCaP Growth Stimulation by Co-Inoculation with Human Cell Lines

Cell Line	Tumours Formed
M5 (osteogenic sarcoma)	8/13 (62%)
rUGM (rat foetal urogenital sinus mesenchyme)	31/51 (61%)
NbF-1 (rat prostate)	3/18 (17%)
3TS (embryonic mouse)	8/12 (67%)
CCD16 (human lung)	0/6
NRK (rat kidney)	0/20

inoculated with different populations of fibroblasts into athymic nude mice. The incidence of tumours formed is described in Table 10.3 (Gleave et al., 1991).

These results show the dramatic increase in oncogenic potential of LNCaP cells with fibroblast co-inoculation. The significance of factors produced by the bone marrow stroma has been further examined in a series of very interesting experiments that throw some insight upon the biological behaviour of this tumour. Short-term cultures of bone marrow were established and the culture media extracted and added to PC3 prostate cancer cell lines. A dose-dependent stimulatory effect on growth was observed and is described in Table 10.4.

A similar effect was observed from culture medium obtained from bone marrow stromal cells and is described in Table 10.5. (Chackal-Roy et al., 1989).

These findings only partly explain the fact that prostate cancer has a predilection for growth in bone. The specific factors causing this predilection remain unknown and require definition.

Table 10.4. Stimulation of PC3 Prostate Cancer by Bone Marrow Factors

[BM Medium] μg/ml	Increase
5	2.5×
15	12×
30	19.7×
65	21×
100	21×

Table 10.5.

[BM SC Medium] μg/ml	Increase
5	1.2×
15	9.4×
30	15.3×
65	23.8×
100	28.6×

MANIPULATING THE ANDROGEN RECEPTOR

Androgen deprivation leads to subjective responses in approximately 80% of patients with prostate cancer and objective evidence for remission is seen in approximately 50% of patients. Remission in metastatic disease is for a median duration of 1 year and is inexorably followed by progression and death. Remission is generally thought to be due to loss of sensitivity to androgen deprivation. It is thought possible that the primary event dictating androgen insensitivity is mutation in the gene encoding the androgen receptor.

This possibility has been investigated by an experiment in which the human androgen receptor cDNA together with the SV40 promotor was transfected into the hormone-insensitive PC3 cell line. This manoeuvre conferred androgen dependence and offers a striking prospect for gene therapy in prostate cancer (Yuan et al., 1993).

MATRIX METALLOPROTEINASES

Tumours are thought to locally invade and metastasize by the release of proteases called metalloproteinases that disrupt the normal extracellular matrix. This matrix is normally regulated by a complex interplay of enzymes and inhibitory proteins that include the metalloproteinases and their specific tissue inhibitors.

The metalloproteinases are defined and named by their substrates and include collagenases, gelatinases, stromelysins and matrilysins. There are four specific tissue inhibitors of metalloproteinases, of which two have been sequenced (Stearns & Wang, 1993).

In one immunohistochemical study, 11 of 26 patients with prostatic cancer had expression of 92-kDa metalloproteinase and no staining was observed in 15 patients with benign hypertrophy (Hamdy et al., 1994).

Using a novel series of antibodies, we have examined a series of 40 patients with prostate cancer and compared levels of collagenase, stromelysin, TIMP-1 and TIMP-2 with 21 patients with rheumatoid arthritis and 56 age-matched controls without arthritis or cancer. Patients with prostate cancer had higher levels of collagenase and TIMP-1 and lower levels of TIMP-2 than controls. Patients with metastatic cancer had significantly higher levels of collagenase than those without metastases. Patients with rheumatoid arthritis had significantly higher levels of stromelysin than either controls or patients with cancer (Baker et al., 1994).

These findings may have clinical relevance, suggesting that there could be a clinical role for the newly synthesized inhibitors of the metalloproteinases in the treatment of cancer.

CONCLUSIONS

Prostate cancer is a remarkable tumour, remarkable for its hormone sensitivity and remarkable also for the limited amount of scientific research into its molecular origins. If one could predict which tumour potentially offers the most chance of providing clues to the molecular mechanisms of hormone-responsive cancer then it must be that prostate cancer is that tumour. It is hoped that in the next few years, the pandemic of prostate cancer that is now facing our community will have become under control and that we will have developed from scientific study, better treatments for this condition. Current research must devolve away from cell lines, which are non-representative of the human condition.

REFERENCES

Baker T., Tickle S., Wasan H., Doherty A., Isenberg D. & Waxman J. (1994) Serum metalloproteinases and their inhibitors: markers for malignant potential. *British Journal of Cancer*, **70**, 506–12.

Bookstein R. & Allred D.C. (1993) Recessive oncogenes. *Cancer*, **71**(3), 1179–86.

Bookstein R., Shew J.Y., Chen P.L., Scully P. & Lee W.H. (1990) Suppression of tumorigenicity of human prostate carcinoma cells by replacing a mutated RB gene. *Science*, **247**, 712–15.

Carter R.S., Epstein J.I. & Isaacs W.B. (1990) *ras* Gene mutations in human prostate cancer. *Cancer Research* **50**, 6830–2.

Chackal-Roy M., Niemeyer C., Moore M. & Zetter B.R. (1989) Stimulation of human prostatic carcinoma cell growth by factors present in human bone marrow. *Journal of Clinical Investigations*, **84**, 43–50.

Fleming W.H., Hamel A., MacDonal R., Ramsey E., Pettigrew N.M., Johnston B., Dodd J.G. & Matusik R. (1986) Expression of the c-*myc* protooncogene in human prostatic carcinoma and benign prostatic hyperplasia. *Cancer Research* **46**, 1535–8.

Fowler J.E., Jr., Lau J.L.T., Ghosh L., Mills S.E. & Mounzer A. (1988) Epidermal growth factor and prostatic carcinoma: an immunohistochemical study. *Journal of Urology*, **139**, 857–61.

Gleave M., Hsieh J.T., Gao C., von Eschenbach A.C. & Chung L.W.K. (1991) Acceleration of human prostate cancer growth in vivo by factors produced by prostate and bone fibroblasts. *Cancer Research*, **51**, 3753–61.

Hamdy F.C., Fadlon E.J., Cottam D., Lawry J., Thurrell W., Silcocks P. B., Anderson J.B., Williams J.L. & Rees R.C. (1994) Matrix metalloproteinase 9 expression in primary human prostatic adenocarcinoma and benign prostatic hyperplasia. *British Journal of Cancer*, **69**, 177–82.

MacDonald A., Chisholm G.D. & Habib F.K. (1990) Production and response of a human prostatic cancer line to transforming growth factor-like molecules. British Journal of Cancer, **62**, 579–84.

Morris G.L. & Green Dodd J. (1990) Epidermal growth factor receptor mRNA levels in human prostatic tumors and cell lines. *Journal of Urology*, **143**, 1272–4.

Nakamoto T., Hang C., Li A. & Chodak G.W. (1992) Basic fibroblast growth factor in human prostate cancer cells. *Cancer Research*, **52**, 571–7.

Partin A.W., Isaacs J.T., Treiger B. & Coffey D.S. (1988) Early cell motility changes associated with an increase in metastatic ability in rat prostatic cancer cells transfected with the v-Harvey-*ras* oncogene. *Cancer Research*, **48**, 6050–3.

Qayum A., Gullick G., Clayton R.C., Sikora K. & Waxman J. (1990) The effects of gonadotrophin releasing hormone analogues in prostate cancer are mediated through specific tumour receptors. *British Journal of Cancer*, **62**, 96–9.

Rijinders A.W.M., van der Korput J.A.G.M., van Steenbrugge G.J., Romijn J.C. & Trapman J. (1985) Expression of cellular oncogenes in human prostatic carcinoma cell lines. *Biochemical and Biophysical Research Communications*, **132**(2), 548–54.

Ross J.S., Nazeer T., Church K., Amato C., Figge H., Rifkin M.D. & Fisher H.A.G. (1993) Contributiuon of HER-2/*neu* oncogene expression to tumor grade and DNA content analysis in the prediction of prostatic carcinoma metastasis. *Cancer*, **72**(10), 3020–8.

Shain S.A., Lin A.L., Koger J.D. & Karaganis A.G. (1990) Rat prostate cancer cells contain functional receptors for transforming growth factor-β. *Endocrinology*, **126**, 818–25.

Stearns M.E. & Wang M. (1993) Type IV collagenase (Mr 72,000) expression in human prostate: benign and malignant tissue. *Cancer Research*, **53**, 878–83.

Treiger B. & Isaacs J. (1988) Expression of a transfected v-Harvey-*ras* oncogene in a Dunning rat prostate adenocarcinoma and the development of high metastatic ability. *Journal of Urology*, **140**, 1580–6.

Uchida T., Wada C., Shitara T., Egawa S. & Koshiba K. (1993) Infrequent involvement of p53 gene mutations in the tumourigenesis of Japanese prostate cancer. *British Journal of Cancer*, **68**, 751–5.

Viola M.V., Fromowitz F., Oravez S., Deb S., Finkel G., Lundey J., Hand P., Thor A. & Schlom J. (1986) Expression of *ras* oncogene p21 in prostate cancer. *New England Journal of Medicine*, **314**(3), 133–7.

Woll P.J. & Rozengurt E. (1990) A neuropeptide antagonist that inhibits the growth of small cell lung cancer *in vitro*. *Cancer Research*, **50**, 3968–73.

Yano T., Pinski J., Groot K. & Schally A.V. (1992) Stimulation by bombesin and inhibition of bombesin/gastrin releasing peptide antagonist RC-3095 of growth of human breast cancer cell lines. *Cancer Research*, **52**, 4545–7.

Zachary I. & Rozengurt E. (1985) High affinity receptors for the bombesin family in Swiss 3T3 cells. *Proceedings of the National Academy of Sciences of the United States of America*, **82**, 7616–20.

Zachary I., Sinnett-Smith J. & Rozengurt E. (1986) Early events elicited by bombesin and structurally related peptides in quiescent Swiss 3T3 cells. *Journal of Cell Biology*, **102**, 2211–22.

Zachary I., Woll P. & Rozengurt E. (1987) A role for neuropeptides in the control of cell proliferation. *Developmental Biology*, **124**, 295–308.

Zachary I., Millar J., Nanberg E., Higgins T. & Rozengurt E. (1987) Inhibition of bombesin-induced mitogenesis by pertussis toxin: dissociation from phosphatase C pathway. *Biochemical and Biophysical Research Communications*, **146**, 456–60.

Zachary I., Gil J., Lehmann W., Sinnett-Smith J. & Rozengurt E. (1991) Bombesin, vasopressin and endothelin rapidly stimulate phosphorylation in intact Swiss 3T3 cells. *Proceedings of the National Academy of Sciences of the United States of America*, **88**, 4577–81.

Zachary I., Sinnett-Smith J. & Rozengurt E. (1991) Stimulation of tyrosine kinase activity in anti-phosphotyrosine immune complexes of Swiss 3T3 cell lysates occurs rapidly after addition of bombesin, vasopressin, and endothelin to intact cells. *Journal of Biological Chemistry*, **266**(35), 24126–33.

Zachary I., Sinnett-Smith J. & Rozengurt E. (1992) Bombesin, vasopressin and endothelin stimulation of tyrosine phosphorylation in Swiss 3T3 cells: identification of a novel tyrosine kinase as a major substrate. *Journal of Biological Chemistry*, **267**, 19031–4.

Zachary I. & Rozengurt E. (1992) Focal adhesion kinase ($p125^{FAK}$): A point of convergence in the action of neuropeptides, integrins and oncogenes. *Cell*, **71**, 891–4.

Zachary I., Sinnett-Smith J., Turner C.E. & Rozengurt E. (1993) Bombesin, vasopressin, and endothelin rapidly stimulate tyrosine phosphorylation of the focal adhesion-associated protein paxillin in Swiss 3T3 cells. *Journal of Biological Chemistry* (in press).

Zurier R.B., Kozma M., Sinnett-Smith J. & Rozengurt E. (1988) Vasoactive intestinal peptide synergistically stimulates DNA synthesis in mouse 3T3 cells: role of cAMP, Ca2+ and protein kinase C. *Experimental Cell Research*, **176**, 155–61.

5

Gonadotrophin-Releasing Hormone and Its Receptor

KARIN A. EIDNE AND LORRAINE ANDERSON

INTRODUCTION

Receptors in the pituitary gland transduce signals from the brain to the peripheral components of the endocrine system. Paracrine and autocrine factors released from within the pituitary itself as well as from the peripheral target organs are also involved. The releasing hormone, gonadotrophin-releasing hormone (GnRH), and its receptor play a pivotal role in the neuroendocrine control of reproduction (Lincoln, 1993). GnRH is released in a pulsatile fashion from the hypothalamus and, following its route down through the portal system, acts on gonadotroph cells of the anterior pituitary gland, via specific recognition sites, to stimulate the secretion of luteinizing hormone (LH) and follicle-stimulating hormone (FSH). This secretion of LH and FSH then activates the release of reproductive steroid hormones from the gonads.

GnRH has a wide range of potential clinical uses. One of the intriguing aspects of this hormone is that in addition to its effect on the hypothalamic-pituitary-gonadal axis, it has been reported to have extrapituitary actions. These extrapituitary effects have important implications for patient therapy. It is generally accepted that neuropeptides are able to act at sites distal to the hypothalamic-pituitary axis, and the concept that GnRH may somehow be involved in autocrine or paracrine control of peripheral tissues has emerged.

The past decade has seen a ferment of activity surrounding GnRH, GnRH analogues and their effects, witnessing the cloning of genes encoding GnRH, and in the last year, its receptor. Discoveries of this nature will provide opportunities to study in greater detail the different mechanisms and sites of action of this important hormone. This chapter deals with the GnRH peptide; the GnRH receptor; and controlling mechanisms of action, highlighting some molecular advances recently made in this field. Some current information regarding the molecular structure of the GnRH receptor and related structure-function studies has been included, as molecular models of the G-protein coupled receptors are of interest, being used by the majority of pharmaceutical companies and some research laboratories as templates for rational drug design. In addition, the direct effects of GnRH analogues on tumour tissues and the putative role of GnRH as an autocrine regulator in extrapituitary tissues will be examined.

GnRH

GnRH Peptide

In the 22 years since the decapeptide structure of GnRH was established, several thousand GnRH analogues have been synthesized. Analogue design has depended in part on the application of empirical and progressive substitutions of the decapeptide. In fact, some of the most powerful antagonists barely resemble the starting material from which they were obtained, in that seven of the ten amino acids have been substituted.

The native GnRH peptide has the following structure:

pyro-Glu^1, His^2, Trp^3, Ser^4, Tyr^5, Gly^6, Leu^7, Arg^8, Pro^9, Gly^{10}-NH_2.

In aqueous solution, GnRH is thought to assume a hairpin configuration in which the COOH terminus is located near the NH_2 terminus (Momany, 1976). Native GnRH is rapidly degraded, with a half-life of approximately 8 minutes. The peptide bond susceptible to cleavage is sited between Tyr^5 and Gly^6, with secondary sites of action between Trp^3 and Ser^4 and at the amino side of Pro^9. Both ends of the molecule are also under attack from desamidases and pyroglutamidases. Modifications of the natural molecule, particularly at positions 6 and 10, result in a more stable peptide with a more potent and prolonged action. Substituting the Gly^6 with a hydrophobic D-amino acid, for example D-Trp, can result in a molecule with a half-life of more than 7 hours. Further substitutions at the COOH-terminal – for example Gly^{10}-amide with ethylamide – also increase the resistance to proteolysis.

The early observation that elimination of His^2 from GnRH resulted in a peptide that had low agonist potency and demonstrated antagonistic properties (Vale et al., 1972) gave rise to the idea that the NH_2-terminal amino acids were important for receptor activation.

Exactly which amino acids are involved is not yet known, but many antagonist analogues with substitutions in positions 1, 2, 3 and 5 together with the D-amino acid in position 6 have been produced (Karten & Rivier, 1986). It is thought that GnRH antagonists operate by binding to the GnRH receptor but are unable to initiate G-protein coupled events associated with the native peptide and its agonists. GnRH antagonists appear to adopt a different orientation at the binding site (Janovick et al., 1993) such that, by mechanisms that are not yet fully understood, they act to block receptor dimerization and some aspect of second messenger activation.

The GnRH Precursor Gene

Both the genomic and cDNA structures of the precursor for GnRH have been characterized (Seeburg & Adelman, 1984). The human GnRH gene has been mapped to the short arm of chromosome 8 (region 8p11.2-p21) (Yang-Feng et al., 1986), whereas in the mouse, this locus is mapped to chromosome 14 (Williamson et al., 1991). Following sequence analysis of clones isolated from human hypothalamic, placental and genomic DNA, it was revealed that the GnRH precursor consisted of a protein of 92 amino acids, encoded by an approximately 600-base mRNA. In the species characterized thus far (human, rat and mouse), the precursor gene comprises four exons and three introns (Adelman et al., 1986; Bond et al., 1989; Mason et al., 1986a). The 92 amino acid protein incorporates a signal peptide of 23 amino acids, the GnRH decapeptide and the 56 amino acid GnRH-associated peptide (GAP). The structure of the promoter elements of the rat GnRH gene, which may be involved in tissue-specific expression and hormonal regulation, have also been determined (Kepa et al., 1992). There is some controversy as to the actual transcription start site of the GnRH gene because, in addition to the well-characterized hypothalamic transcription start site, another major site exists upstream in GnRH genes expressed in human reproductive tissues like placenta, testes, ovary and mammary gland (Dong et al., 1993).

The biological function of the GAP peptide, if any, is not yet fully understood, but it is thought to have an effect on prolactin-releasing activity. Synthetic GAP was described as inhibiting prolactin secretion in rat anterior pituitary cell cultures in vitro (Nikolics et al., 1985). However, data regarding its physiological role in vivo are somewhat equivocal. Another study, investigating the biological function of GAP and truncated versions of GAP, demonstrated that GAP peptides were able to stimulate gonadotrophin release in primate pituitary cell cultures (Millar et al., 1986). The reason why two structurally dissimilar molecules encoded by the same GnRH precursor should both have LH- and FSH-releasing activity remains an enigma.

Clinical Significance of the GnRH Gene The hypogonadal (hpg) mouse is considered a good animal model for the human disorder, hypogonadotrophic hypogonadism. In these animals, a large deletion of the part of the GnRH gene encoding GAP has been described (Mason et al., 1986a). Transcription of this truncated gene in hpg mice results in lower levels of GnRH expression when compared to normal mice. Further experiments showed that gene therapy with full-length GnRH genes was able to restore gonadal function in hpg mice (Mason et al., 1986b).

Hypothalamic deficiency of GnRH is presumed to be the aetiology in patients presenting with idiopathic hypogonadotrophic hypogonadism (IHH). The X chromosome-linked Kallmann's syndrome is an inherited hypogonadotrophic hypogonadism combined with anosmia. The GnRH/GAP gene in IHH patients appears to be normal with no major deletions (Layman, 1991), indicating that the human disorder does not mirror that found in hpg mice. Instead, associated with this syndrome is the apparent loss of GnRH-expressing cells in the brain, even though dense clusters of these cells are apparent in the nose (Schwanzel Fukuda et al., 1989). Normally, GnRH-expressing cells migrate from the olfactory placode up into the brain, and it has been postulated that in patients suffering from Kallmann's, this migration does not occur. This defect occurs at the embryonic stage and an extracellular matrix protein, KAL, has been implicated in this neuronal migratory step (Petit, 1993). KAL appears to guide the embryonic journey of the GnRH-expressing neurons from the olfactory placode to the hypothalamic area. The involvement of the KAL gene, which lies on the X chromosome, makes this a rather complex story in that the interplay of several genetic loci may be necessary before reproductive potential can be fully expressed.

THE GnRH RECEPTOR

The recent cloning of the GnRH receptor can be regarded as the key step towards revealing the complexities of the GnRH receptor ligand recognition and signalling mechanisms.

Structural Aspects of the GnRH Receptor

Molecular Cloning of the GnRH Receptor The cloning of functional GnRH receptors from a variety of species – for example, the mouse gonadotroph cell line αT3-1 (Tsutsumi et al., 1992; Reinhart et al., 1992), rat (Eidne et al., 1992), human (Kakar, 1992) and sheep pituitary (Brooks et al., 1993) – has been reported. The receptor from the αT3-1 cells (Tsutsumi et al., 1992) was cloned using a combination of receptor cloning strategies based on both the polymerase chain reaction (Eidne, 1991) and the inhibition of *Xenopus* oocyte expression by antisense oligonucleotides (hybrid arrest assay; Sumikawa & Miledi, 1988). The *Xenopus* oocyte expression system is described in more detail later.

The characteristic seven-transmembrane-domain structure of the GnRH receptor indicates that it belongs to the superfamily of G-protein coupled receptors (Figure 5.1). The GnRH receptor shows considerable sequence homology and has a number of structural features in common with other members of this receptor superfamily (Probst et al., 1992). The rat pituitary GnRH receptor consists of a single 327 amino acid polypeptide chain incorporating seven hydrophobic stretches of amino acids, two extracellular potential glycosylation

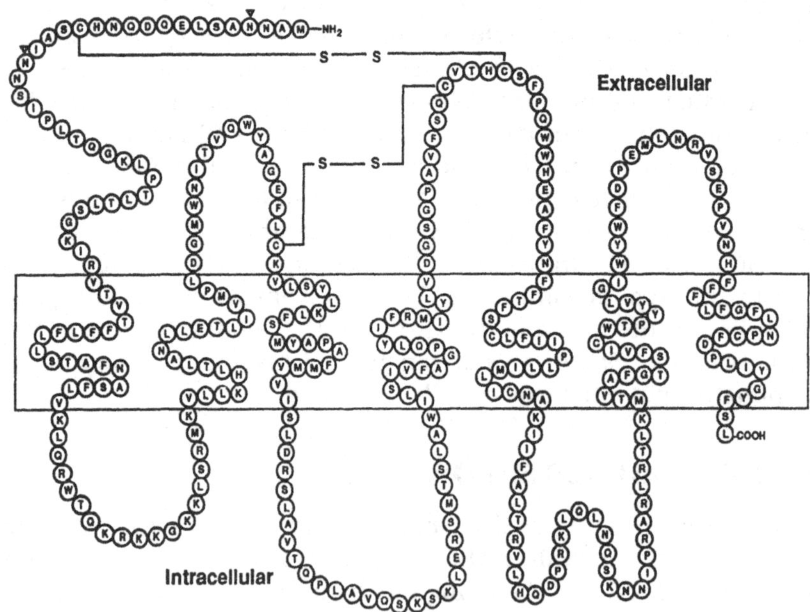

Rat GnRH receptor

Figure 5.1 A schematic representation of the rat pituitary GnRH receptor. The amino acid sequence of the protein is displayed in the one-letter code. Potential N-linked glycosylation sites (▽) are indicated.

sites, and eight intracellular putative phosphorylation sites (Eidne et al., 1992). Other conserved features include a pair of cysteine residues between the second and third extracellular domain and a number of prolines in the transmembrane domains.

The protein sequence of the GnRH receptor is highly conserved between different species (Figure 5.2) and shares significant similarity with other members of this family. However, the GnRH receptor does have certain unusual features. These include (1) the complete absence of the COOH-terminal tail, (2) the interchange of two highly conserved (and therefore potentially critical) amino acids in the second and seventh transmembrane domains and (3) the change of the highly conserved tyrosine in the DRY motif to serine near transmembrane 3. The absence of a COOH-terminal tail is of great interest, because hitherto this region of the receptor has been associated with receptor down-regulation.

Chromosomal Localization To localize the chromosome containing the GnRH receptor, we used cloned human GnRH cDNA probes and fluorescence in situ hybridization (FISH). Southern blots of restriction digests of genomic DNAs electrophoresed in agarose gels were also probed allowing initial characterization of the receptor gene. FISH studies localized the GnRH receptor to human chromosome 4q13.2–13.3 (Morrison et al., 1994). Restriction digests of human genomic DNA showed more hybridizing fragments than predicted from the cDNA sequence for the GnRH receptor, suggesting the presence of introns (unpublished observations). A blot of cleaved genomic DNA from a panel of species (Zooblot, probed with the human GnRH receptor cDNA probe) demonstrated strong cross-reactivity with GnRH receptor genes in monkey and weaker cross-reactivity in rat, mouse, dog, cow and rabbit. Chicken and yeast showed very little cross-reactivity (Duthie et al., unpublished observations).

GnRH Receptor mRNA Regulation During the Oestrous Cycle Until now, little has been known about the endocrine events that control GnRH receptor variation in pituitary gonadotrophs of cycling animals. Using probes based on GnRH receptor sequence information, it has been possible to demonstrate that pituitary GnRH receptor mRNA levels are dynamically regulated during the oestrous cycle of the rat (Bauer-Dantoin et al., 1993) and sheep (Brooks et al., 1993). In preovulatory sheep, both GnRH receptor mRNA and GnRH binding were higher than similar measurements carried out during the luteal phase. Following the LH surge, a significant decline in both GnRH receptor mRNA and binding was seen. The levels of LHβ mRNA

```
                 10        20        30        40        50        60        70        80
                  |         |         |         |         |         |         |         |
Rat     MANNASLEQDQNHCSAINNSIPLTQGKLPTLTLSGKIRVTVTFFLFLLSTAFNASFLVKLQRWTQKRKKGKKLSRMKVLLKH
Mouse   MANNASLEQDPNHCSAINNSIPLIQGKLPTLTVSGKIRVTVTFFLFLLSTAFNASFLLKLQKWTQKRKKGKKLSRMKVLLKH
Sheep   MANGDSPNQNENHCSAINSSILLTPGRLPTLTLSGKIRVTVTFFLFLLSTIFNTSFLLKLQNWAQRKEKRKKLSKMKVLLKH
Man     MANSASPEQNQNHCSAINNSIPLMQGNLPTLTLSGKIRVTVTFFLFLLSATFNASFLLKLQKWTQKKEKGKKLSRMKLLLKH

                90       100       110       120       130       140       150       160
                 |         |         |         |         |         |         |         |
Rat     LTLANLLETLIVMPLDGMWNITVQWYAGEFLCKVLSYLKLFSMYAPAFMMVVISLDRSLAVTQPLAVQSKSKLERSMTSLAW
Mouse   LTLANLLETLIVMPLDGMWNITVQWYAGEFLCKVLSYLKLFSMYAPAFMMVVISLDRSLAITQPLAVQSNSKLEQSMISLAW
Sheep   LTLANLLETLIVMPLDGMWNITVQWYAGELLCKVLSYLKLFSMYAPAFMMVVISLDRSLAITRPLAVKSNSKLGQFMIGLAW
Man     LTLANLLETLIVMPLDGMWNITVQWYAGELLCKVLSYLKLFSMYAPAFMMVVISLDRSLAITRPLALKSNSKVGQSMVGLAW

              170       180       190       200       210       220       230       240
                |         |         |         |         |         |         |         |
Rat     ILSIVFAGPQLYIFRMIYLVDGSGPA-VFSQCVTHCSFPQWWHEAFYNFFTFSCLFIIPLLIMLICNAKIIFALTRVLHQDP
Mouse   ILSIVFAGPQLYIFRMIYLADGSGPT-VFSQCVTHCSFPQWWHQAFYNFFTFGCLFIIPLLIMLICNAKIIFALTRVLHQDP
Sheep   LLSSIFAGPQLYIFGMIHLADDSGQTEGFSQCVTHCSFPQWWHQAFYNFFTFSCLFIIPLLIMLICNAKIIFTLTRVLHQDP
Man     ILSSVFAGPQLYIFRMIHLADSSGQTKVFSQCVTHCSFSQWWHQAFYNFFTFSCLFIIPLFIMLICNAKIIFTLTRVLHQDP

             250       260       270       280       290       300       310       320
               |         |         |         |         |         |         |         |
Rat     RKLQLNQSKNNIPRARLRTLKMTVAFGTSFVICWTPYYVLGIWYWFDPEMLNRVSEPVNHFFFLFGFLNPCFDPLIYGYFSL
Mouse   RKLQMNQSKNNIPRARLRTLKMTVAFATSFVVCWTPYYVLGIWYWFDPEMLNRVSEPVNHFFFLFAFLNPCFDPLIYGYFSL
Sheep   HKLQLNQSKNNIPQARLRTLKMTVAFATSFTVCWTPYYVLGIWYWFDPDMVNRVSDPVNHFFFLFGFLNPCFDPLIYGYFSL
Man     HELQLNQSKNNIPRARLKTLKMTVAFATSFTVCWTPYYVLGIWYWFDPEMLNRLSDPVNHFFFLFAFLNPCFDPLIYGYFSL
```

Figure 5.2 Alignments of the amino acid sequences of the GnRH receptor from different species.

remained constant throughout the oestrous cycle. These changes in GnRH receptor expression and resultant binding capacity are thought to be related to changes in follicle oestradiol production during the follicular phase. Studies of this type therefore indicate that receptor expression and ultimately receptor number are under physiological control.

Functional Aspects of the GnRH Receptor

Electrophysiological Studies in Pituitary Gonadotrophs It has been clearly established that the GnRH-induced stimulation of LH release from pituitary gonadotrophs is calcium dependent (Chang et al., 1986; Leong & Thorner, 1991; Hawes et al., 1992). There is considerable evidence that GnRH mobilizes calcium from both intra- and extracellular stores (Izumi et al., 1990; Anderson et al., 1992). Although pharmacological studies have demonstrated that selective calcium channels are involved in GnRH-induced gonadotrophin secretion, it is not yet clear if these calcium channels are ligand gated, voltage activated or both. Using a whole-cell voltage-clamp technique, electrophysiological studies employing identified pituitary gonadotrophs (Croxton et al., 1988; Mason & Sikdar, 1988) and the gonadotroph cell line αT3-1 (Horn et al., 1991) have attempted to resolve this issue. In pituitary gonadotrophs, the application of GnRH produced delayed, large-amplitude inward pulses of current. The ability of the calcium antagonist D600 to eliminate these effects suggests that these changes are more likely to be generated by voltage-operated calcium channels (Croxton et al., 1988). The nature of this voltage-operated calcium channel response was also investigated in αT3-1 cells. GnRH produced a biphasic inward current response consisting of a transient and sustained phase. The sustained current was high-voltage activated and dihydropyridine sensitive, while the transient current, which was rapidly inactivated, was low-voltage activated (Horn et al., 1991).

Electrophysiological Studies in *Xenopus* Oocytes *Xenopus laevis* oocytes, when injected with foreign mRNA encoding a receptor protein, are capable of translating this RNA into a functional receptor inserted in the oocyte lipid bilayer. This expression system offers a convenient method by which to investigate the ionic mechanisms associated with a variety of G-protein coupled receptors (Eidne, 1994). The GnRH receptor, when expressed in this manner, can couple to G-protein linked second-messenger systems endogenous to the oocyte (Oron et al., 1987; Meyerhof et al., 1988; Yoshida et al., 1989). This system has been successfully used in both the cloning and functional characterization of the GnRH receptor. Whole-cell currents were monitored using either single-electrode membrane potential measurements (Eidne et al., 1988) or two-electrode voltage-clamp measurements (Yoshida et al., 1989; Yoshida & Plant, 1990). Exposure of oocytes to GnRH, injected with either total rat pituitary poly(A^+) mRNA (Yoshida et al., 1989) or capped mRNA transcripts prepared from a GnRH receptor clone (Eidne et al., 1992; Tsutsumi et al., 1992), resulted in a dose-dependent peak of inward depolarizing current. This response involves the activation of ion channels that are endogenous to the oocyte. In the *Xenopus* oocyte system, GnRH-induced depolarizations appears to operate via a calcium-dependent chloride channel as evidenced by antagonism of this depolarization response by a variety of calcium and chloride channel blockers (Yoshida et al., 1989).

Phospholipase C–Mediated Signal Transduction The precise signal transduction mechanisms through which GnRH controls gonadotrophin synthesis and secretion still remain unclear. GnRH communicates with the cell interior via its heptahelical receptor, which in turn is primarily linked to the family of phospholipase C isoenzymes. Receptor activation by GnRH results in a phospholipase C–mediated hydrolysis of the membrane phospholipid phosphatidylinositol 4,5-bisphosphate (PIP_2), producing the second messengers, inositol 1,4,5-trisphosphate (Ins[1,4,5]P_3) and diacylglycerol (DAG) (Limor et al., 1989; Morgan et al., 1987; Naor, 1985). While Ins(1,4,5)P_3 is directly involved in the mobilization of intracellular calcium ($[Ca^{2+}]_i$), DAG activates protein kinase C (PKC), and is therefore indirectly involved in the mobilization of $[Ca^{2+}]_i$. Mobilized calcium is believed to play a pivotal role in hormone secretion (Shangold et al., 1988).

The development of an established gonadotroph cell line, αT3-1 (Windle et al., 1990), highly expressing the GnRH receptor (1.6 pmol/mg protein; Horn et al., 1991), has aided the detailed study of signal transduction pathways associated with the GnRH receptor. Unfortunately, it is not possible to study mechanisms of gonadotrophin secretion in these cells, as they do not synthesize gonadotrophin β subunits and therefore do not secrete LH or FSH in response to GnRH. However, αT3-1 cells are useful for experiments involving the measurement of the upstream signalling events, and in these cells GnRH has been shown to induce a rapid but short-lived rise in Ins(1,4,5)P_3 production (Anderson et al., 1993). Using dual-wavelength fluorescence microscopy combined with dynamic video imaging, this

Ins(1,4,5)P_3 rise was clearly associated with a biphasic increase in $[Ca^{2+}]_i$ in single αT3-1 cells (Figure 5.3) (Anderson et al., 1992). The initial calcium transient appears to involve both an Ins(1,4,5)P_3-mediated rise in cytosolic calcium due to its release from intracellular stores and an influx of extracellular calcium through second-messenger-operated calcium channels. In contrast, the secondary calcium response mainly involves the influx of extracellular calcium through PKC-activated dihydropyridine-sensitive channels (Izumi et al., 1990; Anderson et al., 1992). This biphasic change in $[Ca^{2+}]_i$ is believed to underlie the GnRH-induced pattern of LH release, which similarly consists of an initial spike phase of release followed by a more protracted plateau phase (Davidson et al., 1991).

GnRH Receptor–Associated G Proteins Hormonal activation of PLC is mediated through heterotrimeric GTP-binding (G) proteins. Ligand-binding studies have shown that GnRH binding is altered by guanine nucleotide analogues indicative of G-protein coupling by this receptor (Perrin et al., 1989). GnRH-induced total inositol phosphate (IP) accumulation is pertussis toxin–insensitive, suggesting that the G-protein involved is neither G_i nor G_o, but more probably G_q/G_{11}. Members of this family of G-proteins have been identified in αT3-1 cell membranes using antisera raised against the predicted C-terminal decapeptide of the α subunit of G_q/G_{11} (Hsieh & Martin, 1992; An-

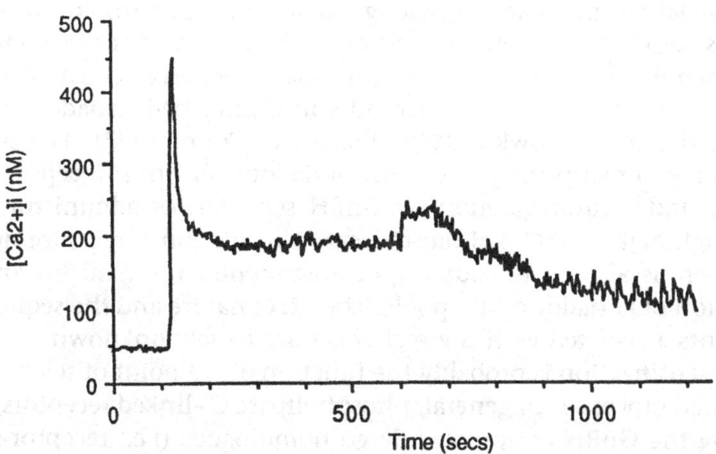

Figure 5.3 Effect of GnRH (10^{-8} M) on intracellular calcium in αT3-1 cells. Cells were labelled with the fluorescent calcium dye, Fura-2 AM (2 μM final concentration for 30 minutes). Ratioed images were captured using dual-wavelength fluorescence microscopy at 340/380 nm wavelength.

derson et al., 1993). Similarly, G_q/G_{11} immune serum inhibited GnRH-stimulated PLC activity in αT3-1 cell membranes (Hsieh & Martin, 1992).

Adenyl Cyclase-Mediated Signal Transduction The role of the adenyl cyclase pathway in the GnRH-induced release of pituitary gonadotrophins has been controversial for many years. Both cAMP and cGMP levels are increased in pituitary cell cultures (Borgeat et al., 1972; Naor et al., 1979) but not in αT3-1 cells (Horn et al., 1991), following stimulation with GnRH. It has been suggested that these second messengers do not transmit the GnRH signal in gonadotroph cells but rather may facilitate GnRH-induced gonadotrophin release (Turgeon et al., 1987; Cronin et al., 1984).

Mechanisms of Receptor Desensitization and Down-Regulation The clinical manifestation of 'chemical castration' following the administration of GnRH analogues results from receptor desensitization. It is therefore important to understand the mechanisms through which this phenomenon occurs. A variety of mechanisms have been proposed in an attempt to explain the antifertility effects of GnRH analogues. These include: GnRH receptor desensitization/down-regulation at the level of the pituitary gonadotroph; secretion of inappropriate amounts or patterns of LH release, leading to gonadal LH receptor desensitization/down-regulation culminating in reduced LH-dependent steroidogenesis; and a direct down-regulation of gonadal receptors and steroidogenic activity. In vitro and in vivo studies show that the pulsatile administration of GnRH is associated with maintenance of gonadotrophin release, whereas constant high doses or rapidly pulsed GnRH results in diminished gonadotrophin release (Conn & Crowley, 1991; Braden & Conn, 1992). The latter results are not surprising given that gonadotroph GnRH receptor levels are under autoregulation by GnRH secretion or administration. Although high-dose GnRH causes a down-regulation of receptor number, there is also an uncoupling of postreceptor mechanisms and a depletion of gonadotrophin pools. The exact nature and the sequence of events associated with these changes are largely unknown.

Desensitization is probably the functional end-point of several interrelated processes. In general, phospholipase C–linked receptors, including the GnRH receptor, undergo homologous (i.e., receptor-specific) desensitization (Wojcikiewicz et al., 1993). The initial step usually involves the uncoupling of the receptor from its intermediary G-protein, with the subsequent loss of downstream second-messenger production. Although low-dose pretreatment of primary pituitary gonadotroph cultures with GnRH results in a marked decrease in LH release, GnRH-induced inositol phosphate (IP) production remains unaltered (Hawes & Conn, 1992). Given that GnRH-induced LH release involves the mobilization of intracellular calcium (McArdle & Poch, 1992), it is possible that an uncoupling of G-protein coupled events beyond IP production (e.g., at the level of calcium mobilization) is involved in the desensitization of GnRH-induced LH release (Smith & Conn, 1984). A single pulse of a high concentration of GnRH results in a rapid desensitization of the GnRH biphasic calcium response in single αT3-1 cells (L. Anderson, unpublished data). Alternatively, the effects of GnRH on IP production and LH release may be mediated through different G-proteins and it may therefore be possible to preferentially uncouple one G-protein but not the other. Several studies have suggested that multiple G-proteins can be stimulated by a single receptor type (Hawes et al., 1992; Milligan, 1993). It has also been proposed that GnRH stimulation of pituitary gonadotrophs causes a movement of LH from a nonreleasable pool to a releasable pool and that this movement is progressively lost as the cells become desensitized (Janovick & Conn, 1993).

Following this initial uncoupling step an additional stage involving receptor sequestration occurs. Sequestration refers to receptor internalization during chronic agonist stimulation and is a process that occurs in minutes to hours. Withdrawal of agonist stimulation results in a recycling of the receptor back to the cell surface where it can once again bind ligand. Chronic GnRH treatment of pituitary gonadotroph cultures results in a temporary loss of measurable amounts of GnRH receptors, with the recovery of receptor number following the removal of GnRH (Conn et al., 1984; Hawes & Conn, 1992). However, prolonged agonist treatment can result in receptor down-regulation. This is a much slower process that can occur from several hours up to several days and involves the internalization and subsequent degradation of receptor protein. These receptors are therefore not available for recycling on withdrawal of agonist; instead, new receptor protein must be synthesized. Agonist-induced receptor phosphorylation is intimately involved in these desensitization processes (Wong et al., 1990; Nussenzveig et al., 1993a, 1993b; Richardson et al., 1993).

GnRH Receptor Structure/Function Studies

Mutational and chimeric receptor studies have been carried out on several members of the G-protein coupled family of receptors. As a result of the alteration of specific regions of these receptors, a general picture can be obtained where discrete areas are associated with ligand binding, G-protein coupling and receptor desensitization (Strader et al., 1987, 1989). Using a strategy based on site-directed mutagenesis, we have demonstrated that specific, single-point mutations can dramatically alter the GnRH receptor's ability to recognize its own ligand as well as its ability to activate the downstream G-protein coupled events (Cook et al., 1993).

Ligand-Binding Domains When considering which regions of a receptor protein are involved in a particular function, like ligand recognition, it is important to remember that the receptor is a three-dimensional structure. The juxtaposition of the alpha helical transmembrane (TM) domains of G-protein coupled receptors, including that of the GnRH receptor, is believed to form a ligand-binding pocket into which the peptide/ligand must slot. Based on the projection map of bacteriorhodopsin and the G-protein coupled rhodopsin (Henderson et al., 1990), a model of the probable arrangement of the TM domains of G-protein coupled receptors has been proposed (Baldwin, 1993). The model infers that these domains lie tilted within the lipid bilayer. By applying the coordinates of the Baldwin model to the GnRH receptor, a helical wheel model of the TM domains of the GnRH receptor has been generated (Eidne et al., unpublished data). This model allows us to identify conserved amino acids within the GnRH receptor and to examine their location with respect to the ligand-binding pocket. It should be noted that this model of the GnRH receptor may differ from other models based on the energy minimization model of receptors, primary sequence comparison and computer simulation of receptor-ligand interactions. Ultimately, only X-ray crystallography of the GnRH receptor will confirm the most appropriate model.

Similarities between the GnRH receptor and other G-protein coupled receptors include the presence of conserved cysteine residues in the extracellular loops. In the GnRH receptor the mutation of the conserved extracellular cysteine residues, Cys^{114}, Cys^{195} and the non-conserved Cys^{14}, and Cys^{199} to serine residues abolished both ligand binding and subsequent G-protein coupled events (Cook et al., unpublished observations). The ability of these residues to form extracellular disulphide bridges, thereby stabilizing the three-dimensional conformation of the receptor, may underlie their obvious importance in ligand recognition and downstream cell signalling events.

As previously mentioned, the GnRH receptor has certain unique features. The GnRH receptor is unlike other G-protein coupled receptors in that the highly conserved amino acids, Asp^{87} in the second

TM region and the Asn^{318} in the seventh TM, are transposed. In an attempt to examine the significance of these changes, mutagenesis studies were carried out in which these residues were mutated back to their normally conserved positions (Cook et al., 1993). Mutation of Asn^{318} to Asp^{318} (Asp^{318Asn}) in TM7 had no effect on ligand receptor binding but abolished GnRH receptor function as assessed by measuring IP accumulation. In contrast, the TM2 mutant, Asn^{87Asp}, in which Asn^{87} was mutated to Asp^{87}, showed a complete loss of GnRH binding and subsequent second messenger events. These results suggest that Asn^{87} is essential for the binding of GnRH to its receptor, whereas Asp^{318}, although not required for binding, is necessary for signal transduction.

G-Protein Coupling Domains All three intracellular loops (IL) of G-protein coupled receptors have varying degrees of importance for efficient G-protein coupling. Of particular importance are membrane regions proximal to the third intracellular loop and possibly the second IL and the COOH-terminal tail. Based on a variety of studies, including those using the wasp venom mastoparan, it has been proposed that these regions form clustered amphipathic alpha-helices (Higashijima et al., 1990). Following ligand binding, these helices, along with the charged intracellular residues of the second and third ILs (e.g., the DRS sequence in the second intracellular loop of the GnRH receptor; Anderson et al., unpublished observations), may cooperatively interact to bind and activate the appropriate G-protein (Strader et al., 1987; Strader et al., 1989).

Receptor Desensitization Domains The process of G-protein uncoupling apparently involves the protein kinase dependent phosphorylation at serine and threonine residues within the third IL and COOH-terminal tail (Bouvier et al., 1988, 1991; Hausdorff et al., 1989; Kennelly & Krebs 1991; Nussenzveig et al., 1993a, 1993b). The lack of a COOH-terminal tail in the GnRH receptor suggests that the third IL may be of particular importance in receptor G-protein uncoupling. Potential PKC phosphorylation sites have also been identified at Thr^{238} and Thr^{264} of the third IL of the GnRH receptor. Further, the substitution of Ser^{140} in the second IL of the GnRH receptor for the conserved tyrosine found in other G-protein coupled receptors (i.e., DRS and not DRY) introduces an additional phosphorylation site and a potential candidate in GnRH receptor phosphorylation and uncoupling (Eidne et al., 1992). It is not yet known whether a specific GnRH receptor kinase akin to the BARK kinase associated with phosphorylation of the β-adrenoreceptor (Benovic et al., 1986) exists for the GnRH receptor. Regardless of the mechanisms involved, it should be noted that this step of G-protein uncoupling occurs without any changes in cell surface receptor number. Although key residues associated with the process of receptor sequestration have been identified in the muscarinic (Wong et al., 1990; Richardson et al., 1993), thyrotrophin-releasing hormone (Nussenzveig et al., 1993a, 1993b) and adrenergic receptors (Strader et al., 1987, 1989), the sites and mechanisms associated with the GnRH receptor have yet to be identified.

GnRH ACTION; ENDOCRINE, PARACRINE AND AUTOCRINE

Clinical Application and Sites of Action

The past decade has seen an expansion in the range of therapeutic applications of GnRH and GnRH superagonists. The clinical value of the GnRH peptides lies in their dual action: the stimulation of gonadal steroid secretion on the one hand, and the loss of steroid hormone release on the other. GnRH, when administered in pulses of appropriate amplitude and interval, can be used to stimulate reproduction in cases of infertility associated with hypothalamic insufficiency. The opposite clinical effect is obtained when GnRH agonists are continuously administered. GnRH receptors become down-regulated, with the result that the secretion of gonadotrophins and gonadal steroids are virtually abolished. This phenomenon, equivalent to a 'chemical castration,' has been exploited for the management of endometriosis, precocious puberty and polycystic ovarian disease. GnRH analogues are also used in the treatment of steroid-dependent neoplasms, such as those of the breast and prostate.

The clinical management of these disorders involves the use of both GnRH agonist and antagonist analogues. Although, GnRH agonists are generally well tolerated, this form of therapy has the drawback that the disease conditions are often aggravated by the initial stimulatory effect sometimes referred to as 'disease flare' observed prior to down-regulation. This flare is due to the early increase in pituitary LH and FSH, which results in the activation of gonadal steroids. In certain cases this activation stage may last up to three weeks in duration before the pituitary-gonadal axis becomes down-regulated. During this time, hormone-sensitive disease may become acutely exacerbated. A more desirable approach would be to administer GnRH antagonists, as the gonads become rapidly suppressed, thereby avoiding the initial stimulatory stage. GnRH antagonists produce a rapid cessation of gonadotrophin release via classical receptor antagonism (Gordon & Hodgen, 1992). Unfortunately, the development of GnRH antagonists for clinical use has been hampered by problems of oedema and anaphylactoid reactions following their subcutaneous administration in humans. In fact, GnRH antagonists have been described as being mast cell secretogogues causing mast cell degranulation and release of histamine (Morgan et al., 1986). New antagonists that have demonstrably less severe side effects are being produced, and a number of antagonists with sufficient affinity and duration have now been produced for clinical trial. An example of the new generation GnRH antagonists is SB-75 or Cetrorelix, ([Ac-3-2-napthyl)-D-Ala^{1}, D-Phe(pCl)^{2}, -(3-pyridyl)-D-Ala^{3}, D-Cit^{6}, D-Ala^{10}]GnRH) (Reissman et al., 1992). This potent antagonist is thought to be free of oedematogenic side effects, and long-acting microcapsule formulations for sustained delivery have been developed.

GnRH Analogue Effects on Extrapituitary and Tumour Tissues

Because of the extensive therapeutic applications of GnRH agonists and antagonists, it is necessary to widen our understanding of the effect of these peptides, particularly since there seems to be more than one mechanism and site of action. Certain studies have documented a direct action of the peptide on extrapituitary target tissues both in vivo and in vitro. GnRH and a number of other peptides have also been shown to have a regulatory effect on tumour cell proliferation (Prevost et al., 1993). The finding that peripheral tissues locally produce both the GnRH (or GnRH-like) peptide and express GnRH binding sites has prompted the idea that these peptides are fulfilling an autocrine or paracrine role at sites distal to the pituitary. This can occur either as a result of direct effects on target tissues via specific receptors or by controlling the secretion of other hormones in a more indirect fashion.

Rat Ovary The direct effects of GnRH in the ovary varies between different species. Whereas in the rat ovary the existence of high-affinity GnRH receptors, similar to those found in the pituitary, has been well documented (Jones et al., 1980; Harwood et al., 1980a, 1980b; Hazum, 1981), generally low-affinity binding sites with differing pharmacological properties have been identified in ovarian as well as other extrapituitary tissues from other species. Rat ovarian GnRH-like peptides have also been isolated (Birnbaumer et al., 1985; Aten et al., 1986). In addition, GnRH has been shown to inhibit FSH-induced steroidogenesis in cultured rat granulosa cells (Hsueh & Ling, 1979). In both hypophysectomized rats and in vitro culture systems, GnRH effects vary according to the gonadotrophin environment, the stage of follicular maturity, and the duration of exposure to the agonists (Fraser & Eidne, 1989). Although GnRH has been shown to have distinct effects in rat ovarian physiology (see later), the evidence in other species is not clear (Wickings et al., 1990).

Human Ovarian Tissue Favourable responses of some patients with refractory ovarian epithelial cancer to GnRH analogues have been reported (Parmar et al., 1985; Waxman, 1987; Kavanagh et al., 1989; Jager et al., 1989; Emons et al., 1993). Adelson and Reece (1993), examining the treatment results of a number of different studies of patients with epithelial ovarian cancers, summarized disease responses from 154 patients following GnRH agonist therapy: 0.6% had complete responses, 11.7% had partial responses, 29.9% had stable disease and 57.8% had progressive disease.

Pituitary gonadotrophins are thought to stimulate ovarian tumour growth. As yet, it is unclear whether these antiproliferative effects are the direct result of a gonadotrophin suppression or involving a direct effect on tumour tissue. Both low- and high-affinity GnRH binding sites have been measured in biopsy samples of human epithelial ovarian cancer tissue and human ovarian cell lines. Although the biological role of these binding sites is unclear, GnRH analogues have been reported to reduce the proliferation of a variety of human ovarian cell lines in vitro (Thompson et al., 1991; Emons et al., 1993). GnRH has also been shown to cause tumour regression of human ovarian epithelial tumours transplanted into nude mice (Schally et al., 1984). A study by Thompson et al. (1991) also reported that in a stable, oestrogen receptor negative ovarian epithelial cell line, 2774, the GnRH analogue, leuprolide acetate, retarded cell growth in a dose-dependent manner. In serum-free medium, leuprolide acetate was able to slow down log growth of these cells by accumulating cells in the resting phase (G_i/G_o) of the cell cycle. However, following long-term culture with leuprolide acetate (three weeks), cells overcame the GnRH agonist's inhibitory effects, plateauing at cell numbers similar to control cultures. These findings concluded that GnRH agonist effects on ovarian cancer were independent of both gonadotrophins and of steroids and involved a cell cycle regulatory event.

Human Breast Cancer Potent GnRH analogues have been used in the clinical management of hormone-dependent breast cancers in premenopausal women (Klijn & De Jong, 1982; Schally et al., 1984;

Manni et al., 1986). Tumour regression is believed to result primarily from a desensitization of the pituitary GnRH receptor, suppressing gonadotrophin release and subsequently gonadal steroid secretion (Nicholson et al., 1984). However, earlier preliminary studies reported that certain postmenopausal women, who have low levels of circulating steroids, respond to GnRH analogue treatment (Harvey et al., 1981; Waxman et al., 1985; Plowman et al., 1986). In an attempt to explain these findings, a mechanism unrelated to pituitary receptor desensitization was proposed; namely, a direct antiproliferative effect of these analogues on tumour cell growth that may or may not involve the GnRH receptor. To address this question, several investigators have reported in vitro studies with a variety of breast cancer cell lines. Data from these studies have been inconsistent in that the growth inhibitory effects of GnRH agonist analogues are not reproducible. In 1985, Miller et al. reported that even at low doses the GnRH agonist Buserelin inhibited the growth of MCF-7 breast cancer cells after two to four days in culture. Contradictory data were later reported by Eidne et al. (1987) where Buserelin did not alter thymidine incorporation of five breast cancer cell lines including MCF-7. Several studies since then either have also failed to reproduce these inhibitory effects (Wilding et al., 1987; Sharoni et al., 1989) or have shown an inconsistent Buserelin-induced stimulation of cell growth under oestrogen-deficient conditions (Segal-Abramson et al., 1992). The reason why these observations are not reproducible has yet to be found. Suggestions have been put forward that clonal variation between cell lines, perhaps reflecting different local environments, may be responsible for these opposing effects of GnRH agonist analogues (Wilding et al., 1987).

Findings from in vitro studies using GnRH antagonists have been more encouraging. In both the hormone-dependent MCF-7 (Eidne et al., 1987; Sharoni et al., 1989; Segal Abramson, 1992) and the hormone-independent human breast cancer cell line MDA-MB-231 (Eidne et al., 1987; Sharoni et al., 1989), a variety of GnRH antagonists, including SB-75, had growth inhibitory effects as measured by either an inhibition of [^{3}H] thymidine uptake into DNA or cell growth. Certain GnRH antagonists had inhibitory effects on human breast cancer cells in culture, while others with different substitutions had no effect (Eidne et al., 1987). We therefore tested a number of GnRH antagonists and found that the following showed the most inhibitory effect (Eidne et al., unpublished observations): antagonist A [Ac-D-Nal(2)^1, D-α-Me-4-ClPhe^2, D-Trp^3, D-Arg^6, D-Ala^{10}]GnRH and antagonist B [Ac-D-Nal(2)^1, D-α-Me-4-ClPhe^2, D-Trp^3, D-Arg^6, D-His^8, D-Ala^{10}]GnRH. Other antagonists with similar structures to these two, but having substitutions in position 5 (other than α-Me-Tyr) were not effective. Another antagonist that was identical to antagonist A, except for Ac-D-α-Me-4-Cl-Phe substituted in position 1, also had no effect on these cells. There was no correlation between these breast cancer cell effects and the potency of antagonist binding to rat pituitaries, their antiovulatory effects in vivo and their ability to release histamine from mast cells. Since this work was carried out, a large number of different GnRH antagonists have been synthesised and studies by Fakete et al. (1989) and Segal-Abramson et al. (1992) showed that these different GnRH antagonists had a wide range of binding and growth inhibitory activities. Some antagonists were more effective than others.

Results from in vivo studies are more difficult to interpret in that inhibitory effects on tumour cell growth can be attributed to GnRH receptor down-regulation and/or blockade at the level of both the pituitary and the tumour. In mice bearing the oestrogen-independent MTX mouse mammary carcinoma (Szepeshazi et al., 1992) or oestrogen-dependent MCF-7 MIII human breast carcinoma (Yano et al., 1992), the GnRH antagonist SB-75 and the agonist [D-Trp^6]-GnRH significantly inhibited tumour cell growth.

If the antiproliferative effects of GnRH antagonists and possibly agonists are the result of a direct interaction with tumour tissue, do these tissues express specific GnRH binding or GnRH-like binding sites? Furthermore, do these cells produce GnRH or GnRH-like peptides, and if so does this imply that under certain conditions GnRH performs an autocrine role influencing tumour cell growth? Certainly, human breast carcinoma cell lines have been shown to produce GnRH-like peptides and GnRH mRNA (Eidne et al., 1985; Harris et al., 1991) and GnRH-like immunoreactivity has also been demonstrated in breast milk (Amarant et al., 1982). The more definitive studies demonstrating that these tissues express both the GnRH peptide and the GnRH receptor genes can be obtained, in part, by molecular approaches. Towards this end, GnRH mRNA transcripts have been demonstrated in human pituitary, cerebral cortex, testes, ovary and mammary gland (Dong et al., 1993), and similarly Kakar et al. (1992) showed a product corresponding in size to that of the GnRH receptor PCR amplified from RNA extracted from human breast and prostate tissue as well as from the MCF-7 breast cancer cell line. Northern analysis was not sensitive enough to identify the presence of receptor mRNA transcripts in these tissues, indicating either low-level expression or insufficient homology with the pituitary receptor probe. Further information regarding the characteristics of the GnRH receptor expressed in these tissues is awaited.

Both high- (Fekete et al., 1989; Segal-Abramson et al., 1992; Baumann et al., 1993; Milovanovic et al., 1993) and low-affinity (Eidne et al., 1987; Fekete et al., 1989; Segal-Abramson et al., 1992; Milovanovic et al., 1993) binding sites have also been reported in a variety of human breast cancer tissue. These high-affinity binding sites were comparable to those reported for human pituitary receptors (Wormald et al., 1987) and apparently represent a functional G-protein coupled receptor, as evidenced by the ability of GnRH to induce IP production (Segal et al., 1987) and guanine nucleotides to compete with GnRH for binding to these sites (Segal-Abramson, 1992). In contrast, low-affinity binding sites were unable to distinguish between various GnRH agonists and superagonists, having similar affinities for both (Eidne et al., 1987). Their functional capacity is also unclear given that guanine nucleotides had no effect on GnRH binding at these sites. In contrast to all of the aforementioned studies, recent work from Miller's group (Mullen et al., 1992) has reported a lack of GnRH or Buserelin binding in human benign and malignant breast tissues as well as in MCF-7 and MDA-MB-231 breast cells. Their interpretation of these findings was that the failure to detect specific binding might be because the GnRH tracer was rapidly inactivated following exposure to homogenates prepared from the two cell lines, although this extensive inactivation was not observed with tracer incubated with breast tissue homogenates. Because this study used crude homogenates rather than purified membrane preparations, it is feasible that the different assay conditions could provide an explanation for the observed discrepancies.

In an effort to specifically target the action of cytotoxic drugs on cancer cells as opposed to noncancerous ones (thereby reducing peripheral toxicity), Schally and co-workers have developed a class of cytotoxic analogues of GnRH presumably for local application. This approach is based on the premise that specific tumour binding sites exist and that GnRH analogues have direct action on tumour tissue. Depending on the route of in vivo administration, these cytotoxic GnRH analogues would also target pituitary gonadotrophs. The specific binding of cytotoxic analogues of GnRH to a range of human breast cancers and a mouse mammary tumour cell line was described (Milovanovic et al., 1992). Cytotoxic GnRH analogues caused a significant inhibition of in vivo tumour growth in oestrogen-dependent MXT mammary tumour cells (Szepeshazi et al., 1992). Similarly, inhibition of experimental prostate cancer in rats following treatment with cytotoxic GnRH analogues has been described (Pinski et al., 1993).

Prostate Cancer In men receiving GnRH agonist therapy for prostate cancer, the resultant chemical castration achieves exactly the same result as a surgical castration would have. The trauma associated with surgical castration can be avoided, as the once-monthly injection of a GnRH analogue depot inhibits testosterone levels, providing a sustained medical castration. Serum acid and alkaline phosphatase levels are reduced, bone pain is relieved and there is a significant remission of metastatic disease (Santen et al., 1986; Waxman, 1987; Decensi et al., 1993). As about 70% of human prostate cancers are testosterone dependent, the treatment of advanced stage C or D is generally based on the inhibition of the pituitary-gonadal axis and subsequent reduction in steroid hormone levels. Similar to the abovementioned findings on GnRH and cancers of the breast and ovary, prostate cancers have also been shown to express both GnRH-like peptides (Qayum et al., 1990b) and GnRH receptors (Qayum et al., 1990a). Once again GnRH has been implicated in prostatic epithelial cell growth and the hypothesis put forward that the effects of GnRH analogues in these cancers are mediated via specific GnRH tumour receptors.

GnRH and Apoptosis

Evidence is mounting that GnRH in extrapituitary tissues may somehow be involved in apoptosis or programmed cell death. Specificity of programmed cell death is mediated by external signals, and a number of diverse hormones including steroids have been implicated in this process (Wyllie, 1980; Compton & Cidlowski, 1992). The involution of endocrine-dependent tissue following hormone withdrawal is an apoptotic-mediated process with involution of lactating mammary gland as an example (Walker et al., 1989). Programmed cell death is associated with DNA degradation, and further examples of endocrine-dependent tissues that undergo this process include, granulosa and luteal cells (Zeleznick et al., 1989), breast cancer cells (Bardon et al., 1987), prostate (Kyprianou & Isaacs, 1988) and uterine epithelium (Rotello et al., 1989). Apoptosis appears to be activated by multiple signals that are capable of converging on one or more signal transduction pathways. A proposed model by Compton and Cidlowski (1992) suggests that programmed cell death is regulated by apoptotic inducers and apoptotic repressors. The inducing signal activates an intracellular transduction pathway, like the elevation of intracellular calcium, which in turn may activate nucleases to cause DNA degradation. The repressing signal inhibits DNA degradation via protein kinase C. Once the nuclease is activated, the genome is systematically cleaved at specific sites on the chromatin, an irreversible process that commits the cell to death.

Hormone-sensitive tissues implicated in apoptosis have been shown to produce both GnRH (or GnRH-like peptides) and binding sites for GnRH. A number of studies have documented the presence of GnRH-like substances and the effects of GnRH analogues on tumours derived from the breast and prostate, both of which are tissues that can be influenced by hormones to undergo apoptosis. The obvious question to address is, Can the manipulation of apoptosis itself be useful in the treatment of diseases like cancers? Schally's group has carried out several similar studies in animal models measuring tumour regression following treatment with GnRH analogues and in some instances in combination with somatostatin analogues. Growth inhibition characteristic of apoptosis was measured in pancreatic tumours (Szende, 1989b). Similarly, apoptotic regression was observed in mammary carcinomas that had been inoculated into female mice following treatment with GnRH and somatostatin analogues (Szende et al., 1989a). The GnRH antagonist SB-75 was shown to inhibit tumour growth and enhance apoptotic cell death in male nude mice bearing human prostate carcinomas (Redding et al., 1992). It is likely, though, that in these whole-animal models the GnRH analogue action was via suppression of the pituitary-gonadal axis with a resultant decline in circulating steroids. A recent study by Billig et al. (1994) has shown that GnRH can directly induce apoptotic cell death in ovaries from hypophysectomized rats. Follicular atresia has been associated with apoptosis, and this study illustrated that treatment with GnRH agonists were able to directly induce DNA degradation. No GnRH agonist-induced apoptosis was detected in granulosa cells of primary follicles or in thecal and interstitial cells. This effect was blocked by a GnRH antagonist, indicating that specific GnRH receptors were involved.

CONCLUSION

GnRH analogues, both agonists and antagonists, are clinically of value in the treatment of a variety of reproductive disorders. They act directly at the level of the pituitary, desensitizing the pituitary gonadotroph GnRH receptor and thereby abolishing LH and FSH release. However, the potential use of GnRH analogues in the management of hormone-independent breast, prostate and ovarian cancers and their mechanism of action remains equivocal. Whether GnRH analogues are able to exert direct extrapituitary actions in species such as primates and humans is unclear. Evidence for the demonstration of extrapituitary GnRH or GnRH-like binding sites is at the very least confusing. Some reports have failed to measure GnRH binding sites, whereas others have reported either low- or high-affinity and in some instances both types of GnRH binding sites. The low-affinity sites may in fact be receptors for some other related peptide, whereas the high-affinity site may indeed represent a fully functional extrapituitary GnRH receptor. Until such time as this receptor is isolated and fully characterized from tissues like breast or prostate cancers, this issue remains to be clarified. The more definitive studies demonstrating that these tissues express the gene for GnRH as well as GnRH receptors can be obtained, in part, by molecular approaches. Further information regarding the characteristics of the GnRH receptor expressed in these tissues is awaited.

Independent of the site of action of GnRH analogues, a clearer understanding of the mechanisms involved in ligand receptor interaction, receptor activation and intracellular communication is essential if we are to rationalize GnRH analogue design. The three-dimensional modelling of the transmembrane regions of the recently cloned GnRH receptor is undoubtedly the first of many important steps that will improve our knowledge of the events involved in the interaction of the GnRH peptide with its receptor. If GnRH analogues are indeed exerting direct extrapituitary effects, then the cloning and modelling of extrapituitary GnRH receptors may enable the design of clinically effective, tissue-specific GnRH analogues offering increased potency but negligible side effects.

Advancing the knowledge of GnRH and GnRH receptor gene structures, their localization and related signalling systems will ultimately contribute to our understanding of the genetic basis of reproductively related disease states and ensure continued interest in both the GnRH peptide and its receptor for many years to come.

REFERENCES

Adelman J.P., Mason A.J., Hayflick J.S. & Seeburg P.H. (1986) Isolation of the gene and hypothalamic cDNA for the common precursor of gonadotropin-releasing hormone and prolactin release-inhibiting factor in human and rat. *Proceedings of the National Academy of Sciences of the United States of America*, **83**, 179–83.

Adelson M.D. & Reece M.T. (1993) Effect of gonadotropin-releasing hormone analogues on ovarian epithelial tumors. *Clinical Obstetrics and Gynecology*, **36**, 690–700.

Amarant T., Fridkin M. & Koch Y. (1982) Luteinizing hormone-releasing hormone and thyrotropin-releasing hormone in human and bovine milk. *European Journal of Biochemistry*, **127**, 647–51.

Voeller H.J., Sugars L.Y., Pretlow T. & Gelmann E.P. (1994) p53 Oncogene mutations in human prostate cancer specimens. *Journal of Urology*, **151**(2), 492–5.

Ware J.L., Maygarden S.J., Koontz W., Jr. & Strom S.C. (1991) Immunohistochemical defection of c-*erb*B-2 protein in human benign and neoplastic prostate. *Human Pathology*, **22**(3), 254–8.

Wolf D.A., Kohlhuber F., Schulz P., Fittler F. & Eick D. (1992) Transcriptional down-regulation of c-*myc* in human prostate carcinoma cells by the synthetic androgen mibolerone. *British Journal of Cancer*, **65**, 376–82.

Yuan S., Trachtenberg J., Mills G.B., Brown T.J., Xu F. & Keating A. (1993) Androgen-induced inhibition of cell proliferation in an androgen-insensitive prostate cancer cell line (PC-3) transfected with a human androgen receptor complementary DNA. *Cancer Research*, **53**, 1304–11.

11

Carcinoid Tumours

S. BLOOM AND P. HAMMOND

INTRODUCTION

Carcinoid tumours were first described in 1888 by Lubarsch (Lubarsch, 1888) and derive their name from the term 'Karzinoide,' first used by Obendorfer in 1907 (Obendorfer, 1907) to characterize gastrointestinal tumours that were carcinoma-like but showed less aggressive malignant behaviour than typical gastrointestinal carcinomas. The classification carcinoid now refers to tumours derived from the diffuse endocrine cells of the embryonic gut which share similar histological characteristics but which are heterogeneous with respect to the products they synthesize and secrete and to their malignant potential. In addition, tumours showing characteristic carcinoid histology have been described, although rarely, in sites with no relationship to the embryonic gut, such as the cervix and kidney, and the mechanism by which these tumours arise in these sites of mesodermal origin is unclear.

Carcinoid tumours can be subdivided according to the region of the embryonic gut from which they arise (Williams & Sandler, 1963), and such a classification partially explains the tumour heterogeneity. The commonest carcinoid tumours arise from the midgut (ampulla of Vater to midtransverse colon) (Godwin, 1975; Feldman, 1987). They characteristically produce excess serotonin (5-hydroxytryptamine (5-HT)), the classical biochemical marker of carcinoid tumours (Maton et al. 1984). The phenol group of the indoleamine serotonin reduces silver salts, the Masson reaction, and as a result these tumours are termed 'argentaffin positive' (Barter & Pearse, 1953; Maton et al., 1984). Foregut carcinoid tumours, including bronchial and pancreatic carcinoids, often have low levels of L-amino acid decarboxylase activity, which converts 5-hydroxytryptophan to serotonin (Figure 11.1) and so characteristically secrete 5-hydroxytryptophan (Maton et al., 1984). Foregut carcinoid tumours are argentaffin negative but show nuclear silver staining in the presence of a reducing agent, a positive Grimelius reaction, and so are termed argyrophilic (Maton et al., 1984; Wilander, Lundqvist & el Salhy, 1985). The basis of the positive Grimelius reaction is not known. Hindgut carcinoids are usually argentaffin and argyrophilic negative and do not secrete either 5-hydroxytryptophan or serotonin (Maton et al., 1984). The biochemical diversity of carcinoid tumours is exemplified by duodenal carcinoids, which produce somatostatin and are often associated with neurofibromatosis type 1 (von Recklinghausen's syndrome) (Griffiths, Williams & Williams, 1987) and bronchial carcinoids, which usually synthesize pro-opiomelanocortin derived peptides (Crosby et al., 1990), particularly adrenocorticotrophic hormone (ACTH), and are frequently associated with Cushing's syndrome (Pass et al., 1990).

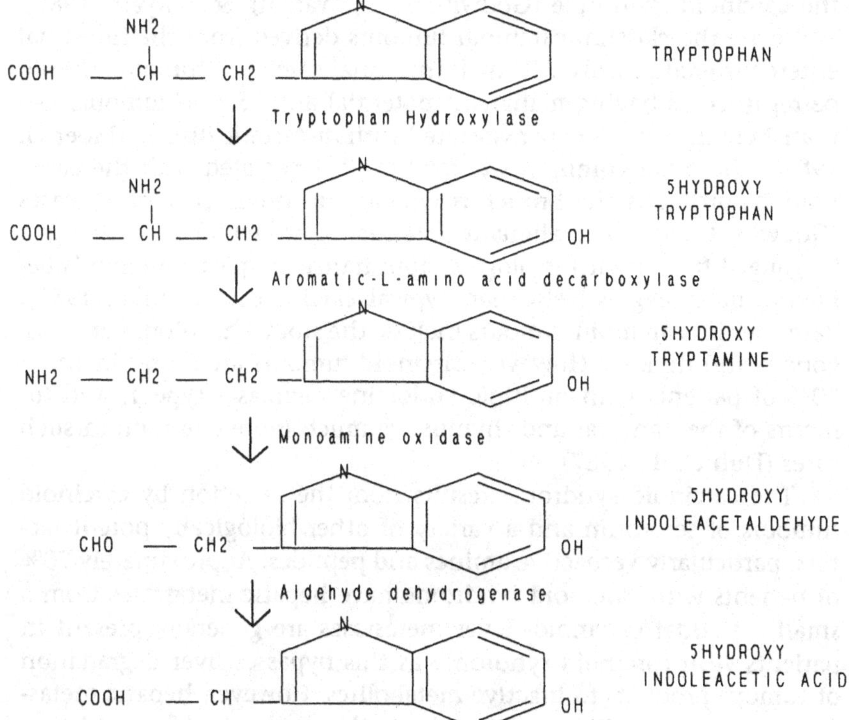

Figure 11.1 Synthesis and degradation of serotonin.

The annual incidence of carcinoid tumours is about 1 per 100,000 of the population (Linell & Mansson, 1966). The commonest site for a carcinoid tumour is the appendix (Godwin, 1975), autopsy studies indicating a prevalence of up to 1% of the population. These tumours are usually found incidentally on histological examinations of appendicectomy specimens and account for 40% of all carcinoid tumours, but they metastasize in less than 2% of cases (Godwin, 1975). Their malignant potential depends on their size, tumours greater than 2 cm in diameter being far more aggressive (Moertel et al., 1987). Carcinoid tumours of the rectum constitute 15% of all carcinoid tumours, and are usually identified incidentally on rectal biopsy specimens (Godwin, 1975; Sauven et al., 1990). Rectal tumours are often multicentric and metastasize in about 20% of cases (Godwin, 1975). Tumours greater than 1 cm in diameter carrying a much greater risk of malignancy (Sauven et al., 1990; Teleky et al., 1992). Metastatic rectal carcinoids are rarely associated with the carcinoid syndrome but carry a poor prognosis and 7% of patients survive two years (Godwin, 1975). Small intestinal, usually ileal, carcinoids represent 25% of all carcinoid tumours, but account for the majority of cases associated with the carcinoid syndrome (Godwin, 1975; Wareing & Sawyers, 1983). These are the classical carcinoid tumours derived from the intestinal enterochromaffin cells. All small intestinal carcinoid tumours should be regarded as having malignant potential and 15% of tumours less than 1 cm in diameter are associated with metastatic disease (Moertel, 1987). The other common site for tumors associated with the carcinoid syndrome is the bronchus which constitutes 10% of all cases (Godwin, 1975). The malignant potential of bronchial carcinoids can be gauged from their histological appearance, atypical carcinoids behaving more aggressively than typical carcinoids (Feldman, 1987). Rare sites for carcinoid tumours include the stomach, colon, pancreas, gonads and thymus. However, carcinoid tumours are found in about 10% of patients with multiple endocrine neoplasia type 1, and tumours of the pancreas and thymus are much more common in such cases (Duh et al., 1987).

The carcinoid syndrome results from the secretion by carcinoid tumours of serotonin and a variety of other biologically potent factors, particularly vasoactive amines and peptides. Approximately 70% of patients with carcinoid syndrome have hepatic metastases from a small intestinal carcinoid. Liver metastases are generally present in patients with carcinoid syndrome as this bypasses liver degradation of tumour products to inactive metabolites. However, hepatic metastases often occur without giving rise to the syndrome. The syndrome can occur in association with large primary intestinal carcinoids, usually greater than 5 cm in diameter, with massive retroperitoneal lymph node involvement (Feldman & Jones, 1982; Haq et al., 1992; Basson et al., 1993), or with a primary tumour, particularly a bronchial carcinoid, which drains directly into the systemic circulation (Basson et al., 1993).

This review will consider the pathophysiology of the carcinoid syndrome and the current therapeutic options, particularly the use of somatostatin analogues and interferons.

PATHOPHYSIOLOGY OF THE CARCINOID SYNDROME

Features of the Carcinoid Syndrome

Flushing Flushing occurs in about 95% of patients with the carcinoid syndrome. The characteristic carcinoid flush is a deep red hue involving the head and neck, occasionally extending to the trunk and limbs (Grahame Smith, 1987). Attacks of flushing are usually paroxysmal and unprovoked, although in some patients attacks may be precipitated by alcohol, food ingestion, stress, emotion or exercise (Sjoerdsma, Terry & Udenfriend, 1957; Davis, Moertel & McIlrath, 1973). Early in the disease flushing attacks are short-lived, lasting up to five minutes (Davis et al., 1973), but as the disease progresses attacks can last for hours and become almost continuous. During these later stages patients develop widespread telangiectasia that give them a plethoric, cyanotic facial hue, and the flush, superimposed on this fixed coloration, has a purple hue (Sjoerdsma et al., 1957). This leonine facies occurs in up to 25% of cases and is particularly common in patients with symptomatic bronchial carcinoids. The latter are frequently associated with a very severe type of flushing (Melmon, Sjoerdsma & Mason, 1965), which can involve the whole body; may be associated with nasal congestion, conjunctival suffusion, lacrimation, facial oedema and explosive diarrhoea; and can be extremely distressing. Such attacks may last several hours. Finally, the release of histamine by gastric carcinoids causes a characteristic wheal-like flush with areas of pallor and erythema, particularly over the neck (Oates & Sjoerdsma, 1962).

Flushing is often associated with hypotension and tachycardia, and in about 20% of patients bronchospasm causes asthmatic episodes. Severe attacks are termed 'carcinoid crises'. They may occur spontaneously or be precipitated (Marsh et al., 1987; Bissonnette et al., 1990) by, for example, anaesthesia, hepatic embolization or autonecrosis of metastases. Hypotension may be profound and patients can become oliguric. Attacks may last for days, with development of confusion and stupor, and rarely may be fatal.

Gastrointestinal Manifestations Secretory diarrhoea occurs in about 75% of patients. This may be profuse, with passage of several litres a day, and occasionally results in electrolyte disturbance. A minority of patients have steatorrhoea. The diarrhoea is not usually temporally related to the flushing. Cramping abdominal pain is frequently associated with the diarrhoea, and nausea and vomiting often occur. Small bowel obstruction from a large ileal carcinoid tumour may rarely be the cause of the diarrhoea. Hepatic metastases can cause right hypochondrial pain, usually as a result of stretching or metastatic infiltration of the liver capsule, and acute exacerbations may occur if metastases become ischaemic and undergo autonecrosis. Weight loss and cachexia may occur as a result of poor dietary intake, malabsorption or increased catabolism.

Cardiac Lesions Over 50% of patients with the carcinoid syndrome have echocardiographic evidence of carcinoid heart disease (Pellikka et al., 1993). This results from endocardial fibrosis, plaques of smooth muscle in collagenous stroma being deposited on the valves (MacDonald & Robbins, 1957). Tricuspid valve involvement is an almost invariable feature, with moderate to severe tricuspid incompetence occurring in about 90% of cases, usually in association with some degree of tricuspid stenosis (Pellikka et al., 1993). Thickening and retraction of the pulmonary valve occurs in over 50% of cases, pulmonary regurgitation being seen in up to 80% of these patients and pulmonary stenosis in about 50% (Pellikka et al., 1993). Left-sided valve lesions occur in about 10% of patients with cardiac involvement and are either due to the presence of a patent foramen ovale or to drainage of tumour products from a bronchial carcinoid into the left atrium. Fibrosis can extend to the vena cavae and pulmonary artery. Other rare cardiac manifestations include variant angina (Petersen et al., 1984; Bluming & Berez, 1988), which may be associated with flushing attacks, myocardial metastasis and pericardial effusion (Pellikka et al., 1993). The commonest symptom resulting from cardiac involvement is dyspnoea, which affects over 50% of patients. Progressive right heart failure may result in marked peripheral oedema and can cause further deterioration in liver function. The presence of echocardiographic evidence of cardiac involvement appears to be associated with a poorer prognosis (Pellikka et al., 1993).

Respiratory Complications Episodes of bronchospasm are usually associated with flushing attacks but can occur independently, and breathlessness is reported by over 25% of patients without evidence of cardiac involvement. Wheeze should never be treated with adrenergic receptor agonists because catecholamines stimulate tumour release of serotonin and tachykinins (Ahlund et al., 1989). A desmoplastic fibrotic reaction, similar to that affecting the endocardium, can occur in other sites such as the skin, mesentery or retroperitoneum (Gupta, Saibil & Kessim, 1985), and it has been reported to affect the pleura in up to 20% of patients (Moss et al., 1993), possibly contributing to dyspnoea. Pulmonary metastases are a rare feature of carcinoid tumours, and lymphatic involvement has been implicated in a case of apparent pulmonary shunting (Amundson & Weiss, 1991). Pulmonary shunting may also occur as a result of the actions of vasodilating tumour products on the pulmonary vasculature.

Other Manifestations The conversion of dietary niacin to tryptophan by tumours can result in nicotinamide deficiency (Figure 11.1), which, in less than 10% of cases, is manifest by pellagra. The characteristic features of this condition are a photosensitive pigmented rash, glossitis and peripheral sensory neuropathy.

Carcinoid arthropathy (Plonk & Feldman, 1974) or myopathy (Lederman, Bukowski & Nickerson, 1987) affects a small number of patients and sclerotic bone metastases are an infrequent finding, although more common in patients with foregut and hindgut tumours.

One of the more puzzling features of patients with carcinoid tumours is the high incidence of synchronous noncarcinoid tumours, particularly adenocarcinoma of the breast and colon, which have been reported to occur in up to 30% of cases (Wareing & Sawyers, 1983).

Carcinoid Tumour Products and Aetiology of the Carcinoid Syndrome

The association of the carcinoid syndrome with carcinoid tumours was first reported by Thorson in 1954 (Thorson et al., 1954). Serotonin had been isolated from carcinoid tumours the previous year (Lembeck, 1953) and elevated levels of 5-hydroxyindoleacetic acid (5-HIAA), which accounts for 95% of the metabolism of serotonin, were demonstrated in patients with the carcinoid syndrome (Udenfriend, Titus & Weissbach, 1955). It has been reported that over 50% of patients with carcinoid tumours have elevated circulating levels of serotonin, but over 20% of these patients had no features of the carcinoid syndrome despite very high circulating levels in some cases (Feldman, 1987). In patients without elevated circulating levels of serotonin, 5% had either diarrhoea or flushing, although none experienced both symptoms (Feldman, 1987). The diarrhoea of the carcinoid syndrome does appear to be principally caused by serotonin (Feldman & Plonk, 1977). Infusion of serotonin increases jejunal tone, motility and secretion (Haverback & Davidson, 1958; Ormsbee & Fondacaro, 1985), and serotonin receptor antagonists, such as cyproheptadine and ketanserin, reduce carcinoid diarrhoea (Vroom et al., 1962; Ahlman et al., 1985). In contrast, pure serotonin antagonists have little effect on the flushing (Vroom et al., 1962) and there is no correlation between circulating serotonin levels and meal- and pentagastrin-stimulated flushing (Richter et al., 1986). Furthermore, despite inducing the carcinoid flush, pentagastrin does not stimulate serotonin release from tumours (Gronstad et al., 1985). The vasoconstrictive actions of serotonin may be responsible for the angina (Willerson et al., 1986) and bronchoconstriction (Herxheimer, 1953) experienced by some patients, and fibrosis (Lundin et al., 1988) appears to be related, at least in part, to the elevation in circulating serotonin. Those patients who develop carcinoid heart disease have been reported to have higher levels of urinary 5-HIAA and circulating tachykinins (Lundin et al., 1988; Pellikka et al., 1993). Thus serotonin is not responsible for all the features of the syndrome, in particular playing little part in the pathogenesis of the flush, and a variety of other tumour products, which may play a role in the pathogenesis of the syndrome, have been identified.

Substance P and other tachykinins (neuropeptide K and neurokinin A), so called because of their rapid action, are derived from the preprotachykinin A and B genes and are synthesized (Yang et al., 1983; Ahlman et al., 1985; Bishop et al., 1989) and secreted (Skrabanek et al., 1978) by carcinoid tumours, resulting in elevated circulating levels. In the gastrointestinal tract these tachykinins are localized to neurones in the myenteric and submucosal plexi (Pearse & Polak, 1975) and to enterochromaffin cells (Heitz et al., 1976), with high concentrations in the duodenum and jejunum (Powell & Skrabanek, 1979). Their principal physiological effects are smooth muscle contraction, vasodilatation and inhibition of intestinal absorption (Powell & Skrabanek, 1979).

Substance P slows gastrointestinal transit (Valdovinos, Thomforde & Camilleri, 1993) and so is unlikely to be involved in the aetiology of carcinoid diarrhoea. It seems more likely that tachykinins are mediators of the carcinoid flush, although their exact role remains controversial. Infusion of substance P induces flushing for two to three minutes in normal individuals (Duner & Pernow, 1960; Schaffalitzky de Muckadell, Aggestrup & Stentoft, 1986). In patients with the carcinoid syndrome, however, substance P is not consistently elevated in meal-induced flushing and suppression of meal-induced flushing by octreotide is associated with only a partial reduction in substance P and neurokinin A (Conlon et al., 1987). Pentagastrin-induced flushing is associated with a rise in circulating tachykinins (Oberg et al., 1989; Balks et al., 1989), which is completely abolished by octreotide despite only partial attenuation of the flush (Oberg et al., 1989; Balks et al., 1989). Thus it seems likely that tachykinins are important in the pathogenesis of the flush but are not wholly responsible for it. The differential suppression by octreotide of tumour cell secretion in response to different secretagogues (Wangberg et al., 1991; Lawrence et al., 1990), such as isoprenaline and pentagstrin, in vitro, provides additional evidence that the relative contribution of different tumour products to the flushing may be stimulus dependent.

Kallikrein is an enzyme which, released into the circulation, converts kininogen to lysylbradykinin, which in turn is converted to bradykinin. Bradykinin is a potent vasoactive peptide but has a very short plasma half-life and thus it is difficult to assess circulating levels. Infusion of bradykinin causes flushing, but this is pinker than the carcinoid flush, with more marked hypotension and tachycardia (Grahame Smith, 1987). It has been reported that bradykinin levels are not elevated during flushing (Gustafsen et al., 1987), but this may be due to rapid inactivation. Other studies have found that carcinoids synthesize and secrete active kallikrein, and elevations in circulating bradykinin, which may correlate with flushing episodes, can be demonstrated in some patients (Oates, Pettinger & Doctor, 1966; Gardner et al., 1967; Adamson et al., 1969).

Histamine causes a very distinctive flush, characterized by wheal-like areas over the neck, and this is usually associated with histamine release from gastric carcinoids (Roberts, Marney & Oates, 1979). Prostaglandins are released by carcinoid tumours (Sandler, Karim & Williams, 1968; Feldman, Plonk & Cornette, 1974) but it seems unlikely that they play an important role in the pathophysiology of the syndrome, since they do not correlate with symptoms (Jaffe & Condon, 1976) and prostaglandin inhibitors have no effect on flushing or diarrhoea (Metz, McRae & Robertson, 1981). Recent studies have implicated transforming growth factors (TGF) in the pathogenesis of fibrosis of the endocardium and elsewhere (Beauchamp et al., 1991; Waltenberger et al., 1993). TGF is synthesized by carcinoid tumours (Beauchamp et al., 1991), stimulates endothelial cell proliferation, and is found in fibroblasts in the fibrotic cardiac lesions (Waltenberger et al., 1993). A variety of other peptides such as adenocorticotrophic hormone, calcitonin, motilin and somatostatin may be produced by carcinoid tumours but do not appear to play a role in the pathogenesis of the carcinoid syndrome.

The growth of carcinoid tumours may be regulated by a number of factors. The most well characterized of these is gastrin, which stimulates growth of enterochromaffin cells in the stomach resulting in the development of gastric carcinoids (Solcia et al., 1993). In man this relationship has been described in patients with achlorhydria and gastrinomas, and in animal models may be provoked by omeprazole treatment. In vitro studies have also implicated insulin-like growth factor (Nilsson et al., 1992), platelet-derived growth factor (Chaudhry et al., 1992), gastrin-releasing peptide (Bostwick et al., 1984) and serotonin itself (Ishizuka et al., 1992) as autocrine growth stimulators.

In making the diagnosis of carcinoid tumours urinary 5-HIAA excretion is the most sensitive and specific marker (Feldman & O'Dorisio, 1986). The plasma concentrations of other peptides such as substance P, motilin, somatostatin, vasoactive intestinal peptide, gastrin-releasing peptide and bradykinin may be elevated, but are not used in routine clinical practice for diagnostic purposes.

THERAPEUTIC OPTIONS

The majority of carcinoid tumours are small, benign lesions. Many are discovered as an incidental finding in surgical specimens, and the rest should be resected if possible. In contrast, tumours associated with the carcinoid syndrome have metastasized in the majority of cases, usually to the liver and local lymph nodes. The therapeutic options available for treating metastatic disease are tumour debulking, by surgery, hepatic embolization, chemotherapy or immunotherapy using interferons; and antisecretory therapy with the somatostatin analogue, octreotide, or the use of specific antagonists to tumour products, particularly serotonin and histamine.

Tumour Debulking

Surgery Surgical debulking involves either radical resection for disease confined to a resectable segment or metastatectomy for single lesions. Curative resection may be attempted, or tumour may be resected to palliate symptoms related to secretion of tumour products or to tumour bulk. In a series from the Mayo Clinic (McEntee et al., 1990) curative resection was attempted in nine symptomatic patients.

Eight patients experienced complete relief of symptoms and five of these were alive at a mean of 26 months without evidence of residual disease. Sixteen patients had palliative resections and 50% of these had complete symptom relief. Recently successful hepatic transplantation has been reported for patients with carcinoid tumours in whom metastases are confined to the liver and the primary tumour has been resected or is resectable (O'Grady et al., 1988; Makowka et al., 1989).

Hepatic Artery Embolization Dearterialization of liver metastases can be achieved by hepatic artery embolization, provided the portal vein is patent. If this is the case, then the normal liver parenchyma, which has a dual blood supply from the hepatic artery and portal vein, is largely preserved, while the metastases become ischaemic due to loss of their sole blood supply. Necrosis of metastases may be associated with massive peptide release, which can provoke a carcinoid crisis, but this can be prevented by using high doses of the somatostatin analogue octreotide to cover the procedure. Symptom relief is achieved in over 70% of cases, with objective response in about 60% as assessed by reduction in hormone levels or a decrease in tumour bulk (Maton et al., 1984; Carrasco et al., 1986). Morbidity may occur due to embolization of adjacent arteries, such as those supplying the gallbladder or pancreas (Mendelson et al., 1989), abscess formation in necrotic metastases or ischaemia of normal liver adjacent to metastases. Mortality has only been reported in patients with severe derangement of liver function (Carrasco et al., 1986) and thus embolization is contraindicated in cases in which more than 50% of the liver parenchyma is replaced by tumour. The procedure can be repeated at six- to nine-month intervals with similar response rates. Hepatic artery embolization is usually most effective when used in combination with chemotherapy, immunotherapy or octreotide and these will be considered in more detail below.

Chemotherapy Many different chemotherapeutic agents have been used in patients with the carcinoid syndrome but most are ineffective. Streptozotocin and 5-fluorouracil (5-FU) have been used because of their efficacy in treating pancreatic islet cell tumours. 5-FU alone given every five weeks has been reported to produce an objective response in between 18 and 26% of cases (Moertel & Hanley, 1979; Moertel, 1983), increasing to 23 to 33% with the addition of streptozotocin (Moertel & Hanley, 1979; Engstrom et al., 1984). Similarly poor response rates have been reported with streptozotocin (Moertel, 1983; Engstrom et al., 1984), doxorubicin (Engstrom et al., 1984), dacarbazine (van Hazel, Rubin & Moertel, 1983), actinomycin

D (Dollinger & Golbey, 1967), cisplatin (Moertel, Rubin & O'Connell, 1986) and the combinations of cyclophosphamide and methotrexate (Moertel et al., 1984), and cyclophosphamide and streptozotocin (Moertel & Handley, 1979). The only trial (Moertel et al., 1985) showing a good response with chemotherapy used dacarbazine, doxorubicin, streptozotocin and 5-FU, given three weeks after hepatic artery embolization. Nine of ten patients had marked or complete symptom relief and urinary 5-HIAA excretion decreased by between 60 and 100%. However, it is unlikely that such a regimen would represent an improvement on the presently available alternatives. More recently, chemoembolization has been successfully employed in patients with carcinoid tumour metastases in the liver (Ruszniewski et al., 1993). Doxorubicin was injected into the vessels supplying the tumour deposits before occlusion of the arteries and this process was repeated every three months. Symptomatic relief was experienced by 72% of patients, 57% had a biochemical response and 33% had significant tumour regression. Two patients had a complete response and the median duration of all responses was 14 months.

Immunotherapy The use of interferon in the treatment of carcinoid tumours was first reported by Obert in 1983 (Oberg, Funa & Alm, 1983). In this study, human lymphoblastoid interferon was used in nine patients with metastatic carcinoid tumours. Six patients with hepatic metastases experienced symptomatic improvement associated with a decrease in urinary 5-HIAA excretion, but only one of three patients with lymph node metastases alone responded.

Since this initial favourable report there has been conflicting evidence in the literature about the benefit of interferon therapy. Oberg and associates have been keen proponents of its use and have studied by far the largest number of patients (Oberg & Eriksson, 1991). In total 111 patients have been treated with either natural or recombinant interferon-α (IFN-α). A partial biochemical response, defined as a reduction in urinary 5-HIAA excretion of greater than 50%, was observed in 42% of patients, and this group included all 15% of patients who demonstrated a greater than 50% decrease in tumour size, a partial tumour response. The median duration of response was 34 months. Symptomatic improvement was experienced by 68% of patients. Stable disease was observed in 39% of patients and progression of disease in 19%. The mean survival of patients treated with IFN-α was over 80 months, compared with a mean survival of eight months amongst 19 patients treated with streptozotocin and 5-FU, only two of whom had an objective response to the treatment. The same group, in a direct comparison of IFN-α-2a alone (12 patients) or in combination with streptozotocin and doxorubicin (11 patients), reported no difference in response at six-month follow-up (Janson et al., 1992). Both treatment modalities caused only a stabilization in disease in the majority of cases (9/12 versus 11/11), although there was one complete remission on IFN-α alone.

The reported response rates in most studies have been similar to those observed by Oberg's group. Partial biochemical response occurred in between 24% and 60% of patients in series including more than ten patients (Smith et al., 1987; Moertel, Rubin & Kvols, 1989; Nobin et al., 1989; Doberauer et al., 1991; Basser et al., 1991; Veenhof et al., 1992; Ahren, Engman & Lindblom, 1992; Joensuu, Kumpulainen & Grohn, 1992; Schoeber et al., 1992; Biesma et al., 1992) and progression of disease was observed in less than 30% of cases. Tumour regression rarely occurs, but in the majority of cases disease remains stable. Symptomatic relief was experienced by between 50 and 68% of patients in most series, with occasional reports of higher subjective response rates (Schober et al., 1992; Biesma et al., 1992). Flushing appears to respond better than diarrhoea to interferon therapy, perhaps indicating that the biochemical response rate, which reflects serotonin production, underestimates the number of patients benefitting from therapy. A particularly poor response rate was reported by Valimaki (Veenhof et al., 1992). Only eight patients were treated, but the biochemical response rate was only 12.5%, symptomatic relief was experienced by only two out of seven patients and progression of disease was observed in 50% of cases.

Controversy over the use of interferon centres on the duration of response and the balance between benefit and adverse effects. Moertel reported a 39% biochemical response rate and a 20% tumour response rate in 27 patients, but with a median duration of four and seven weeks, respectively (Moertel et al., 1989). Similarly, Basser observed a 40% biochemical response rate in 17 patients but with a duration of about eight weeks (Basser et al., 1991) and Doberauer a 66% biochemical response rate in nine patients, with a median duration of four months (Doberauer et al., 1991). Other studies have reported a duration of response of about 15 months (Joensuu et al., 1992; Biesma et al., 1992) but none have found the effect of therapy to be as long lasting as Oberg. Furthermore, Moertel was unable to recommend the use of interferon because of the unacceptability of side effects, both in terms of frequency and severity (Moertel et al., 1989). The principal toxic reactions were chills, fever, fatigue, anorexia, weight loss, bone marrow suppression with leukopenia and thrombocytopenia and deranged liver function.

Moertel qualified his advice by speculating that the use of recombinant interferon containing only one subtype of interferon-α, rather than human leukocyte interferon, which contains a mixture of at least 22 naturally occurring subtypes, might reduce the incidence of adverse events (Moertel et al., 1989). This does not appear to be the case. In two studies using IFN-α-2b, 24 to 42% of patients discontinued the drug because of side effects and almost all patients experienced some drug-related symptoms, usually an influenza-like illness between days three and five of therapy (Basser et al., 1991; Biesma et al., 1992). Other studies have observed that autoimmune phenomena are a frequent occurrence with an increased incidence of antithyroid and antinuclear antibodies, and clinically significant autoimmune thyroid disease (Ronnblom, Alm & Oberg, 1991). Neutralizing antibodies to interferon are responsible for failure of response to therapy in up to 15% of cases, although they occur less frequently with IFN-α-2b than with IFN-α-2a (Grander et al., 1990). Side effects of therapy, however, are almost all dose related (Tiensuu Janson et al., 1992) and a number of studies have concluded that low-dose IFN-α-2b, at 9 MU/week, is as effective as higher dose therapy (Smith et al., 1987; Basser et al., 1991; Veenhof et al., 1992). Most studies have used higher doses, although two unfavourable studies used median doses of 9 MU/week or less (Valimaki et al., 1991; Basser et al., 1991).

The combination of interferon with other therapies may allow the minimum dose to be used while maintaining maximum benefit. Hanssen studied 36 patients and found that those given IFN-α-2b following hepatic artery embolization had a better response than those treated with interferon alone (Hanssen et al., 1991). The biochemical response rates were 60% and 24%; the five-year survival rates, 75% and 40%, respectively. The other reported therapeutic combination, that of octreotide and interferon, will be discussed in detail below.

The mechanism of action of interferon is uncertain; possibilities include inhibition of cell division, induction of cellular differentiation, direct tumour cytotoxicity or modulation of the antitumour immune response. The growth-inhibitory effects of interferon appear to correlate with induction of 2′5′-oligoadenylate synthetase. This enzyme activates an endoribonuclease that can degrade mRNA and rRNA. A greater than threefold increase in enzyme activity in tumour tissue obtained from biopsy of hepatic metastases identified patients who had responded to interferon therapy with 100% sensitivity and 75% specificity (Grander et al., 1990). It remains unclear, however, whether activation of the enzyme is the mechanism for interferon-induced tumour suppression or just represents a marker for the efficacy of interferon therapy. The response to interferon therapy correlates with a decrease in tumour tissue and an increase in connective tissue in biopsied hepatic metastases, the overall size of which remained unchanged (Andersson et al., 1990). This provides further evidence for a direct cytotoxic action of interferon and may explain why a reduction in biochemical parameters following interferon therapy is not paralleled by a decrease in size of hepatic metastases.

Octreotide

Somatostatin was originally isolated from the porcine hypothalamus and was found to inhibit the release of growth hormone. It occurs in 14 and 28 amino acid forms, the relative production of each form being tissue dependent. It is widely distributed in the central and peripheral nervous systems, and is secreted by endocrine cells in the gut, thymus and thyroid. In the gastrointestinal tract somatostatin acts principally as a neurotransmitter and a paracrine agent. It inhibits a wide range of gastrointestinal functions, and blocks both hormone release and the response of the effector tissue.

Paralleling its physiological role, somatostatin proved to be effective at reducing plasma concentrations of many peptides released by neuroendocrine tumours and inhibiting their peripheral action. Early reports demonstrated the efficacy of somatostatin infusion at inhibiting pentagastrin-induced flushing (Frolich et al., 1978; Quatrini et al., 1983) and diarrhoea (Davis et al., 1980; Dharmsathaphorn et al., 1980; Quatrini et al., 1983) in patients with the carcinoid syndrome. To maintain therapeutic benefit, however, continuous infusion proved necessary (Quatrini et al., 1983), since the half-life of native somatostatin is three minutes.

To overcome this problem, octreotide, an eight amino acid analogue preserving the Phe-Trp-Lys-Thr sequence that confers the biological activity of somatostatin, was developed. Octreotide reaches peak plasma concentrations at 30 minutes, has a half-life of 90 to 115 minutes when given intravenously and is effective when administered subcutaneously in two or three divided doses.

Carcinoid tumours have been shown to express somatostatin receptors in over 85% of cases by in vitro autoradiography of tumour specimens using [^{123}I-Tyr^{3}]-octreotide (Reubi et al., 1987) or in vivo visualization using [^{123}I-Tyr^{3}]-octreotide or [^{111}In-DTPA-D-Phe^{1}]-octreotide (Lamberts, Chayvialle & Krenning, 1992), and octreotide reduces peptide and amine synthesis and secretion by carcinoid tumours both in vitro (Lawrence et al., 1990; Wangberg et al., 1991) and in vivo (Balks et al., 1989; Oberg et al., 1989; Stamatis, Freitag & Greschuchna, 1990). Furthermore, it inhibits the actions of tumour products on target tissues and thus ameliorates many of the symptoms of the carcinoid syndrome. Diarrhoea, flushing and wheezing are promptly relieved in 80 to 100% of patients (Kvols et al., 1986; Vinik & Moattari, 1989), and unusual features of the syndrome, such as musculoskeletal symptoms (Smith et al., 1990) and unstable angina (Bluming & Berez, 1988), may also be ameliorated. Creutzfeldt compared octreotide and IFN-α-2c (Creutzfeldt et al., 1991) and reported a biochemical response and symptomatic relief in 100% of patients on octreotide compared with 10% on interferon, although the symptomatic improvement declined with time. Progressive disease occurred in 29% of patients treated with interferon compared with 19% of those treated with octreotide.

Controversy exists over whether octreotide has a direct antitumour effect. Initial studies suggested that it slowed tumour growth (Vinik & Moattari, 1989) and there have been reports of tumour shrinkage in response to octreotide therapy (Wiedenmann et al., 1988). In vitro studies, however, showed no inhibition of growth of cultured carcinoid tumour cells (Wangberg et al., 1991). Recently, a study of 68 patients with carcinoid tumours monitored for at least three months on octreotide therapy observed that 4.4% of patients showed evidence of tumour regression, while in 50% the disease remained stable (Arnold et al., 1992). Octreotide has been shown to reduce tumour blood flow (Cho & Vinik, 1990) and this is one mechanism by which it may inhibit tumour growth.

The side effects of octreotide are pain at the injection site, cholelithiasis as a result of cholestasis, steatorrhoea due to pancreatic exocrine insufficiency and mild glucose intolerance, but they are rarely sufficiently troublesome for therapy to be stopped. The more common problem is tachyphylaxis, possibly due to increased tumour burden or receptor down-regulation or, rarely, antioctreotide antibody formation. In one study of ten patients on octreotide therapy (Wynick et al., 1989), starting at the minimum dosage of 50 μg twice daily, symptoms worsened after five months. This deterioration was reversed by increasing the dose over the next 6 to 12 months to a maximum of 500 μg thrice daily. After a further 24 months at this maximum dosage, however, symptoms recurred. Higher doses or other therapeutic interventions were ineffective and all patients died within five months of entering this resistant phase.

It may be possible to delay or prevent the development of resistance to octreotide by combining it with other antitumour therapies. In eight patients, octreotide, repeated hepatic artery embolization and intra-arterial 5-FU resulted in partial tumour regression in 50% of patients, stable disease in the remainder and complete symptom relief in all patients that persisted at mean follow-up of 22 months (Hajarizadeh et al., 1992).

Octreotide and interferon may act in synergism. Both drugs were needed to control symptoms in one patient, who relapsed if either was stopped (Joensuu, Katka & Kurjari, 1992). Tiensuu-Jansen has recently reported on the addition of IFN-α in 24 patients who were unresponsive or who had become resistant to octreotide (Tiensuu Janson et al., 1992). After starting interferon 77% of patients had a partial biochemical response and 56% noted symptomatic improvement. Another advantage of this regimen was that only 9 MU/week of interferon was given so that adverse reactions were kept to a minimum, although 75% still reported influenza-like symptoms and 62% became fatigued. No regression in tumour size was observed, and in five patients tumour grew despite a biochemical response. These findings are consistent with a study in which rodents were implanted with the human pancreatic carcinoid cell line BON (Evers et al., 1991). Interferon and octreotide prevented growth of freshly implanted tumour but not of established tumour, although the latter responded to these two agents plus α-difluoromethylornithine.

A further therapeutic role for octreotide may be in targeting local radiotherapy to tumour by coupling it to a β-emitting isotope. Local radiotherapy with ^{131}I-methaiodobenzylgaunidine, an agent that visualizes amine synthesizing tumours including carcinoids, has been reported to successfully palliate symptoms in patients with the carcinoid syndrome, although with little effect on tumour size (Colombo et al., 1991; Castellani et al., 1991; Hoefnagel, Taal & Valdes Olmos, 1991; Bestagno et al., 1991). The expression of somatostatin receptors at high density by the majority of carcinoid tumours (Reubi et al., 1987) suggests that it would be a better targeting agent, provided that uptake by normal tissues, particularly the kidney, could be limited.

Other Therapies

Salmon calcitonin has been shown to reduce urinary 5-HIAA excretion and palliate symptoms in patients with the carcinoid syndrome (Antonelli et al., 1987; Antonelli et al., 1992). It appears to be as effective as octreotide therapy (Antonelli et al., 1987) and is not associated with the side effects of steatorrhoea and glucose intolerance, but it has not been widely used. The presence of oestrogen receptors on a few carcinoid tumours (Keshgegian & Wheeler, 1980) led to the use of tamoxifen, with isolated reports of dramatic responses (Myers et al., 1982). This treatment was later shown to be of little value to the majority of patients with carcinoid tumours (Moertel, Engstrom & Schutt, 1984).

Peripheral 5-HT receptor antagonists can palliate symptoms related to serotonin excess. Cyproheptadine is a 5-HT2 receptor blocker that often alleviates the diarrhoea (Vroom et al., 1962). Ketanserin is another 5-HT2 receptor blocker that is largely ineffective in reducing diarrhoea but may be effective in treating flushing, perhaps because of its blockade of histamine H_1 receptors and α-adrenoreceptors (Gustafsen et al., 1986). The 5-HT3 receptor antagonist ondansetron has been reported to alleviate nausea and anorexia (Platt et al., 1992). Inhibitors of 5-HT synthesis such as parachlorphenylalanine, an inhibitor of tryptophan hydroxylase, and chlorpromazine are rarely used. All these alternative medical therapies, with the exception of simple antidiarrhoeal agents, have been largely superseded by the use of octreotide. H_1 and H_2 receptor blockade may be useful in alleviating flushing in patients with histamine-secreting carcinoids (Roberts et al., 1979). Nicotinamide supplements are necessary when patients have pellagra and are often given prophylactically. The treatment of cardiac manifestations is the same as for valve disease and cardiac failure of other aetiologies. Radiotherapy may be beneficial for patients with bony metastases but is not effective in treating carcinoid tumour deposits in other sites.

Conclusion

When considering the treatment options for patients with the carcinoid syndrome, it is worth noting that the five-year survival rate is about 50% regardless of the therapy used. Thus, unless a treatment can be shown to dramatically improve this survival rate, therapy should palliate symptoms with the minimum of adverse effects. Given this aim, the first-line agent for patients with the carcinoid syndrome will usually be octreotide. The duration and degree of response to octreotide may be enhanced by use of an antitumour treatment and, in those patients with significant hepatic metastases, the proven method is hepatic artery embolization. The place of interferon remains unclear; the biochemical and symptomatic response rates are probably no better than for alternative therapies, tumour regression is rarely observed and toxic reactions may be severe. Some patients will be resistant to octreotide therapy or hepatic artery embolization may be contraindicated and interferon may prove valuable in such cases. The ability to identify a subgroup of patients who are likely to respond well to interferon therapy may eventually dictate its role. Newer techniques, such as chemoembolization, may prove useful but require evaluation, and targeted radiotherapy using octreotide may soon be possible.

REFERENCES

Adamson A.R., Grahame Smith D.G., Peart W.S. & Starr M. (1969) Pharmacological blockade of carcinoid flushing provoked by catecholamines and alcohol. *Lancet* **2**, 293–7.

Ahlman H, Dahlstrom A., Gronstad K., Tisell L.E., Oberg K., Zinner M.J. & Jaffe B.M. (1985) The pentagastrin test in the diagnosis of the carcinoid syndrome. Blockade of gastrointestinal symptoms by ketanserin. *Annals of Surgery*, **201**, 81–6.

Ahlund L., Nilsson O., Kling Petersen T., Wigander A., Theodorsson E., Dahlstrom A. & Ahlman H. (1989) Serotonin-producing carcinoid tumour cells in long-term culture. Studies on serotonin release and morphological features. *Acta Oncologica*, **28**, 341–6.

Ahren B., Englman K. & Lindblom A. (1992) Tolerance to long-term treatment of malignant midgut carcinoid with a highly purified human leukocyte alpha-interferon. *Anticancer Research*, **12**, 881–4.

Amundson D.E. & Weiss P.J. (1991) Hypoxemia in malignant carcinoid syndrome: A case attributed to occult lymphangitic metastatic involvement. *Mayo Clinic Proceedings*, **66**, 1178–80.

Andersson T., Wilander E., Eriksson B., Lindgren P.G. & Oberg K. (1990) Effects of interferon on tumor tissue content in liver metastases of human carcinoid tumors. *Cancer Research*, **50**, 3413–15.

Antonelli A., Del Guerra P., Fierabracci A., Gori E. & Baschieri L. (1987) Effect of salmon calcitonin on symptoms and urinary excretion of 5 hydroxyindoleacetic acid in the carcinoid syndrome. *British Medical Journal*, **295**, 961.

Antonelli A., Gambuzza C., Bertoni F. & Baschieri L. (1992) Treatment of the carcinoid syndrome with somatostatin, salmon calcitonin, or octreotide. *Clinical Therapeutics*, **14**, 178–84.

Arnold R., Benning R., Neuhaus C., Rolwage M. & Trautmann M.E. (1992) Gastroenteropancreatic endocrine tumors: effect of Sandostatin on tumor growth. *Metabolism*, **41**, 116–18.

Balks H.J., Conlon J.M., Creutzfeldt W. & Stockmann F. (1989) Effect of a long-acting somatostatin analogue (octreotide) on circulating tachykinins and the pentagastrin-induced carcinoid flush. *European Journal of Clinical Pharmacology*, **36**, 133–7.

Barter R. & Pearse A.G. (1953) Detection of 5-hydroxytryptamine in mammalian cells. *Nature*, **172**, 810.

Basser R.L., Lieschke G.J., Sheridan W.P., Fox R.M. & Green M.D. (1991) Recombinant alpha-2b interferon in patients with malignant carcinoid tumour. *Australia and New Zealand Journal of Medicine*, **21**, 875–8.

Basson M.D., Ahlman H., Wangberg B. & Modlin I.M. (1993) Biology and management of the midgut carcinoid. *American Journal of Surgery*, **165**, 288–97.

Beauchamp R.D., Coffey R.J.J., Lyons R.M., Perkett E.A., Townsend C.M.J. & Moses H.L. (1991) Human carcinoid cell production of paracrine growth factors that can stimulate fibroblast and endothelial cell growth. *Cancer Research*, **51**, 5253–60.

Bestagno M., Pizzocaro C., Pagliaini R., Rossini P.L. & Guerra P. (1991) Results of [131I]metaiodobenzylguanidine treatment in metastatic carcinoid. *Journal of Nuclear Biology and Medicine*, **35**, 343–5.

Biesma B., Willemse P.H., Mulder N.H., Verschueren R.C., Kema I.P., de Bruijn H.W., Postmus P.E., Sleijfer D.T. & de Vries E.G. (1992) Recombinant interferon alpha-2b in patients with metastatic apudomas: effect on tumours and tumour markers. *British Journal of Cancer*, **66**, 850–5.

Bishop A.E., Hamid Q.A., Adams C., Bretherton Watt D., Jones P.M., Denny P., Stamp G.W., Hurt R.L., Grimelius L., Harmar A.J., Cedermark B., Legon S., Ghatei M.A., Bloom S.R. & Polak J.M. (1989) Expression of tachykinins by ileal and lung carcinoid tumors assessed by combined in situ hybridization, immunocytochemistry, and radioimmunoassay. *Cancer*, **63**, 1129–37.

Bissonnette R.T., Gibney R.G., Berry B.R. & Buckley A.R. (1990) Fatal carcinoid crisis after percutaneous fine-needle biopsy of hepatic metastasis: case report and literature review. *Radiology*, **174**, 751–2.

Bluming A.Z. & Berez R.R. (1988) Successful treatment of unstable angina in malignant carcinoid syndrome. *American Journal of Medicine*, **85**, 872–4.

Bostwick D.G., Roth K.A., Barchas J.D. & Bensch K.G. (1984) Gastrin-releasing peptide immunoreactivity in intestinal carcinoids. *American Journal of Clinical Pathology*, **82**, 428–31.

Carrasco C.H., Charnsangavej C., Ajani J., Samaan N.A., Richli W. & Wallace S. (1986) The carcinoid syndrome: palliation by hepatic artery embolizaiton. *American Journal of Roentgenology*, **147**, 149–54.

Castellani M.R., Di Bartolomeo M., Maffioli L., Zilembo N., Gasparini M. & Buraggi G.L. (1991) [131I]metaiodobenzylguanidine therapy in carcinoid tumors. *Journal of Nuclear Biology and Medicine*, **35**, 349–51.

Chaudhry A., Papanicolaou V., Oberg K., Heldin C.H. & Funa K. (1992) Expression of platelet-derived growth factor and its receptors in neuroendocrine tumors of the digestive system. *Cancer Research*, **52**, 1006–12.

Cho K.J. & Vinik A.I. (1990) Effect of somatostatin analogue (octreotide) on blood flow to endocrine tumors metastatic to the liver: angiographic evaluation. *Radiology*, **177**, 549–53.

Colombo L., Vignati A., Lomuscio G. & Dottorini M.E. (1991) Preliminary results of [131I]metaiodobenzylguanidine treatment in metastatic carcinoid tumors. *Journal of Nuclear Biology and Medicine*, **35**, 352–4.

Conlon J.M., Deacon C.F., Richter G., Stockmann F. & Creutzfeldt W. (1987) Circulating tachykinins (substance P, neurokinin A, neuropeptide K) and the carcinoid flush. *Scandinavian Journal of Gastroenterology*, **22**, 97–105.

Creutzfeldt W., Bartsch H.H., Jacubaschke U. & Stockmann F. (1991) Treatment of gastrointestinal endocrine tumours with interferon-alpha and octreotide. *Acta Oncologica*, **30**, 529–35.

Crosby S.R., Stewart M.F., Farrell W.E., Gibson S. & White A. (1990) Comparison of ACTH and ACTH precursor peptides secreted by human pituitary and lung tumour cells in vitro. *Journal of Endocrinology*, **125**, 147–52.

Davis G.R., Camp R.C., Raskin P. & Krejs G.J. (1980) Effect of somatostatin infusion on jejunal water and electrolyte transport in a patient with secretory diarrhea due to malignant carcinoid syndrome. *Gastroenterology*, **78**, 346–9.

Davis Z., Moertel C.G. & McIlrath D.C. (1973) The malignant carcinoid syndrome. *Surgery, Gynecology and Obstetrics*, **137**, 637–4.

Dharmsathaphorn K., Sherwin R.S., Cataland S., Jaffe B. & Dobbins J. (1980) Somatostatin inhibits diarrhea in the carcinoid syndrome. *Annals of Internal Medicine*, **92**, 68–9.

Doberauer C., Mengelkoch B., Kloke O., Wandl U. & Niederle N. (1991) Treatment of metastatic carcinoid tumors and the carcinoid syndrome with recombinant interferon alpha. *Acta Oncologica*, **30**, 603–5.

Dollinger M. & Golbey R. (1967) Actinomycin D in the treatment of the carcinoid tumors. *Clinical Research*, **15**, 335.

Duh Q.Y., Hybarger C.P., Geist R., Gamsu G., Goodman P.C., Gooding G.A. & Clark O.H. (1987) Carcinoids associated with multiple endocrine neoplasia syndromes. *American Journal of Surgery*, **154**, 142–8.

Duner R. & Pernow B. (1960) Circulatory studies on substance P in man. *Acta Physiologica Scandinavica*, **49**, 261–6.

Engstrom P.F., Lavin P.T., Moertel C.G., Folsch E. & Douglas H.O. (1984) Streptozotocin plus fluorouracil versus doxorubicin therapy for metastatic carcinoid tumor. *Journal of Clinical Oncology*, **2**, 1255–9.

Evers B.M., Hurlbut S.C., Tyring S.K., Townsend C.M.J., Uchida T. & Thompson J.C. (1991) Novel therapy for the treatment of human carcinoid. *Annals of Surgery*, **213**, 411–16.

Feldman J.M. (1987). Carcinoid tumors and syndrome. *Seminars in Oncology*, **14**, 237–46.

Feldman J.M. & Jones R.S. (1982) Carcinoid syndrome from gastrointestinal carcinoids without liver metastasis. *Annals of Surgery*, **196**, 33–7.

Feldman J.M. & O'Dorisio T.M. (1986) Role of neuropeptides and serotonin in the diagnosis of carcinoid tumors. *American Journal of Medicine*, **81**, 41–8.

Feldman J.M. & Plonk J.W. (1977) Gastrointestinal and metabolic function in patients with the carcinoid syndrome. *American Journal of the Medical Sciences*, **273**, 43–54.

Feldman J.M., Plonk J.W. & Cornette J.C. (1974) Serum prostaglandin F-2 alpha concentration in the carcinoid syndrome. *Prostaglandins*, **7**, 501–6.

Frolich J.C., Bloomgarden Z.T., Oates J.A., McGuigan J.E. & Rabinowitz D. (1978) The carcinoid flush. Provocation by pentagastrin and inhibition by somatostatin. *New England Journal of Medicine*, **299**, 1055–7.

Gardner B., Dollinger M., Silen W., Back N. & O'Reilly S. (1967) Studies of the carcinoid syndrome: its relationship to serotonin, bradykinin, and histamine. *Surgery*, **61**, 846–52.

Godwin D.J. (1975) Carcinoid tumours: an analysis of 2837 cases. *Cancer*, **36**, 560–9.

Grahame Smith D.G. (1987) What is the cause of the carcinoid flush? (editorial). *Gut*, **28**, 1413–16.

Grander D., Oberg K., Lundqvist M.L., Janson E.T., Eriksson B. & Einhorn S. (1990) Interferon-induced enhancement of 2′,5′-oligoadenylate synthetase in mid-gut carcinoid tumours. *Lancet*, **336**, 337–40.

Griffiths D.F., Williams G.T. & Williams E.D. (1987) Duodenal carcinoid tumours, phaeochromocytoma and neurofibromatosis: islet cell tumour, phaeochromocytoma and the von Hippel-Lindau complex: two distinctive neuroendocrine syndromes. *Quarterly Journal of Medicine*, **64**, 769–82.

Gronstad K.O., Nilsson O., Hedman I., Skolnik G., Dahlstrom A. & Ahlman H. (1985) On the mode of action of the pentagastrin test in the carcinoid syndrome: *Scandinavian Journal of Gastroenterology*, **20**, 508–11.

Gupta A., Saibil F. & Kessim O. (1985) Retroperitoneal fibrosis caused by carcinoid tumour. *Quarterly Journal of Medicine*, **56**, 367–75.

Gustafsen J., Boesby S., Nielsen F. & Giese J. (1987) Bradykinin in carcinoid syndrome. *Gut*, **28**, 1417–19.

Gustafsen J., Lendorf A., Raskov H. & Boesby S. (1986) Ketanserin versus placebo in carcinoid syndrome. *Scandinavian Journal of Gastroenterology*, **21**, 816–18.

Hajarizadeh H., Ivancev K., Mueller C.R., Fletcher W.S. & Woltering E.A. (1992) Effective palliative treatment of metastatic carcinoid tumors with intra-arterial chemotherapy/chemoembolization combined with octreotide acetate. *American Journal of Surgery*, **163**, 479–83.

Hanssen L.E., Schrumpf E., Jacobsen M.B., Kolbenstvedt A.N., Kolmannskog F., Bergan A. & Dolva L.O. (1991) Extended experience with recombinant alpha-2b interferon with or without hepatic artery embolization in the treatment of midgut carcinoid tumours. A preliminary report. *Acta Oncologica*, **30**, 523–7.

Haq A.U., Yook C.R., Hiremath V. & Kasimis B.S. (1992) Carcinoid syndrome in the absence of liver metastasis: a case report and review of literature. *Medical and Pediatric Oncology*, **20**, 221–3.

Haverback B.J. & Davidson J.D. (158) Serotonin and the gastrointestinal tract. *Gastroenterology*, **35**, 570–8.

Heitz P., Polak J.M., Timson D.M. & Pearse A.G. (1976) Enterochromaffin cells as the endocrine source of gastrointestinal substance P. *Histochemistry*, **49**, 343–7.

Herxheimer H. (1953) Influence of 5-hydroxytryptamine on bronchial function. *Journal of Physiology*, **122**, 49P–50P.

Hoefnagel C.A., Taal B.G. & Valdes Olmos R.A. (1991) Role of [131I]metaiodobenzylguanidine therapy in carcinoids. *Journal of Nuclear Biology and Medicine*, **35**, 346–8.

Ishizuka J., Beauchamp R.D., Townsend C.M.J., Greeley G.H.J. & Thompson J.C. (1992) Receptor-mediated autocrine growth-stimulatory effect of 5-hydroxytryptamine on cultured human pancreatic carcinoid cells. *Journal of Cellular Physiology*, **150**, 1–7.

Jaffe B.M. & Condon C. (1976) Prostaglandin E and F in endocrine diarrheogenic syndromes. *Annals of Surgery*, **184**, 516–24.

Janson E.T., Ronnblom L., Ahlstrom H., Grander D., Alm G., Einhorn S. & Oberg K. (1992) Treatment with alpha-interferon versus alpha-interferon in combination with streptozotocin and doxorubicin in patients with malignant carcinoid tumors: a randomized trial. *Annals of Oncology*, **3**, 635–8.

Joensuu H., Katka K. & Kujari H. (1992) Dramatic response of a metastatic carcinoid tumour to a combination of interferon and octreotide. *Acta Endocrinologica (Copenhagen)*,, **126**, 184–5.

Joensuu H., Kumpulainen E. & Grohn P. (1992) Treatment of metastatic carcinoid tumour with recombinant interferon alfa. *European Journal of Cancer*, **28A**, 1650–3.

Keshgegian A.A. & Wheeler J.E. (1980) Estrogen receptor protein in malignant carcinoid tumor: a report of 2 cases. *Cancer*, **45**, 293–6.

Kvols L.K., Moertel C.G., O'Connell M.J., Schutt A.J., Rubin J. & Hahn R.G. (1986) Treatment of the malignant carcinoid syndrome. Evaluation of a long-acting somatostatin analogue. *New England Journal of Medicine*, **315**, 663–6.

Lamberts S.W., Chayvialle J.A. & Krenning E.P. (1992) The visualization of gastroenteropancreatic endocrine tumors. *Metabolism*, **41**, 111–15.

Lawrence J.P., Ishizuka J., Haber B., Townsend C.M.J. & Thompson J.C. (1990) The effect of somatostatin on 5-hydroxytryptamine release from a carcinoid tumor. *Surgery*, **108**, 1131–4.

Lederman R.J., Bukowski R.M. & Nickerson P. (1987) Carcinoid myopathy. *Cleveland Clinic Journal of Medicine*, **54**, 299–303.

Lembeck F. (1953) 5-hydroxytryptamine in a carcinoid tumour. *Nature,* **172**, 910–11.

Linell F. & Mansson K. (1966) On the prevalence and incidence of carcinoids in Malmo. *Acta Medica Scandinavica,* **179**, 377–82.

Lubarsch O. (1888) Uber den primaren krebs des ileum nebst bemerkungen uber das gleichzeitige vonkommen von krebs und tuberculose. *Virchows Archiv. A, Pathological Anatomy and Histopathology,* **111**, 281–8.

Lundin L., Norheim I., Landelius J., Oberg K. & Theodorsson Norheim E. (1988) Carcinoid heart disease: relationship of circulating vasoactive substances to ultrasound-detectable cardiac abnormalities. *Circulation,* **77**, 264–9.

MacDonald R.A. & Robbins S.L. (1957) Pathology of the heart in the carcinoid syndrome. *Archives of Pathology,* **63**, 103–12.

Makowka L., Tzakis A.G., Mazzaferro V., Teperman L., Demetris A.J., Iwatsuki S. & Starzl T.E. (1989) Transplantation of the liver for metastatic endocrine tumors of the intestine and pancreas. *Surgery, Gynecology and Obstetrics,* **168**, 107–11.

Marsh H.M., Martin J.K.J., Kvols L.K., Gracey D.R., Warner M.A., Warner M.E. & Moertel C.G. (1987) Carcinoid crisis during anesthesia: successful treatment with a somatostatin analogue. *Anesthesiology,* **66**, 89–91.

Maton P.N., Camilleri M., Griffin G., Allison D.J., Hodgson H.J.F. & Chadwick V.S. (1984) The role of hepatic artery embolisation in the carcinoid syndrome. *British Medical Journal,* **287**, 932–5.

McEntee G.P., Nagorney D.M., Kvols L.K., Moertel C.G. & Grant C.S. (1990) Cytoreductive hepatic surgery for neuroendocrine tumors. *Surgery,* **108**, 1091–6.

Melmon K.L., Sjoerdsma A. & Mason D.T. (1965) Distinctive clinical and therapeutic aspects of the syndrome associated with bronchial carcinoid tumors. *American Journal of Medicine,* **39**, 568–81.

Mendelson D.S., Rubinoff S.W., Dan S.J. & Jones R.B. (1989) Inadvertent pancreatic embolization as a complication of hepatic carcinoid treatment – computed tomography appearance. *Clinical Imaging,* **13**, 212–14.

Metz S.A., McRae J.R. & Robertson P.R. (1981) Prostaglandins as mediators of paraneoplastic syndromes. Review and update. *Metabolism,* **30**, 299–316.

Moertel C.G. (1983) Treatment of the carcinoid tumor and the malignant carcinoid syndrome. *Journal of Clinical Oncology,* **1**, 727–40.

Moertel C.G. (1987) An odyssey in the land of small tumors. *Journal of Clinical Oncology,* **5**, 1503–22.

Moertel C.G., Engstrom P.F. & Schutt A.J. (1984) Tamoxifen therapy for metastatic carcinoid tumor: a negative study. *Annals of Internal Medicine,* **100**, 531–2.

Moertel C.G. & Hanley J.A. (1979) Combination chemotherapy trials in metastatic carcinoid tumor and the malignant carcinoid syndrome. *Career Clinical Trials,* **2**, 327–34.

Moertel C.G., May G.R., Martin J.K., Rubin J. & Schutt A.J. (1985) Sequential hepatic artery occlusion (HAO) and chemotherapy for metastatic carcinoid tumor and islet cell carcinoma (ICC). *Proceedings of the American Society of Clinical Oncology,* **4**, 80.

Moertel C.G., O'Connell M.J., Reitemeier R.J. & Rubin J. (1984) An evaluation of combined cyclophosphamide and methotrexate therapy in the treatment of metastatic carcinoid tumor and the malignant carcinoid syndrome. *Cancer Treatment Reports,* **68**, 665–7.

Moertel C.G., Rubin J. & Kvols L.K. (1989) Therapy of metastatic carcinoid tumor and the malignant carcinoid syndrome with recombinant leukocyte interferon A. *Journal of Clinical Oncology,* **7**, 865–8.

Moertel C.G., Rubin J. & O'Connell M.J. (1986) A phase II study of cisplatin therapy in patients with metastatic carcinoid tumor and the malignant carcinoid syndrome. *Cancer Treatment Reports,* **70**, 1459–60.

Moertel C.G., Weiland L.H., Nagorney D.M. & Dockerty M.B. (1987) Carcinoid tumor of the appendix: treatment and prognosis. *New England Journal of Medicine,* **317**, 1699–701.

Moss S.F., Lehner P.J., Gilbey S.G., Kennedy A., Hughes J.M., Bloom S.R. & Hodgson H.J. (1993) Pleural involvement in the carcinoid syndrome. *Quarterly Journal of Medicine,* **86**, 49–53.

Myers C.F., Ershler W.B., Tannenbaum M.A. & Barth R. (1982) Tamoxifen and carcinoid tumor. *Annals of Internal Medicine,* **96**, 383.

Nilsson O., Wangberg B., Theodorsson E., Skottner A. & Ahlman H. (1992) Presence of IGF-I in human midgut carcinoid tumours – an autocrine regulator of carcinoid tumour growth? *International Journal of Cancer,* **51**, 195–203.

Nobin A., Lindblom A., Mansson B. & Sundberg M. (1989) Interferon treatment in patients with malignant carcinoids. *Acta Oncologica,* **28**, 445–9.

O'Grady J.G., Polson R.J., Rolles K., Calne R.Y. & Williams R. (1988) Liver transplantation for malignant disease. Results in 93 consecutive patients. *Annals of Surgery,* **207**, 373–9.

Oates J.A., Pettinger W.A. & Doctor R.B. (1966) Evidence for the release of bradykinin in carcinoid syndrome. *Journal of Clinical Investigation,* **45**, 173–8.

Oates J.A. & Sjoerdsma A. (1962) A unique syndrome associated with secretion of 5-hydroxytryptophan by metastatic gastric carcinoids. *American Journal of Medicine,* **32**, 333–44.

Obendorfer S. (1907) Karzinoide tumoren des Dunndarms. *Frankfurt Zeitschrift fur Pathologie,* **1**, 426–32.

Oberg K. & Eriksson B. (1991) The role of interferons in the management of carcinoid tumors. *Acta Oncologica,* **30**, 519–22.

Oberg K., Funa K. & Alm G. (1983) Effects of leukocyte interferon on clinical symptoms and hormone levels in patients with mid-gut carcinoid tumors and carcinoid syndrome. *New England Journal of Medicine,* **309**, 129–33.

Oberg K. Norheim I., Theodorsson E., Ahlman H., Lundqvist G. & Wide L. (1989) The effects of octreotide on basal and stimulated hormone levels in patients with carcinoid syndrome. *Journal of Clinical Endocrinology and Metabolism,* **68**, 796–800.

Ormsbee H.S. & Fondacaro J.D. (1985) Action of serotonin on the gastrointestinal tract. *Proceedings of the Society for Experimental Biology and Medicine,* **178**, 333–8.

Pass H.I., Doppman J.L., Nieman L., Stovroff M., Vetto J., Norton J.A., Travis W., Chrousos G.P., Oldfield E.H. & Cutler G.B., Jr. (1990) Management of the ectopic ACTH syndrome due to thoracic carcinoids. *Annals of Thoracic Surgery,* **50**, 52–7.

Pearse A.G. & Polak J.M. (1975) Immunocytochemical localization of substance P in mammalian intestine. *Histochemistry,* **41**, 373–5.

Pellikka P.A., Tajik A.J., Khandheria B.K., Seward J.B., Callahan J.A., Pitot H.C. & Kvols L.K. (1993) Carcinoid heart disease. Clinical and echocardiographic spectrum in 74 patients. *Circulation,* **87**, 1188–96.

Petersen K.G., Seemann W.R., Plagwitz R. & Kerp L. (1984) Evidence for coronary spasm during flushing in the carcinoid syndrome. *Clinical Cardiology*, **7**, 445–8.

Platt A.J., Heddle R.M., Rake M.O. & Smedley H. (1992) Ondansetron in carcinoid syndrome. *Lancet*, **339**, 1416.

Plonk J.W. & Feldman J.M. (1974) Carcinoid arthropathy. *Archives of Internal Medicine*, **134**, 651–4.

Powell D. & Skrabanek P. (1979) Brain and gut. *Clinics in Endocrinology and Metabolism*, **8**, 299–312.

Quatrini M., Basilisco G., Conte D., Bozzani A., Bardella M.T. & Bianchi P.A. (1983) Effects of somatostatin infusion in four patients with malignant carcinoid syndrome. *American Journal of Gastroenterology*, **78**, 149–51.

Reubi J.C., Maurer R., von Werder K., Torhorst J., Klijn J.G. & Lamberts S.W. (1987) Somatostatin receptors in human endocrine tumors. *Cancer Research*, **47**, 551–8.

Richter G., Stockmann F., Conlon J.M. & Creutzfeld W. (1986) Serotonin release into blood after food and pentagastrin. Studies in healthy subjects and in patients with metastatic carcinoid tumors. *Gastroenterology*, **91**, 612–18.

Roberts L.J., Marney S.R. & Oates J.A. (1979) Blockade of the flush associated with metastatic gastric carcinoid by combined histamine H1 and H2 receptor antagonists: evidence for an important role of H2 receptors in human vasculature. *New England Journal of Medicine*, **300**, 236–8.

Ronnblom L.E., Alm G.V. & Oberg K. (1991) Autoimmune phenomena in patients with malignant carcinoid. *Acta Oncologica*, **30**, 537–40.

Ruszniewski P., Rougier P., Roche A., Legmann P., Sibert A., Hochlaf S., Ychou M. & Mignon M. (1993) Hepatic arterial chemoembolization in patients with liver metastases of endocrine tumors. A prospective phase II study in 24 patients. *Cancer*, **71**, 2624–30.

Sandler M., Karim S.M. & Williams E.D. (1968) Prostaglandins in amine-peptide-secreting tumours. *Lancet*, **2**, 1053–4.

Sauven P., Ridge J.A., Quan S.H. & Sigurdson E.R. (1990) Anorectal carcinoid tumors. Is aggressive surgery warranted? *Annals of Surgery*, **211**, 67–71.

Schaffalitzky de Muckadell O.B., Aggestrup S. & Stentoft P. (1986) Flushing and plasma substance P concentration during infusion of synthetic substance P in normal man. *Scandinavian Journal of Gastroenterology*, **21**, 498–502.

Schober C., Schmoll E., Schmoll H.J., Poliwoda H., Schuppert F., Stahl M., Bokemeyer C., Wilke H. & Weiss J. (1992) Antitumour effect and symptomatic control with interferon 2b in patients with endocrine active tumours. *European Journal of Cancer*, **28A**, 1664–6.

Sjoerdsma A., Terry L.L. & Udenfriend S. (1957) Malignant carcinoid. A new metabolic disorder. *Archives of Internal Medicine*, **99**, 1009–12.

Skrabanek P., Cannon D., Kirrane J. & Powell D. (1978) Substance P secretion by carcinoid tumours. *Israel Journal of Medical Sciences*, **147**, 47–9.

Smith D.B., Scarffe J.H., Wagstaff J. & Johnston R.J. (1987) Phase II trial of rDNA alfa 2b interferon in patients with malignant carcinoid tumor. *Cancer Treatment Reports*, **71**, 1265–6

Smith S., Anthony L., Roberts L.J., Oates J.A. & Pincus T. (1990) Resolution of musculoskeletal symptoms in the carcinoid syndrome after treatment with the somatostatin analog octreotide. *Annals of Internal Medicine*, **112**, 66–8.

Solcia E., Rindi G., Silini E. & Villani L. (1993) Enterochromaffin-like (ECL) cells and their growths: relationships to gastrin, reduced acid secretion and gastritis. *Baillieres Clinical Gastroenterology*, **7**, 149–65.

Stamatis G., Freitag L. & Greschuchna D. (1990) Limited and radical resection for tracheal and bronchopulmonary carcinoid tumour. Report on 227 cases. *European Journal of Cardiothoracic Surgery*, **4**, 527–32.

Teleky B., Herbst F., Langle F., Neuhold N. & Niederle B. (1992) The prognosis of rectal carcinoid tumours. *International Journal of Colorectal Disease*, **7**, 11–14.

Thorson A., Bjork G., Bjorkman G. & Waldenstrom J. (1954) Malignant carcinoid of the small intestine with metastases to the liver, valvular disease of the right heart (pulmonary stenosis and tricuspid regurgitation without septal defect), peripheral vasomotor symptoms, bronchoconstriction and an unusual type of cyanosis. *American Heart Journal*, **47**, 795–817.

Tiensuu Janson E.M., Ahlstrom H., Andersson T. & Oberg K.E. (1992) Octreotide and interferon alfa: a new combination for the treatment of malignant carcinoid tumours. *European Journal of Cancer*, **28A**, 1647–50.

Udenfriend S., Titus E. & Weissbach H. (1955) The identification of 5-hydroxyindoleacetic acid in normal urine and a method for its assay. *Journal of Biological Chemistry*, **21**, 499–505.

Vandovinos M.A., Thomforde G.M. & Camilleri M. (1993) Effect of putative carcinoid mediators on gastric and small bowel transit in rats and the role of 5-HT receptors. *Alimentary Pharmacology and Therapeutics*, **7**, 61–6.

Valimaki M., Jarvinen H., Salmela P., Sane T., Sjoblom S.M. & Pelkonen R. (1991) Is the treatment of metastatic carcinoid tumor with interferon not as successful as suggested. *Cancer*, **67**, 547–9.

van Hazel G.A., Rubin J. & Moertel C.G. (1983) Treatment of metastatic carcinoid tumor with dactinomycin or decarbazine. *Cancer Treatment Reports*, **67**, 583–5.

Veenhof C.H., de Wit R., Taal B.G., Dirix L.Y., Wagstaff J., Hensen A., Huldij A.C. & Bakker P.J. (1992) A dose-escalation study of recombinant interferon-alpha in patients with a metastatic carcinoid tumour. *European Journal of Cancer*, **28**, 75–8.

Vinik A. & Moattari A.R. (1989) Use of somatostatin analog in management of carcinoid syndrome. *Digestive Diseases and Sciences*, **34**, 14S–27S.

Vroom F.Q., Brown R.E. & Dampsey H. (1962) Studies on several possible antiserotonin compounds in patients with the functioning carcinoid syndrome. *Annals of Internal Medicine*, **56**, 941–5.

Waltenberger J., Lundin L., Oberg K., Wilander E., Miyazono K., Heldin C.H. & Funa K. (1993) Involvement of transforming growth factor-beta in the formation of fibrotic lesions in carcinoid heart disease. *American Journal of Pathology*, **142**, 71–8.

Wangberg B., Nilsson O., Theodorsson E., Dahlstrom A. & Ahlman H. (1991) The effect of a somatostatin analogue on the release of hormones from midgut carcinoid tumour cells. *British Journal of Cancer*, **64**, 23–8.

Wareing T.H. & Sawyers J.L. (1983) Carcinoids and the carcinoid syndrome. *American Journal of Surgery*, **145**, 769–72.

Wiedenmann B., Rath U., Radsch R., Becker F. & Kommerell B. (1988) Tumor regression of an ileal carcinoid under the treatment with the somatostatin analogue SMS 201-995. *Klinische Wochenschrift*, **66**, 75–7.

Wilander E., Lundquist M. & el Salhy M. (1985) Serotonin in foregut carcinoids. *Journal of Pathology*, **145**, 251–8.
Willerson J.T., Hillis L.D., Winniford M. & Buja L.M. (1986) Speculation regarding mechanisms responsible for acute ischemic heart disease. *Journal of the American College of Cardiology*, **8**, 245–50.
Williams E.D. & Sandler M. (1963) The classification of carcinoid tumours. *Lancet*, **i**, 238–9.
Wynick D., Anderson J.V., Williams S.J. & Bloom S.R. (1989) Resistance of metastatic pancreatic endocrine tumours after long-term treatment with the somatostatin analogue octreotide (SMS 201-995). *Clinical Endocrinology (Oxford)*, **30**, 385–8.
Yang K., Ulich T., Cheng L. & Lewis K.J. (1983) The neuroendocrine products of intestinal carcinoids. *Cancer*, **51**, 1918–26.

PART 4

Endocrine Complications of Cancer Treatment

12

Humoral Hypercalcaemia

JOHN J. WYSOLMERSKI AND ARTHUR E. BROADUS

INTRODUCTION

Malignancy-associated hypercalcaemia (MAHC) was first noted in the 1920s, not long after the measurement of serum calcium was introduced into clinical medicine (Zondek, Petow & Siebert, 1924). The first large series of patients was reported by Gutman in 1936 (Gutman, Tyson & Gutman, 1936); these patients suffered from myeloma and breast cancer, and almost all of them had extensive tumour involvement of their skeletons. Thus, it was assumed at the time that MAHC was uniformly the result of localized skeletal destruction caused by primary or metastatic tumour in bone. In 1941, Fuller Albright first suggested that in some patients with MAHC, hypercalcaemia might be the result of a circulating humor (Case Records of the Massachusetts General Hospital Case 17461, 1941). Several series reported in the 1950s and 1960s confirmed Albright's suspicions by describing patients with cancer who had little or no skeletal tumour burden but who were nonetheless hypercalcaemic, and in whom resection or debulking of the tumour corrected the hypercalcaemia (Connor, Thomas & Howard, 1956; Plimpton & Gelhorn, 1956). In 1966, Lafferty reported a series of 50 patients with cancer who were hypercalcaemic in the absence of any bone involvement and noted that the majority of this group of patients had squamous, renal or urothelial tumours. In contrast, he observed that most of the patients with extensive bony involvement and hypercalcaemia tended to have myeloma or breast cancer (Lafferty, 1966). He thought that the tumours causing hypercalcaemia via an apparent humoral mechanism were producing parathyroid hormone, and coined the term 'pseudohyperparathyroidism' to describe this syndrome.

Thus, by the late 1960s it had been established that distinct subsets of tumours could cause MAHC either through local or systemic effects on the skeleton. Today, we refer to these two subtypes of MAHC as local osteolytic hypercalcaemia (LOH) and humoral hypercalcaemia of malignancy (HHM), and it is now clear, contrary to initial beliefs, that the humoral mechanism is the dominant one (Burtis et al., 1990; Stewart et al., 1980).

Our current understanding of both forms of MAHC follows from several sets of observations made in the 1980s. Firstly, various lymphokines were found to have bone resorbing activity in vitro, and these were implicated as paracrine mediators of local osteoclastic bone resorption in LOH. Secondly, a new hormone, parathyroid hormone-related peptide (PTHrP), was discovered to be the systemic activator of diffuse osteoclastic bone resorption in the syndrome of HHM. In the first part of this chapter, we shall briefly consider LOH and then explore in some detail HHM and the discovery of PTHrP. In the second section, we shall discuss the molecular biology of PTHrP and the molecular pathogenesis of HHM. Finally, we will consider some potential normal biological functions of PTHrP.

LOCAL OSTEOLYTIC HYPERCALCAEMIA

LOH refers to a syndrome of hypercalcaemia caused by osteoclastic bone resorption occurring in close proximity to tumour deposits in the skeleton. It accounts for 20 to 30% of all patients with MAHC (Budayr et al., 1989; Burtis et al., 1990; Stewart et al., 1980). These patients characteristically have extensive skeletal tumour involvement, but sites free of tumour do not show excessive bone resorption. Typically, patients with LOH suffer from myeloma, breast cancer or lymphoma. By definition, the serum calcium is elevated, but the serum phosphorus concentration and the renal phosphate threshold are typically normal. The levels of PTH, nephrogenous c'AMP and 1,25-dihydroxyvitamin D_3 (1,25-$(OH)_2D$) are reduced, secondary to the hypercalcaemia. Urinary calcium excretion is markedly increased, both because of the increased filtered load and because of diminished distal tubular calcium reabsorption as a result of the suppressed PTH concentrations. At the same time, intestinal calcium absorption is decreased as a consequence of the low 1,25-$(OH)_2D$ levels. Therefore, these patients are in markedly negative calcium balance.

Although some cancer cells seem to be capable of resorbing bone directly (Eilon & Mundy, 1978), the primary pathophysiological mechanism in LOH is the secretion by tumour cells of paracrine factors that stimulate neighbouring osteoclasts to resorb bone. This has been best characterized for myeloma. As early as 20 years ago, it was known that conditioned media from cultured myeloma cells contained a soluble factor, termed 'osteoclast activating factor' (OAF), that could stimulate bone resorption in vitro (Mundy et al., 1974). Subsequently, it was shown that several lymphokines, including interleukin-1α, interleukin-1β, tumor necrosis factor alpha (TNF-α), tumor necrosis factor beta (TNF-β; lymphotoxin), and transforming growth factor alpha (TGF-α) can stimulate osteoclastic bone resorption in vitro and cause hypercalcaemia when infused into mice (Mundy, 1989). However, it remains unclear as to which of these factors or combination of factors is actually responsible for the hypercalcaemia in most patients. It appears that the predominant bone-resorbing substance in cultures of normal monocytes is interleukin-1β (Dewhirst et al., 1985), and there are data to suggest that either interleukin-1β (Kawano et al., 1989; Yamamoto et al., 1989) or lymphotoxin (Garrett et al., 1987) is the major osteoclast-stimulating factor in myeloma. A tight causal link has yet to be established between any one cytokine and hypercalcaemia in haematological malignancies.

Breast cancer has traditionally been thought to cause hypercalcaemia exclusively via local osteolysis, but recently there has been a reassessment of the mechanisms involved. It now appears that PTHrP may play an important role in causing hypercalcaemia in breast cancer either by acting systemically as a hormone or by acting locally in a paracrine fashion. In a prospective study, Isales and co-workers found that a substantial minority of hypercalcaemic patients with breast cancer, perhaps as many as 35%, display the typical biochemical profile of HHM (see below) (Isales, Carcangiu & Stewart, 1987). Despite traditional dogma, this is not particularly surprising, as previous series of patients with HHM always included some patients with breast cancer (Stewart et al., 1980), and one of the tumours that our group used to purify PTHrP was, in fact, a breast carcinoma. As for the potential paracrine role for PTHrP in breast cancer, Vargas et al. (Vargas et al., 1992) have demonstrated that 70 to 90% of metastatic lesions in bone express the PTHrP gene and produce the peptide, compared with only 60% PTHrP positivity in the primary tumours. It is possible that the bone microenvironment may activate or up-regulate PTHrP gene expression in some breast carcinoma cells. It is known that PTHrP is a natural product of mammary epithelial cells, especially during pregnancy and lactation, and that very high levels of the peptide are found in milk (Burtis et al., 1990; Strewler & Nissenson, 1990). Therefore, it may be that some breast cancers produce enough PTHrP to produce prototypical HHM, whereas other tumours may secrete only enough to act locally, in a paracrine fashion, and cause LOH. The second part of this hypothesis, while attractive, remains conjectural and has yet to be systematically studied.

HUMORAL HYPERCALCAEMIA OF MALIGNANCY

HHM refers to a syndrome of diffuse osteoclastic bone resorption, classically as a result of a tumour distant from the skeleton. Although it is now recognized that there may be some skeletal involvement by tumour in patients with this syndrome (e.g., those with breast cancer), the hypercalcaemia is the result of hormone secretion into the systemic circulation affecting the entire skeleton rather than only a part of the skeleton. This syndrome is now recognized to be the dominant form of MAHC, causing up to 75 to 80% of consecutive, non-selected cases of hypercalcaemia occurring in the setting of malignancy (Burtis et al., 1990; Stewart et al., 1980). As is the case with LOH, patients with this syndrome also present with a distinct subset of tumour types, with the majority of cases being accounted for by squamous, renal and urothelial malignancies. In addition, virtually 100% of hypercalcaemic patients with HTLV-1–associated adult T-cell leukemia/lymphoma have HHM (Watanabe et al., 1990).

The first careful biochemical characterization of HHM was published by Stewart and co-workers in 1980 (Stewart et al., 1980), and this study established a characteristic constellation of laboratory findings that defines HHM (Figure 12.1). These findings include an elevated serum calcium, a low serum phosphorus, a low PTH level, low 1,25 $(OH)_2D$ levels and an elevated nephrogenic c'AMP excretion rate. This profile is in part similar to that of patients with primary hyperparathyroidism, especially the elevation in nephrogenic c'AMP, which was previously considered to be a specific test of PTH action, as it reflects activation of the renal proximal tubular PTH receptor. However, there are key differences between hyperparathyroidism and HHM, these being the low PTH levels, low levels of 1,25-$(OH)_2D$, and the reduced distal tubular calcium reabsorption seen in HHM. Another characteristic feature described in subsequent histomorphometric studies of bone is the uncoupling of bone resorption and bone formation in HHM (Figure 12.2) (Stewart et al., 1981). As would be expected, osteoclast activity is increased, which leads to the hypercalcaemia, but unlike hyperparathyroidism, where bone turnover is increased in a coupled fashion, bone formation is suppressed in HHM. Since the PTH and vitamin D axes are appropriately suppressed, gut absorption of calcium is diminished and calcium clearance by the kidney is increased in patients with HHM. Since bone resorption is

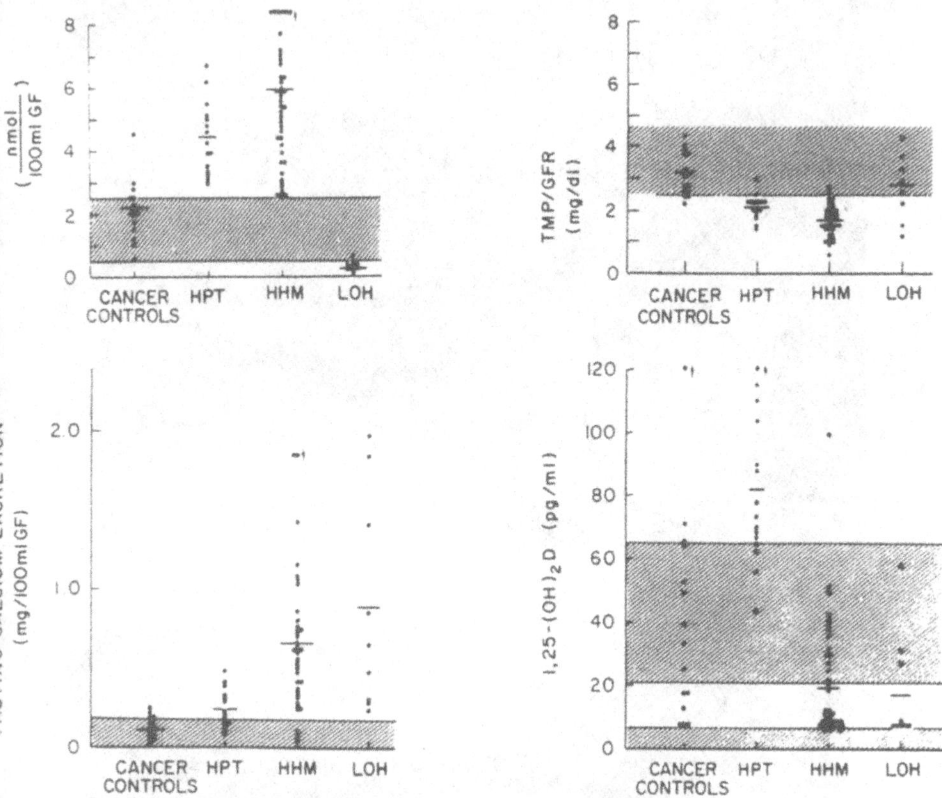

Figure 12.1 Biochemical characterization of patients with cancer and normal serum calcium concentrations (Cancer Controls), primary hyperparathyroidism (HPT), humoral hypercalcemia of malignancy (HHM), and local osteolytic hypercalcemia (LOH). NcAMP indicates nephrogenous cyclic adenosine monophosphate excretion, and TMP/GFR denotes the renal tubular threshold for phosphorus. (From Stewart et al., 1980. Used by permission).

occurring unopposed, these patients are typically severely hypercalcaemic and in profoundly negative calcium balance.

Discovery and Characterization of PTHrP

The studies cited above had established, by the early 1980s, that HHM was not caused by ectopic production of PTH but by another factor that seemed to be able to mimic some actions of PTH. In fact, the PTH-like nature of this factor with respect to its ability to increase

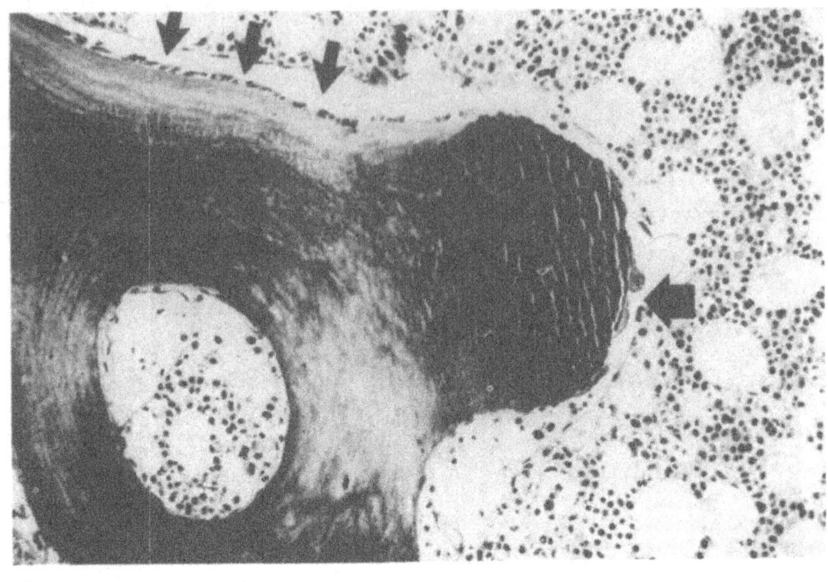

A

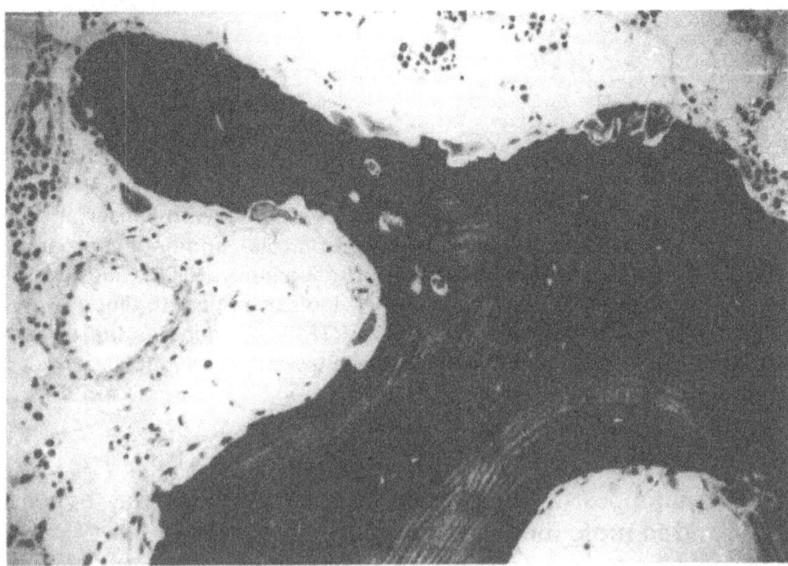

B

Figure 12.2 Photomicrographs of bone biopsy specimens from representative patients with either hyperparathyroidism (A) or HHM (B). Note the presence of active osteoblasts lining an osteoid seam in (A) marked by the smaller arrows; the larger arrow points out an osteoclast, which are seen in abundance in (B). (From Stewart et al., 1982. Used by permission).

nephrogenic c'AMP production proved to be the key characteristic that allowed its isolation and characterization. In the early 1980s, investigators in several laboratories used PTH-sensitive, c'AMP-generating bioassays to demonstrate that tumour extracts or media conditioned by tumour cells taken from patients with HHM contained a PTH-like bioactivity, whereas tumours taken from patients with LOH contained no such activity (Stewart et al., 1983; Strewler, Williams & Nissenson, 1983). This activity could be abolished by specific competitive inhibitors of PTH binding, but it was not affected by PTH antisera (Stewart et al., 1983). The results of these studies were taken as confirmation of the results from the previous clinical studies that a factor similar to, but distinct from, PTH was secreted by malignant tumours associated with the syndrome of HHM. These observations led several of the same laboratories to use the c'AMP-generating assays to guide attempts at purification of this factor. This effort required some five years and a 20,000- to 60,000-fold purification that led to the discovery of a new peptide hormone termed 'parathyroid hormone-related peptide' (PTHrP) (Burtis et al., 1987; Moseley et al., 1987; Strewler et al., 1987). Soon after PTHrP was purified to homogeneity and partial sequence was available, two groups isolated c'DNAs for PTHrP (Mangin et al., 1988b; Suva et al., 1987) and shortly thereafter, the genomic structure of the PTHrP gene was elucidated (Mangin et al., 1989; Suva et al., 1989; Yasuda et al., 1989).

The structure and expression of the PTHrP gene are explored at some length below and will not be discussed here except to say that the deduced primary amino acid sequence of PTHrP, when it became available, was truly enlightening with respect to the pathogenesis of HHM. c'DNAs encoding proteins of 139, 141 and 173 amino acids were isolated, all of which shared identical amino acid sequence through the first 139 residues. At its amino terminus PTHrP has sequence identity to PTH at 8 of the first 13 amino acids. After amino acid 13, the PTHrP sequence was noted to be unique and to share no homology to PTH. However, although amino acids 20 through 34 of PTHrP and PTH are not alike in their primary amino acid sequence, it has been suggested that they share similar secondary structure in this region (see Figure 12.3). These regions of shared primary and secondary structure correspond to the regions of PTH that were known previously to be important for receptor binding and activation. Indeed, many studies have now shown that N-terminal fragments of PTHrP are equipotent with PTH in binding to and activating classical PTH receptors (Orloff & Stewart, 1989). Thus, it is now clear that the majority of the biochemical features of HHM result from the secretion by tumours of PTHrP into the systemic circulation, with

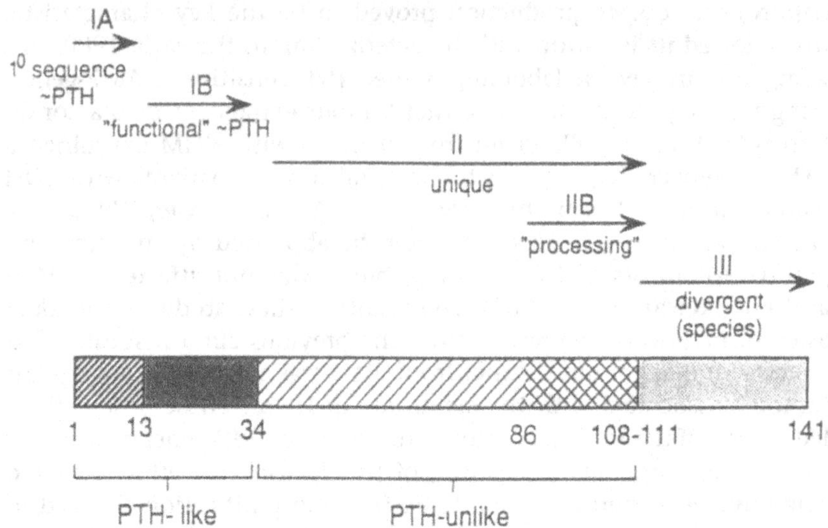

Figure 12.3 Diagrammatic representation of parathyroid hormone-related protein demonstrating the regions of homology with either the primary or secondary structure of parathyroid hormone. PTHrP isoforms are all well conserved between species up to amino acid 111, after this point they diverge. (From Broadus & Stewart, in press. Used by permission).

subsequent interaction or cross-reaction with PTH receptors located in bone and kidney.

In the past several years, a series of studies have further cemented the causal relationship of PTHrP to the syndrome of HHM. Firstly, soon after c'DNAs for PTHrP were cloned, PTHrP mRNA was documented in tumours associated with HHM (Ikeda et al., 1988a). Secondly, synthetic N-terminal fragments of PTHrP have been shown to cause severe hypercalcaemia, hypophosphatemia, and elevated nephrogenic c'AMP levels when infused into rodents (Kemp et al., 1987; Stewart et al., 1988). Thirdly, studies using sensitive immunoassays have shown that patients with HHM have elevated circulating levels of PTHrP (Budayr et al., 1989; Burtis et al., 1990). Finally, it has been shown that neutralizing antibodies to PTHrP can reverse the hypercalcaemia caused by HHM-associated human tumours grown in nude mice (Kukreja et al., 1988). It thus appears that PTHrP is both necessary and sufficient to explain the key PTH-like features of the syndrome of HHM.

Certain pathophysiological features of the syndrome, however, remain incompletely understood. These include the uncoupling of bone turnover, the inhibition of 1,25-$(OH)_2D$ production, and the apparent reduced potency of PTHrP in increasing distal tubular calcium reabsorption as compared to PTH. As opposed to the clinical findings in studies of HHM in humans, several studies employing the infusion of synthetic N-terminal fragments of PTHrP into rodents have shown an increase in bone formation and in 1,25-$(OH)_2D$ levels (Kitazawa et al., 1991; Rizzoli et al., 1989; Rosol, Capen & Horst, 1988). In addition, N-terminal PTHrP fragments have been shown to cause an increase in renal calcium resorption in studies using isolated perfused kidneys (Ebeling et al., 1990; Scheinman, Mitnick & Stewart, 1990). In contrast to these infusion studies, in the athymic mouse model it has been shown that HHM-associated tumours suppress bone formation parameters in the murine skeleton and that the infusion of neutralizing antisera to PTHrP increases bone formation in addition to lowering resorption parameters (Kukreja et al., 1990). Previous reviews should be consulted for a thorough discussion of these issues (Strewler & Nissenson, 1990), but several possible explanations for these conflicting data will be presented briefly here. Firstly, there may be species differences in responsiveness to PTHrP. Secondly, most studies have used short N-terminal PTHrP fragments in their designs, and it is possible that other regions of the PTHrP molecule are important in this regard; the actual secretory and/or circulating form of PTHrP has yet to be determined in patients with HHM. Thirdly, it has been suggested that tumours may co-secrete other factors that inhibit bone formation and/or 1,25-$(OH)_2D$ formation. Finally, it may be that coexistent debilitation and/or the severity of the hypercalcaemia may somehow suppress bone formation and 1,25-$(OH)_2D$ synthesis in these patients independent of the direct effects of PTHrP. These points remain areas of active investigation and are of some importance, given the reproducibility of the biochemical and clinical phenotype in patients with HHM.

Humoral Hypercalcaemia of Malignancy Associated with Factors Other Than PTHrP

Since the discovery of PTHrP, there have been three reported cases of true ectopic PTH production in malignancy, each documented by modern molecular techniques (Nussbaum, Gaz & Arnold, 1990; Strewler et al., 1987; Yoshimoto et al., 1989). These patients suffered from small-cell lung cancer, ovarian cancer and an undifferentiated neuroectodermal tumour. In the patient with ovarian cancer, there appeared to be a clonal rearrangement of the 5′ regulatory region of the PTH gene in the tumour, probably resulting in the activation of its expression (Nussbaum, Gaz & Arnold, 1990). Thus although 'pseudohyperparathyroidism' does exist after all, this remains a reportable cause of HHM.

Another rare humoral cause of hypercalcaemia in malignancy is the overproduction of 1,25-dihydroxyvitamin D by lymphomas (Adams et al., 1989; Breslau et al., 1984). This syndrome clearly differs from HHM as defined earlier, since the hypercalcaemia results to a large extent from the hyperabsorption of calcium in the intestine. In a recent study, it was reported that up to 50% of hypercalciuric patients with lymphoma had an elevated 1,25-$(OH)_2D$ level (Adams et al., 1989). Presumably, this is either the result of factors secreted by the lymphoma that stimulate the renal 1-α-hydroxylase or, more likely, extrarenal hydroxylation of 25-hydroxyvitamin D by lymphoma cells or by macrophages, similar to the situation seen in granulomatous diseases.

Finally, there are several growth factors and lymphokines that have been shown to have bone-resorbing activity in vitro. Although these factors are more likely to play a paracrine role in the pathogenesis of LOH, it remains possible that occasional patients may have tumours that secrete these factors in sufficient quantities to act in a humoral fashion. However, there have been no such patients described to date, and these growth factors seem to be relatively weak hypercalcaemic factors when administered systemically (Strewler & Nissenson, 1990)

MOLECULAR BIOLOGY OF PTHrP

The PTHrP Gene

The human PTHrP gene consists of eight exons spanning more than 15 kb of genomic DNA (Mangin et al., 1989; Suva et al., 1989; Yasuda et al., 1989). It is a complex transcriptional unit that gives rise, through alternative splicing, to several different classes of mRNAs coding for three protein isoforms: one of 139 amino acids, one of 141 amino acids and one of 173 amino acids. The first four exons (1A, 1B, 1C and 2) are noncoding and are subject to alternative splicing (Figure 12.4). Exon 3 encodes the majority of the prepro region of the peptide, except for the dibasic endoproteolytic cleavage sight, which is carried on exon 4. Exon 4 encodes the bulk of the PTHrP coding region, that which is common to all three PTHrP isoforms. It also contains a common stop codon-splice donor sequence and a 3′ UTR that define the 139 amino acid isoform of PTHrP. Finally, exons 5 and 6 contain the sequences that encode the C-terminal regions of the 173 and 141 amino acid peptides, respectively. Each of these exons

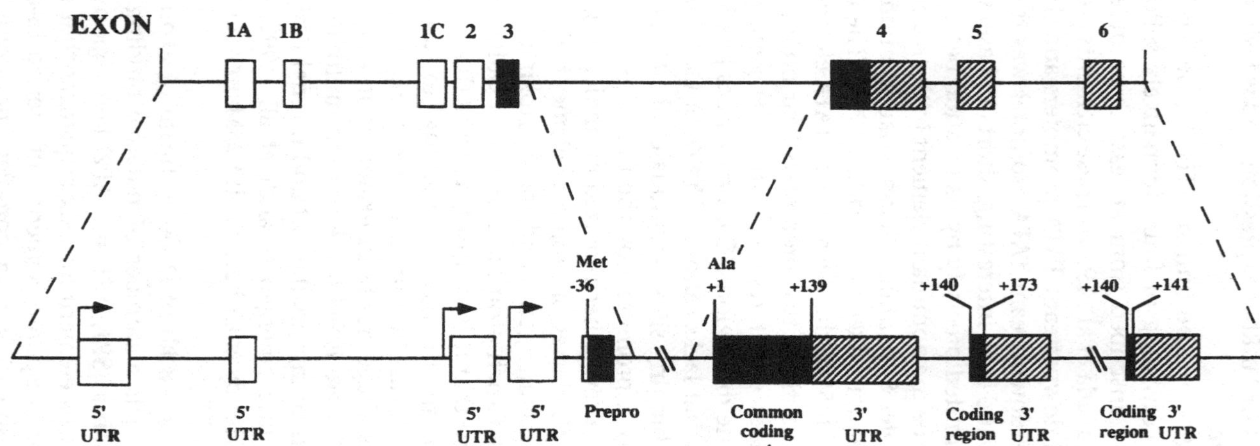

Figure 12.4 Organization of the human PTHrP gene. The open boxes represent 5′ untranslated (5′ UTR) sequences, the solid boxes coding sequences, and the hatched boxes 3′ untranslated (3′ UTR) sequences. The arrows define the start sites used by the three promoter elements. The initiating methionine (Met), the first amino acid of the mature peptide (Ala), and the C termini of the three PTHrP isoforms are indicated.

also contains a stop codon and a unique 3′ UTR. The structure of the PTHrP gene, especially its 5′ flank and 3′ UTRs, provides some insight into critical aspects of PTHrP mRNA expression, and we will elaborate on these regions further.

The 5′ flanking region of the human PTHrP gene has a highly complex organization, consisting of four alternatively spliced, non-coding exons that are transcribed from at least three independent promoter elements (Vasavada et al., 1993). These elements are referred to as the upstream and downstream TATA promoters and the midregion GC promoter. The downstream TATA promoter was the first element to be recognized and is an interesting, short (45-base) structure, the size of which is delimited precisely by its location between exons 1C and 2. This seems to be the dominant element in the rodent PTHrP genes, which have simpler 5′ flanking regions than the human gene (Karaplis et al., 1990; Mangin, Ikeda & Broadus, 1990). The upstream TATA promoter lies 2.7 kb 5′ of the downstream TATA element. Apart from the TATA consensus, these two promoters bear no resemblance to one another, nor does either resemble the PTH gene promoter (Mangin et al., 1990). The midregion GC promoter lies just 5′ of exon 1C in a GC-rich region that lacks canonical TATA or CAAT sequences but is enriched in SP1 binding sites (Vasavada et al., 1993). The use of both TATA and GC-rich promoters by the PTHrP gene is very unusual, there being only a few other reported examples of genes that are transcribed from both classes of promoter elements (Vasavada et al., 1993). Many housekeeping genes and some cytokine/growth factor genes operate from GC-rich promoters (Hendy & Goltzman, 1992; Vasavada et al., 1993), so that it is tempting to infer that the GC-rich PTHrP gene promoter might have something to do with its widespread expression, at least in human tissues. To date, preferential or cell-specific promoter usage has been examined in only a limited number of studies, and there is evidence of both multiple and preferential promoter use in certain malignant and normal tissues, without a clear pattern having emerged (Brandt et al., 1992; Campos, Wang & Drucker 1992; Hendy & Goltzman, 1992; Mangin et al., 1990; Vasavada et al., 1993).

A computer search of 4.8 kb of DNA upstream of exon 2 of the human PTHrP gene reveals a number of putative binding sites for transcription factors such as SP1, AP1 and AP2, two regions that resemble a c′AMP consensus element and six sequences that are identical to a steroid hormone response element half-site; no 15-base consensus sequences corresponding to a complete hormone response element are present, even allowing for three-base mismatches. However, it is clear that steroid hormones are among the host of influences that seem to regulate PTHrP mRNA expression; these controls are summarized in Table 12.3 and in the following section. Possibly because of the complexity of the 5′ flanking region of the PTHrP gene, only a limited number of functional studies of basal promoter activity and/or regulated transcription have appeared (Campos et al., 1992; Kremer et al., 1991; Suva et al., 1991; Vasavada, 1992; Vasavada et al., 1993). An important aspect of control that has been only recently recognized is that of negative regulation or inhibition of basal PTHrP gene transcription. For example, there appear to be multiple negative regulatory or 'silencer' sequences located upstream of the midregion GC promoter (see below for additional detail) (Vasavada et al., 1992). In essence, the general picture that is beginning to emerge is that the complex structure of the human PTHrP gene 5′ flanking region correlates with an equivalent complexity in terms of control and that the transcription of the gene is subject to finely tuned checks and balances in the form of both positive and negative controls.

The human PTHrP gene contains three alternatively spliced 3′ exons that give rise to three mRNA classes encoding three PTHrP isoforms, each with a unique C-terminus (Figure 12.5) (Mangin et al., 1988b; Mangin et al., 1988a; Suva et al., 1987; Thiede et al., 1988). The splicing pattern here is unusual, in that exon 4 can either remain unspliced to generate the mRNA encoding one of the PTHrP isoforms or be alternatively spliced to exons 5 or 6 to generate the other two; the common coding region for 139 amino acids from exon 4 is included in all three products (Figures 12.4 and 12.5). The key 'hinge' sequence in this regard occurs at the end of the coding region in exon 4. This four-base sequence, GTAA, plays the dual role of splice donor site (GT consensus) or a stop codon (TAA). Although there is Northern blotting evidence for apparent tumour-specific preferential splicing (Mangin et al., 1988a; Ikeda et al., 1989), virtually nothing is known with respect to possible cell-specific preferential splicing patterns or the regulation of splice choices in normal human tissues. All three

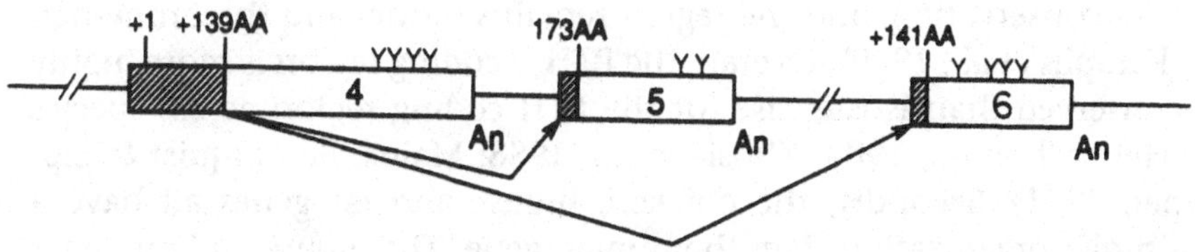

Figure 12.5 Schematic representation of the alternatively spliced 3′ exons of the human PTHrP gene. Coding regions are hatched, and the locations of the ATTTA motifs are designated by the Ys.

mRNA species seem to exist in similar abundance in normal human keratinocytes (Mangin et al., 1988b), but the mRNA encoding the 139 amino acid product appears to be relatively enriched in amnion (Brandt et al., 1992).

Although the three PTHrP mRNA classes encode different isoforms, examination of their 3′ UTRs reveals an important common feature, in that each is AU-rich and contains multiple copies of an AUUUA 'instability' motif (indicated by the Y symbols in Figure 12.5) or AU-rich element (ARE) that has been shown previously to confer rapid turnover on a number of cytokine and proto-oncogene mRNAs (Hargrove & Schmid, 1989; Shaw & Kamen, 1986). Several aspects of the presence of these AREs in the 3′ ends of PTHrP mRNAs are noteworthy from an evolutionary perspective. First, this AU-rich, multiple AUUUA motif sequence is highly conserved in all PTHrP mRNAs from chicken to man (Karaplis et al., 1990; Mangin et al., 1988c; Mangin, Ikeda & Broadus, 1990; Suva et al., 1987; Schermer et al., 1991; Thiede & Rutledge, 1990). Second, the chicken, mouse and rat PTHrP genes have a somewhat simpler organization than the human gene, so that the unspliced 3′ end of human exon 4 or its equivalent seems to have evolved separately, and it is clear that human exon 5 has evolved quite recently. Nevertheless, all of these 3′ ends are AU-rich and bear multiple copies of the AU motif. Finally, comparison of the three human 3′ ends with each other as well as across species reveals no significant sequence similarity apart from the AREs. These findings would be anticipated only if rapid mRNA turnover is critical for proper regulation of PTHrP mRNA expression and PTHrP biological function.

PTHrP c'DNAs and/or the gene have been isolated from three additional species (Karaplis et al., 1990; Mangin et al., 1990; Schermer et al., 1991; Thiede et al., 1990). These structures are informative in several ways. First, the PTHrP coding region is highly conserved (98%) to amino acid residue 111, whereas distal to residue 112 there is significant divergence and only 25% sequence homology. However, if this C-terminal region is realigned with gaps, there is a 60% amino acid conservation, and the region remains serine- and threonine-rich (Karaplis et al., 1990). Overall, the PTHrP coding region is more highly conserved than is the case for the PTH coding region across species (Heinrich et al., 1984; Khosla et al., 1988; Mains, Bloomquist & Eipper, 1991). Secondly, the chicken, mouse and rat genes all have a simpler organization than the human gene. The mouse and rat genes seem to use predominantly the downstream TATA promoter element (Karaplis et al., 1990; Mangin et al., 1990); exon 1–like sequences are present upstream of the mouse gene but are represented in mouse

PTHrP mRNA in such low abundance that it has been impossible to map a putative upstream promoter (Mangin et al., 1990). With respect to available 3′ splice choices, the mouse and rat genes seem to use exclusively the equivalent of the human exon 4 to 6 splicing pattern (Figure 12.5) to generate a single major PTHrP mRNA species; these genes do not contain the equivalents of human exon 5 or the 3′ UTR of exon 4 (Karaplis et al., 1990; Mangin et al., 1990). In contrast, while the chicken gene appears to use predominantly the exon 4–6 splicing pattern, it also contains sequences equivalent to the 3′ UTR of human exon 4 (Schermer et al., 1991; Thiede et al., 1990). These findings have been taken as evidence that the avian and rodent genes probably evolved in parallel rather than in a linear sequence.

Distribution of PTHrP Expression

Unlike the PTH gene, whose expression is limited to parathyroid chief cells, the PTHrP gene is widely expressed. Tables 12.1 and 12.2 list the adult and foetal tissues in which PTHrP mRNA and/or protein have been documented. It is beyond the scope of this review to discuss each of these sites, but some generalizations can be made.

Firstly, PTHrP expression is widespread, having been documented in a diverse collection of foetal and adult and endocrine and nonendocrine tissues representing structures derived from each of the three embryonic germ layers. This pattern of widespread expression has suggested that PTHrP may normally play a predominantly local role as a paracrine and/or autocrine factor (Broadus & Stewart, 1994). This notion is supported by the fact that despite the widespread production of this secretory peptide, little or no PTHrP can be measured in the circulation in normal subjects (Burtis et al., 1990).

Secondly, PTHrP mRNA and peptide are present in low adundance and require sensitive techniques for their detection. Finally, although there are few studies carefully examining the developmental profile of PTHrP expression in specific tissues, the gene does appear to be developmentally regulated. For example, foetal parathyroid and liver cells express the PTHrP gene, while their adult counterparts do not (Burton et al., 1990; Ikeda et al., 1988; Moniz et al., 1990; Senior, Heath & Beck, 1991). In addition, changes in the pattern of PTHrP production during development have been documented in skin, kidney, dental lamina and bone (Broadus & Stewart, in press). These observations have led to the speculation that PTHrP may contribute to the control of cellular proliferation and/or differentiation during development. As will be discussed below, recent studies using transgenic technology have lent support to this notion.

Table 12.1. PTHrP Gene Expression in Adult Mammalian Tissues

Adrenal cortex
Adrenal medulla
Amnion
Bone
Brain
Endothelium
Epidermis and other epithelia
Heart
Kidney
Lung
Mammary gland
Ovary
Pancreatic islets
Parathyroid
Pituitary
Placenta
Prostate
Skeletal muscle
Small intestine
Smooth muscle
Vascular
Uterine
Bladder
Gastric
Spleen
Stomach mucosa
Testis
Thyroid
Thymus
Urothelium
Uterus (endometrium)

Regulation of PTHrP Gene Expression

There have been two recent studies that have attempted to define in some detail sequences important to the basal expression of the human PTHrP gene. Vasavada et al. found that approximately 500 bp of DNA flanking the midregion GC-rich promoter contained sequences critical for expression of the PTHrP gene in renal carcinoma cells (Vasavada et al., 1993). This region, as might be expected, is very GC rich and contains many SP1 consensus binding sequences. From these studies it is unclear whether this region is important for expression originating from all three promoter elements or simply for that originating from the GC-rich promoter. Campos et al. have re-

Table 12.2. PTHrP Gene Expression During Embryogenesis

I. Chicken
Day 3–10 embryo
Body and head
Allantois
Yolk sac
Chorioallantoic membrane
Day 15 embryo
Brain
Gizzard
Intestine
Liver
Lung
Skeletal muscle
Chorioallantoic membrane and yolk sac
II. Human and Rat
Nervous system
Brain
Spinal cord
Dorsal root ganglion
Developing eye
Epithelia
Epidermis and hair follicles
Pharynx and larynx
Bronchial epithelium
Stomach and intestine
Pancreatic acini
Liver
Salivary ducts
Endocrine glands
Parathyroid
Thyroid
Adrenal
Gonad
Muscle
Cardiac muscle
Striated muscle
Smooth muscle
Urogenital tract (human)
8–10 weeks: glomeruli, mesonephros and metanephros
20 weeks and beyond: proximal tubule, distal tubule, collecting duct and urothelium
Bone and teeth
Dental lamina
Immature chondrocytes
Mature chondrocytes
Osteoblast-like cells

Table 12.3. Regulation of PTHrP Gene Expression

Agent	Effect
Physiological stimuli	
Suckling	Up-regulates
Uterine occupancy	Up-regulates
Stretch	Up-regulates
Differentiation	Up-regulates
Pharmacological stimuli	
Glucocorticoids	Down-regulates
Vitamin D	Down-regulates
Oestrogen	Up-regulates or down-regulates
Serum	Up-regulates
EGF	Up-regulates
TGF-β	Up-regulates
Prolactin	Up-regulates
Calcitonin	Up-regulates
Cyclohexamide	Up-regulates
Forskolin	Up-regulates
Phorbal ester	Up-regulates
Endothelin I	Up-regulates
Angiotensin II	Up-regulates

ported similar findings regarding this region of the 5′ flank, although they did not recognize the presence of the midregion promoter element (Campos, Wang & Drucker, 1992). However, they did find that an additional 350-bp region just 5′ of the upstream TATA-containing promoter acted to up-regulate transcription of this promoter when cloned in isolation. This 350-bp region contains several consensus sequences for common transcription factors such as AP1, AP2 and SP1.

In the basal state, PTHrP mRNA has generally been found in low abundance as previously discussed. It appears that this results from a combination of negative regulatory elements found in the promoter region of the gene that may keep transcription in check, as well as the inherently unstable nature of the mRNAs. Both of the aforementioned studies found evidence for the existence of strong negative regulatory domains within the 5′ flank of the PTHrP gene. The addition of anywhere from 300 bp to 1 kb of 5′ sequences beyond the positive regulatory region flanking the midregion promoter significantly reduces the transcription of transiently transfected PTHrP-CAT hybrid genes (Vasavada et al., 1993). In a preliminary report, Vasavada et al. have found that this region of the gene can also down-regulate the transcription of the heterologous promoter, suggesting the presence of true silencer sequences within this portion of the gene (Vasavada et al., 1992). Again, Campos et al. have extended these findings to the upstream TATA-containing promoter, sequences 5′ to the initial 350-bp region discussed above have a strong inhibitory effect on transcription from this promoter cloned in isolation (Campos et al., 1992). Therefore, it seems quite likely that transcription of the PTHrP gene may be held under tonic negative tone governed through specific regions of the 5′ flanking DNA. This type of control may operate in trans, through the binding of specific proteins to these sequences, or it may operate through cis-modifications of the promoter region DNA such as methylation. Indeed, as will be discussed below, Holt et al. have found evidence for sequence-specific methylation of the PTHrP promoter upstream of the positive regulatory region flanking and midregion GC-rich promoter (Holt et al., 1993).

Another feature of PTHrP expression that contributes to the low constitutive level of PTHrP mRNA is its rapid turnover. The half-life of PTHrP mRNA has been found to range from 30 minutes to several hours, both in vivo and in vitro (Broadus & Stewart, 1994; Holt et al., 1994). In addition, modulation of PTHrP mRNA expression is often seen over a narrow range, with a rapid peak followed by a rapid decay of mRNA (Holt et al., 1994). This pattern of unstable mRNAs and rapid induction/deinduction kinetics is shared by many cytokine, lymphokine, and proto-oncogenes and, as in the case with mRNA encoding these molecules, PTHrP mRNAs contain ARE 'instability' sequences in their 3′ UTRs. Our group has recently found that the source of PTHrP mRNA instability resides, as expected, in these 3′ UTR instability sequences (W. Philbrick, unpublished data).

A great number of physiological and pharmacological stimuli have now been shown to modulate PTHrP expression and protein production (Broadus & Stewart, 1994). These factors are described in Table 12.3. We will not discuss this literature in any great detail and the reader is referred to recent reviews for a more complete discussion (Broadus & Stewart, 1994; Hendy & Goltzman, 1992). Apart from the effects of suckling and prolactin administration on PTHrP expression in lactating breast (Thiede & Rodan, 1988; Thiede, 1989), the best studied physiological stimuli are the efects of stretch on smooth muscle. Mechanical stretch has been shown to cause a prolonged induction of PTHrP mRNA in rat myometrium, rat bladder and the chicken oviduct during the egg-laying cycle (Daifotis et al., 1992; Thiede et al., 1991; Yamamoto et al., 1992). The pharmacological observations generally involve the effects of steroid hormones and growth factors on various cells in culture (Broadus & Stewart, 1994). It is clear from this literature that there exist two different characteristic patterns of PTHrP mRNA response. One, as generally seen in response to growth factors, has the rapid induction/deinduction kinetics discussed above and presumably involves a short burst of transcriptional activity followed by rapid decay of the mRNA. The other type, as seen in response to stretch of smooth muscle and in response to TGF-β in certain renal and squamous carcinoma lines, is defined by a slower rise in mRNA levels followed by a prolonged plateau (Kirayama et al., 1993; Zakalik et al., 1992). This pattern of response must involve both a more prolonged increase in transcription rate and also a stabilization of the mRNA through post-transcriptional events. It is interesting to ponder whether these different types of responses have a functional correlate, but the study of the mechanisms responsible for these responses and any biological implications that each may have remain largely unexplored.

PTHrP Expression in Tumours: The Molecular Pathogenesis of Humoral Hypercalcaemia of Malignancy

Unlike many classical hormones that are stored in secretory granules and are released in response to a stimulus, PTHrP appears to be secreted constitutively, with the secretory rate being a direct function of its production (Broadus & Stewart, 1994). Since this, in turn, is a reflection of its steady-state mRNA levels, it follows that any attempt to understand why certain tumours cause HHM and others do not quickly reduces to the study of PTHrP gene expression in HHM-related tumour cells.

The general problem of hormone production by tumours has become in most instances a question of gene regulation, and there are growing numbers of reports on the mechanisms involved. For instance, selective stabilization of the normally labile transcripts for basic fibroblast growth factor and granulocyte-macrophage colony-stimulating factor (GM-CSF) has recently been shown to cause their overexpression in astrocytoma and lymphoid tumour lines, respectively (Murphy, Guo & Friesen, 1990; Schuler & Cole, 1988). The ectopic expression of adrenocorticotrophic hormone (ACTH) by several tumours has been shown to involve a shift in pro-opiomelanocortin promoter usage to one mimicking the pattern normally restricted to the pituitary (Texier et al., 1991). This shift has been correlated with changes in the methylation status of specific regions of the pro-opiomelanocortin promoter (Lavender, 1991). Finally, the excessive activity of trans-acting factors and the lack of a specific trans-repressing factor have been shown to be responsible for the overexpression of the G-CSF and α-fetoprotein genes, respectively, in carcinoma cells (Nakabayashi et al., 1991; Nishizawa et al., 1990). As seen by these examples, there appears to be a great deal of heterogeneity in the mechanisms responsible for 'ectopic' hormone production, and it is likely that most of the normal regulatory mechanisms that control expression of a given peptide hormone gene may be targets for dysregulation in malignancy. The mechanisms underlying PTHrP gene expression by HHM-associated tumour cells are only beginning to be carefully examined, but there are three tumour systems that have begun to shed some light on this process. Given the comments above regarding the precedent for multiple molecular mechanisms for hormone production by tumours, it comes as no particular surprise that a different mechanism appears to apply in each of these three systems.

The first involves PTHrP production by HTLV-1–infected T cells in patients with the adult T cell leukaemia syndrome. This is a common neoplasm in Japan, and some 70% of affected patients develop HHM during their course. PTHrP appears to be responsible for all instances of HHM (Fukumoto et al., 1988; Motokuta et al., 1989; Watanabe et al., 1990), and there is evidence that the PTHrP gene is expressed by virtually 100% of HTLV-1–infected T cells (Watanabe et al., 1990). Here, it has been proposed on the basis of transfection studies that the PTHrP gene is being overexpressed because it is being activated or stimulated in trans by tax, a viral product that is a known transactivator of other cellular genes (Watanabe et al., 1990). This is an appealing mechanism, but the initial report did not include appropriate controls (Watanabe et al., 1990), and a subsequent preliminary report could not reproduce these findings (Prager et al., 1991). Nevertheless, given the specificity of HTLV-1 infection to the pathogenesis of this syndrome, it is likely that some viral protein is directly or indirectly responsible for stimulating PTHrP gene expression in infected T cells.

The second tumour system to be studied involves PTHrP gene expression in human renal carcinomas. Renal carcinoma is second only to squamous carcinoma as a cause of HHM, and about 25% of cultured renal carcinoma cells appear to be capable of producing PTHrP (Weir et al., 1988). Working with six examples each of PTHrP-producing (PTHrP+) and nonproducing (PTHrP−) renal carcinoma cell lines as defined by RNase protection analysis, Holt et al. found that the status of PTHrP gene expression in these cells correlated absolutely with the methylation status of four CpG dinucleotides in a 550-bp region located upstream of the midregion GC promoter (Figure 12.6) (Holt et al., 1993). The promoter itself is contained in a 900-bp CpG island, which is found to be unmethylated in all cells (Figure 12.6). This analysis was carried out using a series of methylation-sensitive and -insensitive isoschizomers that either fail to cleave or cleave DNA as a function of methylation of CpG residues in their recognition sequences. Holt et al. further demonstrated that demethylation of PTHrP− cells by 5-azacytidine converted them to a PTHrP+ phenotype, although the level of PTHrP mRNA expression achieved was less than that seen in the native PTHrP+ cells (Holt et al., 1993). Methylation is an important means of silencing gene expression, and the results in this system clearly indicate that this cis modification is the functional equivalent of an 'off-on' switch in terms of PTHrP gene expression. This phenotypic characterization is directly relevant to the clinical syndrome, in that these same cell lines have been previously shown to be capable (PTHrP+ cells) or incapable (PTHrP− cells) of inducing HHM in nude mice on the basis of their PTHrP phenotype (Weir et al., 1988). It is unclear how these data might bear on the 'eutopic-ectopic' question, and there are two possibilities. One is that the methylation status of the PTHrP gene in renal carcinoma cells might reflect the status of the gene in the untransformed cell of origin and that PTHrP+ cells are basically expressing the gene in a eutopic fashion. The other is that methylation of the gene might change as a function of transformation and that this is a dysregulated mechanism that is actually responsible for PTHrP gene expression.

The third system involves PTHrP gene expression in human squamous carcinoma cells, the most common cause of HHM. The data here are preliminary (Wysolmerski et al., 1992), but it is clear that the

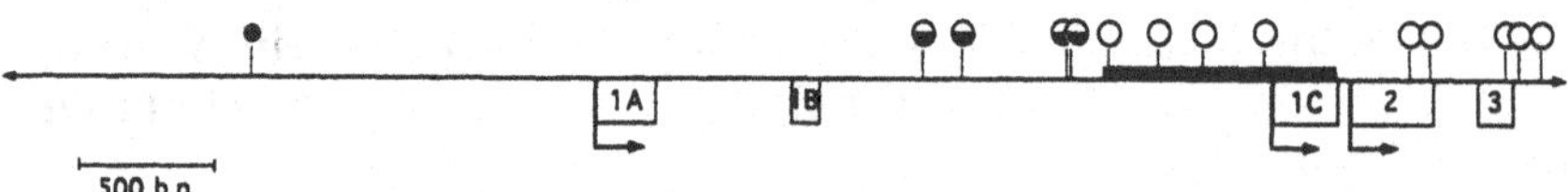

Figure 12.6 Methylation pattern of the PTHrP gene in human renal carcinoma cell lines. The exons and start sites are as designated in Figure 12.4. The half-filled circles correspond to CpG dinucleotides that were found to be unmethylated in renal carcinoma cells that express the PTHrP gene and methylated in cells that do not express the gene; these are located just upstream of a CpG island (bold horizontal bar). Other CpG dinucleotides were found to be methylated (solid circle) or unmethylated (open circles) in all cells examined and did not correlate with PTHrP expression. (From Holt et al., 1993. Used by permission).

findings in this system are very different from those in the renal carcinoma system just described. Whereas renal carcinoma cells seem to fall into two clear phenotypic subpopulations with respect to PTHrP gene expression, squamous carcinoma cells display a continuum of PTHrP mRNA expression covering an approximately 20-fold range, from barely detectable expression to abundant expression. As with the renal cell carcinoma lines, there is a good correlation between the level of PTHrP expression in an individual cell line and its ability to cause HHM (J. Wysolmerski, unpublished data). In addition, there appears to be a dosage effect as regards the production of HHM in athymic mice, reflecting the spectrum of expression seen in cultured squamous cancer cells. That is, there is a threshold level of expression necessary for the production of hypercalcaemia, and above this level of PTHrP expression hypercalcaemia is seen with smaller and smaller tumour burdens. Initial transfection studies indicate that the activity of PTHrP-CAT constructs correlates with endogenous gene activity, suggesting that dysregulation of PTHrP gene expression in squamous carcinoma cells resides in one or another trans-acting mechanism (Wysolmerski et al., 1992). The working hypothesis here is that the potential of a given malignant squamous cell for producing HHM may reside in the quantitative capacity of that cell to express the PTHrP gene, which in turn may be determined by the activity of specific trans-activating transcription factors interacting with the PTHrP promoter region.

Physiological Functions of PTHrP

Since the discovery of PTHrP and its widespread expression in normal tissues, there has been much work directed towards trying to understand its normal physiological function. There have been many functions suggested, but there is direct evidence to support a role in three areas. Firstly, it appears that PTHrP may contribute to the control of foetal and neonatal calcium metabolism, since PTHrP has been shown to stimulate transplacental calcium transport (Rodda, Caple & Martin, 1992). Secondly, in a variety of smooth muscle systems, PTHrP has been shown to be induced by mechanical stretch and to act as a relaxant (Daifotis et al., 1992; Thiede et al., 1991; Yamamoto et al., 1992). Therefore, the peptide may play a role in local control of smooth muscle tone. Finally, given the expression of PTHrP in many foetal sites (see Table 12.2), there has been much speculation that PTHrP may play an important role as an autocrine/paracrine factor during development (Broadus & Stewart, in press). We will not attempt to review this growing literature in a systematic fashion; rather, we will discuss several recent experiments that address the potential developmental role of PTHrP, the one that is most relevant to malignancy.

There have been a pair of reports suggesting that PTHrP may play a role early in mouse development, during embryogenesis. Both studies documented the induction of PTHrP with initiation of the differentiation of F-9 teratocarcinoma cells or embryonic stem cells (Chan et al., 1990; de Stolpe et al., 1993). In addition, PTHrP has been detected in developing trophoectoderm cells in the late morula stage of mouse embryos, and it has been suggested that the peptide may play a role in the control of parietal endoderm differentiation (de Stolpe et al., 1993). Any role that PTHrP has at this early stage must be as part of a redundant system, for as will be discussed below 'PTHrP-knockout mice' engineered through homologous recombination techniques survive until birth (Karaplis et al., 1992).

The first study to document a role for PTHrP during organogenesis was the targeted disruption of the PTHrP gene through homologous recombination. These mice display a form of chondrodysplasia and die at birth because of acute respiratory distress and/or the impingement of craniofacial abnormalities on the brain stem (Karaplis et al., 1992). The animals appear to lack other obvious abnormalities, although the window of observation is very limited because the mice do not survive. Grossly, the mice have a foreshortened and domed cranium, greatly foreshortened long bones, and a fixed chest wall. Histologically, two abnormalities are seen. The first is disruption of the normal architecture of the epiphyseal growth plate. This abnormality is manifest early, before the onset of ossification in endochondral bone, and consists of a decrease in the numbers of resting and proliferative chondrocytes; the numbers of prehypertrophic and hypertrophic chondrocytes appear to be normal (Karaplis et al., 1992). This finding accounts for the dwarfing. The second abnormality is abnormal endochondral/perichondral ossification in a number of locations, including the costal cartilages and the base of the skull. It is these two abnormalities that seem to account for the perinatal mortality (Karaplis et al., 1992).

These findings clearly implicate PTHrP in the developmental program that controls the orderly sequence of events associated with epiphyseal growth and cartilaginous mineralization. PTH has previously been shown to stimulate the proliferation of chondrocytes and to inhibit the mineralization of cartilage mediated by hypertrophic chondrocytes (Kato et al., 1990; Koike et al., 1990). Since cartilage is avascular and presumably removed from the influences of circulating

PTH, PTHrP produced locally is likely to mediate these effects in vivo. If one makes this assumption, then the removal of PTHrP, as in the knock-out experiment, might be expected to lead to a failure of chondrocyte proliferation and to premature calcification at the growth plate, which would explain the observed phenotype.

The second experiment supporting a role for PTHrP in organogenesis is the overexpression of PTHrP in transgenic mice, using the human keratin 14 (K14) promoter to target skin (Wysolmerski et al., 1994). These mice display an interesting cutaneous phenotype characterized by a delay or failure in the induction of embryonic hair follicles (Figure 12.7). In addition, the native K14 gene as well as the K14-PTHrP transgene are expressed in myoepithelial cells of the breast, and some of these transgenic mice display breast hypoplasia and an impairment or failure in their ability to nurse their pups. A preliminary examination of breast development in these mice reveals defects both in ductular proliferation during adolescence and pregnancy and in lobuloalveolar development during pregnancy and lactation (Wysolmerski et al., 1993). Therefore, local overexpression of PTHrP in skin and breast appears to result in the retardation or failure of the development of their characteristic structures.

Bone, breast and hair follicles are similar in the sense that their development is dependent on a rich exchange of information between neighbouring cells that regulates the orderly progression of pluripotent cells through a program of proliferation and differentiation. If one views the results of the above experiments in this context, one can make the case that the knock-out mice suffer from an acceleration of such a program in bone while the K14-PTHrP mice display a delay or failure of such programs in hair follicles and breast tissue. Hence it may be that PTHrP helps to regulate the pace with which these developmental programs proceed. Although this is admittedly speculative, and may prove to be overly simplistic, it appears that PTHrP most definitely contributes to the control of cellular proliferation and/or differentiation during organogenesis in bone breast and skin and perhaps also in the many other sites in which it is found in the foetus.

CONCLUSION

PTHrP has been shown to be the cause of humoral hypercalcaemia associated with malignancy. Recent observations have defined a much broader role for the PTHrP gene with the finding of its involvement in the normal development of bone, and the possibility of its implication in organogenesis. A greater understanding of the molecular

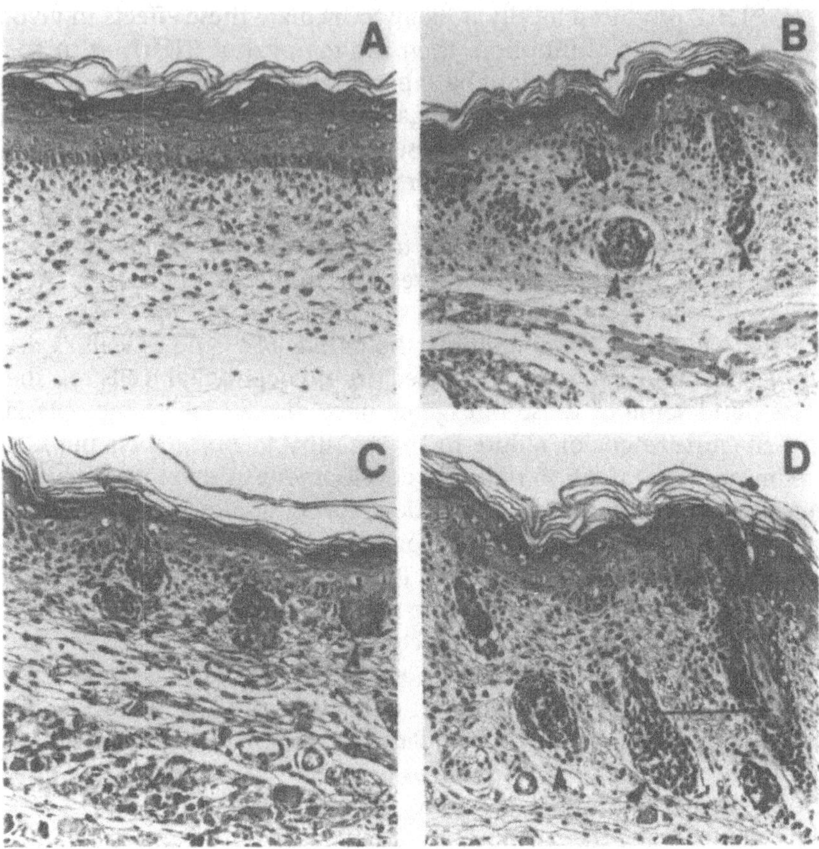

Figure 12.7 Histological sections taken from the ventral (A and B) or dorsal (C and D) surface of newborn K14-PTHrP transgenic mice (A and C) or normal littermates (B and D). The arrowheads highlight developing follicles; the arrow in D points to a growing hair shaft. Note the absence (A) or delay (C) in follicle development in transgenics as compared to controls (B and D). (From Wysolmerski et al., in press. Used by permission.)

mechanisms controlling the expression of the PTHrP gene may allow us to develop new methods of controlling humoral hypercalcaemia of malignancy.

REFERENCES

Adams J.S., Fernandez M., Gacad M.A., Gill P.S., Endres D.B., Rasheed S. & Singer F.R. (1989) Vitamin D metabolite-mediated hypercalcaemia and hypercalciuria in patients with AIDS- and non-AIDS-associated lymphoma. *Blood,* **73**, 235.

Brandt D.W., Bruns M.E., Bruns D.W., Ferguson J.E., Burton D.W. & Deftos L.J. (1992) The parathyroid hormone-related protein (PTHrP) gene preferentially utilizes a GC-rich promoter and the PTHrP 1-139 coding pathway in normal human amnion. *Biochemical and Biophysical Research Communications,* **189**, 938–43.

Breslau N.A., McGuire J.L., Zerwekh J.E., Frenkel E.P. & Pak C.Y. (1900) Hypercalcemia associated with increased serum calcitriol levels in three patients with lymphoma. *Annals of Internal Medicine,* **100**, 1.

Broadus A.E. & Stewart A.F. (1994) PTHrP structure, processing and physiologic actions. In J.P. Bilezikian, M. Levine & R. Marcus (Eds.) *The Parathyroids.* New York, Raven Press.

Budayr A.A., Nissenson R.A., Klein R.F., Pun K.K., Clark G.H., Diep D., Arnaud C.D. & Strewler G.J. (1989) Increased serum levels of a parathyroid hormone-like protein in malignancy-associated hypercalcemia. *Annals of Internal Medicine,* **111**, 807.

Burtis W.J., Wu T., Bunch C., Wysolmerski J.J., Insogna K.L., Weir E.C., Broadus A.E. & Stewart A.F. (1987) Identification of a novel 17,000-dalton parathyroid hormone-like adenylate cyclase-stimulating protein from a tumor associated with humoral hypercalcemia of malignancy. *Journal of Biological Chemistry,* **262**, 7151–6.

Burtis W.J., Brady T.G., Orloff J.J., Ersbak J.W., Warrell R.P., Jr., Olson B.R., Wu T., Mitnick M.E., Broadus A.E. & Stewart A.F. (1990) Immunochemical characterization of circulating parathyroid hormone-related protein in patients with humoral hypercalcemia of cancer. *New England Journal of Medicine,* **322**, 1106–1112.

Burton P.B.J., Moniz C., Quirke P. et al. (1990) Parathyroid hormone-related peptide in the human urogenital tract. *Molecular and Cellular Endocrinology,* **69**, R13–17.

Campos R.V., Wang C. & Druckers D.J. (1992) Regulation of parathyroid hormone-related peptide (PTHrP) gene transcription: cell- or tissue-specific promoter utilization mediated by multiple positive and negative cis-acting DNA elements. *Molecular Endocrinology,* **6**, 1642–52.

Case Records of the Massachusetts General Hospital (Case 17461). (1941) *New England Journal of Medicine,* **225**, 789–91.

Chan S.D.H., Strewler G.S., King K.L. & Nissenson R.A. (1990) Expression of a parathyroid hormone-like protein and its receptor during differentiation of embryonal carcinoma cells. *Molecular Endocrinology,* **4**, 638–6.

Connor T.B., Thomas W.C. & Howard J.E. (1956) The etiology of hypercalcemia associated with lung carcinoma. *Journal of Clinical Investigation,* **35**, 597.

Cretien S., Duhart A., Beaupain D., Raich N., Grandchamp B., Rosa J., Goussens M. & Romeo P. (1988) Alternative transcription and splicing of the human porphobilinogen deaminase gene results either in tissue-specific or in housekeeping expression. *Proceedings of the National Academy of Sciences of the United States of America,* **85**, 6.

Daifotis A.G., Weir E.C., Dreyer B.E. & Broadus A.E. (1992) Stretch-induced parathyroid hormone-related peptide gene expression in the rat uterus. *Journal of Biological Chemistry,* **267**, 23455–8.

de Stolpe A., Karperian M., Lowik C.W.G.M., Juppner H., Segre G.V., Abou-Samra A.B., deLaat S.W. & Delize L.H.K. (1993) Parathyroid hormone-related peptide as an endogenous inducer of parietal endoderm differentiation. *Journal of Cell Biology,* **120**, 235–43.

Dewhirst F.E., Stashenko P.P., Mole J.E. & Tsurumachi T. (1985) Purification and partial sequence of human osteoclast activating factor: identity with interleukin 1B. *Journal of Immunology,* **135**, 2562.

Ebeling P.R., Adam W.R., Moseley J.M. & Martin T.J. (1990) Actions of synthetic PTHRP(1-34) on the isolated rat kidney. *Journal of Endocrinology,* **120**, 45.

Eilon G. & Mundy G.R. (1978) Direct resorption of bone by human breast cancer cells *in vitro. Nature,* **276**, 726–8.

Fukumoto S., Matsumoto T., Ikeda K., Yamashita T., Watanabe T., Yamaguchi K., Kiyokawa T., Tatatsuki K., Shibuya N. & Ogata E. (1988) Clinical evaluation of calcium metabolism in adult T-cell leukemia/lymphoma. *Archives of Internal Medicine,* **148**, 921–5.

Garrett I.R., Burie B.G.M., Nedwin G.E., Gillespie A., Bringman T., Sabatini M., Bertolini D.R. & Mundy G.R. (1987) Production of lymphotoxin, a bone-resorbing cytokine, by cultured human myeloma cells. *New England Journal of Medicine,* **317**, 526.

Gutman A.B., Tyson T.L. & Gutman E.B. (1936) Serum calcium, inorganic phosphorus and phosphatase activity in hyperparathyroidism, Paget's disease, multiple myeloma and neoplastic disease of the bones. *Archives of Internal Medicine,* **57**, 379–413.

Hargrove J.L. & Schmidt F.H. (1989) The role of mRNA and protein stability in gene expression. *FASEB Journal,* **3**, 2360–70.

Heinrich G., Kronenberg H.M., Potts J.T., Jr. & Habener J.F. (1984) Gene encoding parathyroid hormone. Nucleotide sequence of the rat gene and deduced amino acid sequence of rate preproparathyroid horone. *Journal of Biological Chemistry,* **259**, 3320–9.

Hendy G.N. & Goltzman D. (1992) Molecular biology of parathyroid hormone-like peptide. In *Parathyroid hormone-related protein—normal physiology and its role in cancer,* pp. 25–55. Boca Raton, CRC Press.

Holt E.H., Lu C., Dreyer B.E., Dannies P.S. & Broadus A.E. (1994) Regulation of parathyroid hormone-related peptide gene expression by estrogen in GH_4C_1 rat pituitary cells has the pattern of a primary response gene. *Journal of Neurochemistry,* **62**, 1239–46.

Holt E.H., Vasavada R., Broadus A.E. & Philbrick W.M. (1993) Region-specific methylation of the PTH-related peptide gene determines its expression in human renal carcinoma cell lines. *Journal of Biological Chemistry,* **268**, 20639–45.

Ikeda K., Mangin M., Dreyer B.E., Webb A.C., Posillico J.T., Stewart A.F., Bander N.H., Weir E.C., Isogna K.L. & Broadus A.E. (1988a) Identification of transcripts encoding a parathyroid hormone-like peptide in messenger RNAs from a variety of human and animal tumors associated with humoral hypercalcemia of malignancy. *Journal of Clinical Investigations,* **81**, 2010–14.

Ikeda K., Weir E.C., Mangin M., Dannies P.S., Kinder B., Deftos L.F., Brown E.M. & Broadus A.E. (1988b) Expression of messenger ribonucleic acids encoding a parathyroid hormone-like peptide in normal human and animal tissues with abnormal expression in human parathyroid ademomas. *Molecular Endocrinology,* **2**, 1230–6.

Ikeda K., Arnold A., Mangin M., Kinder B., Vydelingum N.A., Brennan M.F. & Broadus A.E. (1989) Expression of transcripts encoding a parathyroid hormone-related peptide in abnormal human parathyroid tissues. *Journal of Clinical Endocrinology and Metabolism,* **69**, 1240–8.

Isales C., Carcangiu M.L. & Stewart A.F. (1987) Hypercalcemia in breast cancer: reassessment of the mechanism. *American Journal of Medicine*, **82**, 1143.

Karaplis A.C., Yasuda T., Hendy G.N., Goltzman D. & Banville D. (1990) Gene encoding parathyroid hormone-like peptide: nucleotide sequences of the rat gene and comparison with the human homologue. *Molecular Endocrinology*, **4**, 441–6.

Karaplis A., Tybulewicz V., Mulligan R.C. & Kronenberg H.M. (1992) Disruption of parathyroid hormone-related peptide gene leads to multitude of skeletal abnormalities and perinatal mortality. *Journal of Bone and Mineral Research*, **7**, S93.

Kato Y., Shimazu A., Nakashima K., Suzuki F., Jikko A. & Iwamoto M. (1990) Effects of parathyroid hormone and calcitonin on alkaline phosphatase activity and matrix calcification in rabbit growth plate chondrocyte cultures. *Endocrinology*, **127**, 114–18.

Kawano M., Yamamoto I., Iwato K., Tanaka H., Asaoku H., Tanabe O., Ishikawa H., Nobuyoshi M., Ohmoto Y., Hirai Y. & Kuramoto A. (1989) Interleukin-1β rather than lymphotoxin as the major bone resorbing activity in human multiple myeloma. *Blood*, **73**, 1646–9.

Kemp B.E., Moseley J.M., Rodda C.P., Ebeling P.R., Wettenhall R.E.H., Stapelton D., Diefenbach-Jagger H., Ure F., Michelangeli V.P., Simmons H.A., Raisz L.G. & Martin T.J. (1987) Parathyroid hormone-related protein of malignancy: active synthetic fragments. *Science*, **238**, 1568–70.

Khosla S., Demay M., Pines M., Hurwitz S., Potts J.T. & Kronenberg H.M. (1988) Nucleotide sequence of cloned cDNAs encoding chicken preparathyroid hormone. *Journal of Bone and Mineral Research*, **3**, 689–98.

Kirayama T., Gillespie M.T., Glutz J.A., Fukumoto S., Moseley J.M. & Martin T.J. (1993) Transforming growth factor beta stimulation of parathyroid hormone-related peptide: a paracrine regulator? *Molecular and Cellular Endocrinology*, **92**, 55–62.

Kitazawa R., Imai Y., Fukase M. & Fujita T. (1991) Effect of continuous infusion of PTH and PTHRP on rat bone *in vivo*. *Bone and Mineral*, **12**, 157.

Koike T., Iwamoto M., Shimazu A., Nakashima K., Suzuki F. & Kato Y. (1990) Potent mitogenic effects of parathyroid hormone (PTH) on embryonic chick and rabbit chondrocytes. *Journal of Clinical Investigation*, **95**, 626–31.

Kremer R., Karaplis A.C., Henderson J., Gulliver W., Banville D., Hendy G.N. & Goltzman D. (1991) Regulation of parathyroid hormone-like peptide in cultured normal human keratinocytes. *Journal of Clinical Investigation*, **87**, 884–93.

Kukreja S.C. et al. (1988) Antibodies to parathyroid hormone-related protein lower serum calcium in athymic mouse models of malignancy-associated hypercalcemia due to human tumors. *Journal of Clinical Investigation*, **82**, 1798.

Kukreja S.C., Rosol R.J., Wimbiscus S.A., Shevrin D.H., Grill V., Barengolts E. & Martin T.J. (1990) Tumor resection and antibodies to parathyroid hormone-related protein cause similar changes on bone histomorphology in hypercalcemia of cancer. *Endocrinology*, **127**, 305.

Lafferty F.W. (1966) Pseudohyperparathyroidism. *Medicine* (Baltimore), **45**, 247.

Lavender P., Clark A., Besser G. & Rees L. (1991) Variable methylation of the 5′-flanking DNA of the human pro-opiomelanocortin gene. *Journal of Molecular Endocrinology*, **6**, 53–61.

Mains R.E., Bloomquist B.T. & Eipper B.A. (1991) Manipulation of neuropeptide biosynthesis through the expression of antisense RNA to PAM. *Molecular Endocrinology*, **5**, 187–93.

Mangin M., Webb A.C., Dreyer B.E., Posillico J.T., Ikeda K., Weir E.C., Stewart A.F., Bander N.H., Milstone L., Barton D.E., Francke U. & Broadus A.E. (1988b) An identification of a cDNA encoding a parathyroid hormone-like peptide from a human tumor associated with humoral hypercalcemia of malignancy. *Proceedings of the National Academy of Sciences of the United States of America,* **85**, 597–601.

Mangin M., Ikeda K., Dreyer B.E., Milstone L. & Broadus A.E. (1988a) Two distinct tumor-derived parathyroid hormone-like peptides result from alternative ribonucleic acid splicing. *Molecular Endocrinology,* **2**, 1049–55.

Mangin M., Ikeda K., Dreyer B.E. & Broadus A.E. (1989) Isolation and characterization of the human parathyroid hormone-like peptide gene. *Proceedings of the National Academy of Sciences of the United States of America,* **86**, 2408–12.

Mangin M., Ikeda K. & Broadus A.E. (1990a) Structure of the mouse gene encoding the parathyroid hormone-related peptide. *Gene,* **95**, 195–202.

Mangin M., Ikeda K., Dreyer B.E. & Broadus A.E. (1990b) Identification of an upstream promoter of the human parathyroid hormone-related peptide gene. *Molecular Endocrinology,* **4**, 851.

Moniz C., Burton P.B.J., Malik A.N., Dixit M., Banga J.P., Nicolaides K., Quirke P., Knight P.E. & McGregor A.M. (1990) Parathyroid hormone-related peptide in normal human fetal development. *Journal of Molecular Endocrinology,* **5**, 259–66.

Moseley J.M., Kubota M., Diefenbach-Jagger H., Wettenhall E.H., Kemp B.E., Suva L.J., Rodda C.P., Ebeling P.R., Hudson P.J. & Martin T.J. (1987) Parathyroid hormone-related protein purified from a human lung cancer cell lines. *Proceedings of the National Academy of Sciences of the United States of America,* **84**, 5048–52.

Motokuta T., Fukumoto S., Matsumoto T., Takahashi S., Fujita A., Yamashita T., Igarashi T. & Ogata E. (1989) Parathyroid hormone-related protein in adult T-cell leukemia-lymphoma. *Annals of Internal Medicine,* **111**, 000.

Mundy G.R., Raisz L.G., Cooper R.A., Schechter G.P. & Salmon S.E. (1974) Evidence for the secretion of an osteoclast stimulating factor in myeloma. *New England Journal of Medicine,* **291**, 1041.

Mundy G.R. (1989) Hypercalcemic factors other than parathyroid hormone-related protein. *Endocrinology and Metabolism Clinics of North America,* **18**, 795–805.

Murphy P.R., Guo J.Z. & Friesen H.G. (1990) Messenger RNA stabilization accounts for elevated basic fibroblast growth factor transcript levels in a human astrocytoma cell line. *Molecular Endocrinology,* **4**, 196–200.

Nakabayashi H., Hashimoto T., Kiyao Y., Tjong K., Chan J. & Tamaoki T. (1991) A position-dependent silencer plays a major role in repressing α feto-protein expression in human hepatoma. *Molecular and Cellular Biology,* **11**, 5885–93.

Nishizawa M., Tsuchiya M., Watanabe-Fukunaga R. & Nagata S. (1990) Multiple elements in the promoter of granulocyte colony-stimulating factor gene regulate its constitutive expression in human carcinoma cells. *Journal of Biological Chemistry,* **265**, 5897–902.

Nissenson R.A. & Strewler G.I. (1992) Molecular mechanism of action of PTHrP. In B.P. Halloran & R.A. Nissenson (Eds.) *Parathyroid hormone-related protein: normal physiology and its role in cancer,* pp. 145-00.

Nussbaum S., Gaz R. & Arnold A. (1990) Hypercalcemia and ectopic secretion of parathyroid hormone by an ovarian carcinoma with rearrangement of the gene for parathyroid hormone. *New England Journal of Medicine*, **323**, 1324–8.

Orloff J.J. & Stewart A.F. (1989) Parathyroid hormone-like proteins: biochemical responses and receptor interactions. *Endocrine Reviews*, **10**, 476–95.

Plimpton D.H. & Gelhorn A. (1956) Hypercalcemia in malignant disease without evidence of bone destruction. *American Journal of Medicine*, **21**, 750.

Prager D., Massari M., Gebremedhin S., Yamasaki H., Hendy G.N. & Clemens T.L. (1991) Transcriptional hormone-related protein gene in T lymphocytes. *Journal of Bone and Mineral Research*, **6**, S225.

Rizzoli R., Caversazio J., Chapuy M.C., Martin T.J. & Bonjour J.P. (1989) Role of bone and kidney in PTHRP-induced hypercalcemia in rats. *Journal of Bone and Mineral Research*, **4**, 759.

Rodda C.P., Caple I.W. & Martin T.J. (1992) Role of PTHrP in fetal and neonatal physiology. In *Parathyroid hormone-related protein: normal physiology and its role in cancer*, pp. 169–96. Boca Raton, CRC Press.

Rosenthal N., Insogna K.L., Godsall J.W., Smaldone L., Waldron J.A. & Stewart A.F. (1985) Elevations in circulating 1,25-dihydroxyvitamin D in three patients with lymphoma-associated hypercalcemia. *Journal of Clinical Endocrinology and Metabolism*, **60**, 29.

Rosol T.J., Capen C.C. & Horst R.L. (1988) Effect of infusion of human parathyroid hormone-related protein (1-40) in nude mice: histomorphometric and biochemical evaluation. *Journal of Bone and Mineral Research*, **3**, 699.

Scheinman S.J., Mitnick M.A. & Stewart A.F. (1990) Direct effects of synthetic parathyroid hormone-like peptides on renal calcium transport. *Journal of Bone and Mineral Research*, **5**, 653.

Schermer P.T., Chan S.D.H., Bruce R., Nissenson R.A., Wood W.I. & Strewler G.J. (1991) Chicken parathyroid hormone-related protein and its expression during embryologic development. *Journal of Bone and Mineral Research*, **6**, 149–55.

Schulter G.D. & Cole M.D. (1988) GM-CSF and oncogene mRNA stabilities are independently regulated in trans in a mouse monocytic tumor. *Cell*, **55**, 1115–22.

Senior P.V., Heath D.A. & Beck F. (1991) Expression of parathyroid hormone-related protein mRNA in the rat before birth: demonstration by hybridization histochemistry. *Journal of Molecular Endocrinology*, **6**, 281–90.

Shaw G. & Kamen R. (1986) A conserved AU sequence from the 3′ untranslated region of GM-CSF mRNA mediates selective mRNA degradation. *Cell*, **46**, 659–67.

Stewart A.F., Horst R., Deftos L.J., Cadman E.C., Lang R. & Broadus A.E. (1980) Biochemical evaluation of patients with cancer-associated hypercalcemia: evidence for humoral and nonhumoral groups. *New England Journal of Medicine*, **303**, 1377–83.

Stewart A.F., Vignery A., Silvergate A., Ravin N.D., LiVolsi V., Broadus A.E. & Baron R. (1981) Quantitative bone histomorphometry in humoral hypercalcemia of malignancy: uncoupling of bone cell activity. *Journal of Clinical Endocrinology and Metabolism*, **55**, 219–27.

Stewart A.F., Insogna K.L., Goltzman D. & Broadus A.E. (1983) Identification of adenylate cyclase-stimulating activity and cytochemical glucose-6-phosphate dehydrogenase-stimulating activity in extracts of tumors from patients with humoral hypercalcemia of malignancy. *Proceedings of the National Academy of Sciences of the United States of America*, **80**, 1454.

Stewart A.F., Mangin M., Wu T., Goumas D., Insogna K.L., Burtis W.J. & Broadus A.E. (1988) Synthetic human parathyroid hormone-like protein stimulates bone resorption and causes hypercalcemia in rats. *Journal of Clinical Investigation*, **81**, 596–600.

Strewler G.J., Williams R.D. & Nissenson R.A. (1983) Human renal carcinoma cells produce hypercalcemia in the nude mouse and a novel protein recognized by parathyroid hormone receptors. *Journal of Clinical Investigation*, **71**, 769.

Strewler G.J., Budayr A.A., Bruce R.J., Clark O.H. & Nissenson R.A. (1987a) Secretion of authentic parathyroid hormone by a malignant tumor. *Clinical Research*, **38**, 461A.

Strewler G.J., Stern P.J., Jacobs J.W., Evelott J., Klein R.F., Leung S.C., Rosenblatt M. & Nissenson R.A. (1987b) Parathyroid hormone-like protein from human renal carcinoma cells. Structural and functional homology with parathyroid hormone. *Journal of Clinical Investigation*, **80**, 1803–7.

Strewler G.J. & Nissenson R.A. (1980) Hypercalcemia in malignancy. *Western Journal of Medicine*, **153**, 635–40.

Suva L.J., Winslow G.A., Wettenhall E.H., Hammonds R.G., Moseley J.M., Diefenbach-Jagger H., Rodda C.P., Kemp B.E., Rodriguez H. & Chen E.Y. (1987) A parathyroid hormone-related protein implicated in malignant hypercalcemia: cloning and expression. *Science*, **237**, 893–6.

Suva L.J., Mather K.A., Gillespie M.T., Webb G.C., Ng K.W., Winslow G.A., Wood W.I., Martin T.J. & Hudson P.J. (1989) Structure of the 5′ flanking region of the gene encoding human parathyroid hormone-related protein (PTHrP). *Gene*, **77**, 5–105.

Suva L.J., Gillespie M.T., Center R.J., Gardner R.M., Rodan G.A., Martin T.J. & Thiede M.A. (1991) A sequence in the human PTHrP gene promoter responsiveness to estrogen. *Journal of Bone and Mineral Research*, **6**, S196.

Texier P., DeKeyzer R., Laeave A., Vieau F., Leuve F., Rojas-Miranda A., Verley J., Luton J., Kahn A. & Bertagna X. (1991) Proopiomelanocortin gene expression in normal and tumoral human lung. *Journal of Clinical Endocrinology and Metabolism*, **73**, 414–20.

Thiede M.A. & Rodan G.A. (1988) Expression of a calcium-mobilizing parathyroid hormone-like peptide in lactating mammary tissue. *Science*, **242**, 278–80.

Thiede M.A., Strewler G.J., Nissenson R.A., Rosenblatt M. & Rodan G.A. (1989b) Human gene carcinoma expresses two messages encoding a parathyroid hormone-like peptide: evidence for the alternative splicing of a single-copy gene. *Proceedings of the National Academy of Sciences of the United States of America*, **85**, 4605–9.

Thiede M.A. (1989) The mRNA encoding a parathyroid hormone-like peptide is produced in mammary tissue in response to elevations in serum prolactin. *Molecular Endocrinology*, **3**, 14434–47.

Thiede M.A. & Rutledge S.U. (1990) Nucleotide sequence of a parathyroid hormone-related peptide expressed by the 10 day chicken embryo. *Nucleic Acids Research*, **18**, 3062.

Thiede W.A., Harm S.C., McKee R.L., Grasser W.H., Duong M.T. & Leach R.M. (1991) Expression of the parathyroid hormone-related protein gene in the avian oviduct: potential role as a local modulator of vascular smooth muscle tension and shell gland motility during the egg-laying cycle. *Endocrinology*, **129**, 1958–66.

Vargas S.J., Gillespie M.T., Powell G.J., et al. (1992) Localization of parathyroid hormone-related protein mRNA expression in breast cancer and metastatic lesions by *in situ* hybridization. *Journal of Bone and Mineral Research,* **7**, 971–9.

Vasavada R., Wysolmerski J.J., Philbrick W.M. & Broadus A.E. (1992) A negative regulatory element in the PTHrP gene promoter. *Journal of Bone and Mineral Research,* **7**, S118.

Vasavada R., Wysolmerski J.J., Broadus A.E. & Philbrick W.M. (1993) Identification and characterization of a GC-rich promoter of the human parathyroid hormone-related peptide gene. *Molecular Endocrinology,* **7**, 273–82.

Watanabe T., Yamaguchi K., Takatsuki K., Osama M. & Yoshika M. (1990) Constitutive expression of parathyroid hormone-related protein gene in human T cell leukemia virus type 1 (HTLV-1) carriers and adult T cell leukemia patients that can be trans-activated by HTLV-1 tax gene. *Journal of Experimental Medicine,* **172**, 795–65.

Weir E.C., Insogna K.L., Brownstein D.G., Bander N.H. & Broadus A.E. (1988) *In vitro* adenylate cyclase-stimulating activity predicts the occurrence of humoral hypercalcemia of malignancy in nude mice. *Journal of Clinical Investigation,* **81**, 818–21.

Wysolmerski J.J., Vasavada R., Burtis W.J., Broadus A.E. & Philbrick W.M. (1992) PTHrP gene expression in human squamous carcinoma cells. *Journal of Bone and Mineral Research,* **7**, S231.

Wysolmerski J.J., Broadus A.E., Zhou J., Fuchs E., Milstone L.M. & Philbrick W.M. (1994) Overexpression of parathyroid hormone-related protein in the skin of transgenic mice interferes with hair follicle development. *Proceedings of the National Academy of Sciences of the United States of America,* **91**, 1133–7.

Wysolmerski J.J., Daifotis A., Broadus A., Milstone L. & Philbrick W. (1993) Overexpression of PTHrP in transgenic mice results in breast hypoplasia. *Journal of Bone and Mineral Research* (Suppl. 1), S149.

Yamamoto I., Kawano M., Sone T., Iwato K., Tanaka H., Ishikawa H., Kitamura N., Lee K., Shigeno C. & Konishi J. (1989) Production of interleukin 1β, a potent bone resorbing cytokine, by cultured human myeloma cells. *Cancer Research,* **49**, 4242–6.

Yamamoto M., Harm S.C., Grasser W.A. & Thiede M.A. (1992) Parathyroid hormone-related protein in rat urinary bladder: a smooth muscle relaxant produced locally in response to mechanical stretch. *Proceedings of the National Academy of Sciences of the United States of America,* **89**, 5326–30.

Yashuda T., Banville D., Hendy G.N. & Goltzman D. (1989) Characterization of the human parathyroid hormone-like peptide gene. *Journal of Biological Chemistry,* **264**, 7720–5.

Yoshimoto K., Yamasaki T., Sakai H., Tezuka U., Takahashi M., Iizuka M., Seikiya T. & Saito S. (1989) Ectopic production of parathyroid hormone by small cell lung cancer in a patient with hypercalcemia. *Journal of Clinical Endocrinology and Metabolism,* **68**, 976–81.

Zakalik D., Diep D., Hooks M.A., Nissenson R.A. & Strewler G.J. (1900) Transforming growth factor beta increases stability of parathyroid hormone-related protein messenger RNA. *Journal of Bone and Mineral Research,* **7**, S118.

Zondek H., Petow H. & Siebert W. (1924) Die bedeutund der calciumbestimmung im blute für niereninsuffizientz. *Zeitschrift fur Medizine,* **99**, 129.

13

Anaemia of Cancer

CAROLE B. MILLER AND JERRY L. SPIVAK

INTRODUCTION

Erythropoiesis is the continuous process through which committed erythroid progenitor cells differentiate into mature circulating erythrocytes responsible for oxygen transport from the lungs to the tissues. Normally, the circulating red cell mass is maintained at a constant level in each of us, although that level may vary amongst individuals of the same age and gender by more than 10%. Under ambient oxygen tension, two factors determine the circulating red cell mass; the lifespan of the erythrocyte and the rate of effective erythrocyte production. Red cell lifespan in humans is finite and averages 120 days. Therefore, to maintain a constant red cell mass, approximately 0.8% (or 20 ml) of the circulating red cells must be replaced each day to compensate for the erythrocytes lost through senescence. The continuous production of erythrocytes is dependent on an adequate supply of nutrients of which iron, folic acid and vitamin B_{12} are particularly important, owing to the central role of haemoglobin and DNA synthesis in red cell production.

In the presence of an adequate supply of nutrients, the rate of erythropoiesis is regulated by the glycoprotein hormone erythropoietin. Erythropoietin is unique amongst the haematopoietic growth factors, since it is the only factor that behaves like a hormone. Erythropoietin is produced in the kidneys and the liver (Koury, Bondurant & Koury, 1988; Lacombe et al., 1988; Koury et al., 1991) and interacts with primitive erythroid progenitor cells in the bone marrow to promote their proliferation and maintain their survival (Koury & Bondurant, 1990; Spivak et al., 1991). Erythropoietin is not the only growth factor that influences the growth of erythroid progenitor cells, although it is clearly the most important (Spivak, 1992).

ERYTHROPOIETIN AND HAEMATOPOIETIC DIFFERENTIATION

Within the bone marrow, haematopoietic progenitor cells are organized in a hierarchy according to their capacity for self-renewal and lineage-specific commitment (Ogawa, Porter & Nakahata, 1983). Pluripotent haematopoietic stem cells, the most primitive of all haematopoietic progenitor cells, are capable of both self-renewal and differentiation into multipotent progenitor cells. The latter can differentiate into myeloid, erythroid or megakaryocytic progenitor cells but have only a limited capacity for self-renewal. At each stage in the differentiation cascade, haematopoietic progenitor cells become more restricted with respect to their ability to differentiate along lineage-specific pathways and at the same time lose the capacity for self-renewal. In keeping with these changes, the proportion of the particular haematopoietic progenitor cell population, which is in active cell cycle, increases. Thus, for example, only a minority of pluripotent haematopoietic progenitor cells are in cell cycle, whilst the majority of committed erythroid progenitor cells are actively cycling (Becker et al., 1965; Iscove, 1977).

At each level within the haematopoietic progenitor cell hierarchy, specific haematopoietic growth factors are required to maintain the viability of these progenitor cells and permit their differentiation. Like their target cell populations, the haematopoietic growth factors can also be organized into a hierarchy according to whether they are multipotent or restricted with respect to their cellular interactions (Walker et al., 1985). Thus, receptors for interleukin-3 (IL-3) and granulocyte-macrophage colony-stimulating factor (GM-CSF) are expressed not only by pluripotent stem cells but also by committed haematopoietic progenitor cells, while receptors for erythropoietin and CSF-1 are expressed primarily by committed haematopoietic progenitor cells (Nicola, 1989).

Haematopoietic growth factors appear to largely play a permissive role in the proliferation and survival of haematopoietic progenitor cells (Suda, Suda & Ogawa, 1983). Thus, individual growth factors do not initiate dormant target cells into cycle but rather maintain the viability of these cells until they enter cell cycle, which appears to occur on a random basis. In various combinations, which may be the more physiologic situation, these growth factors can shorten the period of dormancy of haematopoietic progenitor cells and also enhance their capacity for proliferation (Leary et al., 1992). They do not, however, alter the capacity for lineage-specific differentiation. That is to say, an overabundance of one growth factor with a resulting disproportionate increase in expansion of one type of progenitor cell does not diminish the capacity for or rate of production of other types of progenitor cells. Stated in other terms, the lineage-specific commitment of haematopoietic progenitor cells is apparently a random event not influenced by haematopoietic growth factors (Nakahata, Gross & Ogawa, 1982).

With respect to the erythroid system, the earliest erythroid progenitor cell as identified by in vitro clonal assays is the erythroid burst-forming unit (BFU-E) (Axelrad et al., 1900). This primitive progenitor cell is initially erythropoietin independent and responds to IL-3 and GM-CSF (Iscove, 1978; Metcalf, Johnson & Burgess, 1980). It also appears to require insulin-like growth factor I (IGF-I) (Merchau, Tatarsky & Hochberg, 1988). BFU-E are largely not in active cell cycle but have a high proliferative capacity, giving rise in vitro to colonies containing thousands of erythroid cells. As they mature, BFU-E lose proliferative capacity and become more responsive to erythropoietin as indicated by an increase in their expression of erythropoietin receptors (Sawada et al., 1990). The maturing BFU-E appears to represent an important transition point in erythroid differentiation, since it is at this stage that erythroid progenitor cells are susceptible to infection by certain viruses (Kost et al., 1979), that endotoxin interrupts erythropoiesis (Udupa & Reissman, 1977) and that clonal suppression occurs in polycythemia vera (Adamson et al., 1980).

The next stage in erythropoiesis is represented in clonal cultures by the erythroid colony forming unit (CFU-E), a cell with limited proliferative capacity that is largely in cycle, requires erythropoietin for its survival and which terminally differentiates into the recognizable nucleated erythroid precursors seen in stained preparations of bone marrow aspirates (Stephenson & Axelrad, 1971). The CFU-E also represents an important transition phase during erythropoiesis, since it is after this phase that iron and folic acid deficiency interrupt erythropoiesis (Kimura, Finch & Adamson, 1986; Antony et al., 1987), while the CFU-E are sensitive to growth inhibition by IL-I, tumor necrosis factor (TNF) and α-interferon (Schooley, Kullgren & Allison, 1987; Johnson et al., 1989; Mamus, Beck-Schroeder & Zanjani, 1985).

THE REGULATION OF ERYTHROPOIETIN

The continuous production of new red cells requires a constant supply of erythropoietin, since the hormone is responsible for not only promoting the proliferation of erythroid progenitor cells but also maintaining their viability. For this reason, erythropoietin is constitutively produced in both the kidneys and the liver, and plasma erythropoietin is maintained at a constant level in each individual just as the red mass is maintained at a constant level. There are no preformed stores of erythropoietin, and when additional hormone is required, more cells are recruited in an exponential fashion to synthesize it (Koury et al., 1989). In the kidneys, erythropoietin is primarily produced in peritubular interstitial cells of the inner renal cortex (Koury, Bondurant & Koury, 1988; Lacombe et al., 1988). Erythropoietin production is maximal in each cell and with progressive tissue hypoxia, more cells initiate its synthesis (Koury et al., 1989). In the liver, erythropoietin is produced in both hepatocytes and interstitial cells, but production in liver cells is regulated and not an all-or-none phenomenon (Koury et al., 1991). However, the threshold for initiating erythropoietin production in the liver is much higher than in the kidneys, and liver production does not compensate for impaired renal erythropoietin production except under unusual circumstances (Klassen & Spivak, 1990).

Erythropoietin production is controlled at the level of its gene. Tissue hypoxia stimulates erythropoietin production and erythrocytosis suppresses it, but never completely (Spivak & Hogans, 1987). The oxygen sensor that transduces the hypoxic signal is thought to be a rapidly turning-over heme protein (Goldberg, Dunning & Bunn, 1988). In addition to increasing erythropoietin gene transcription, hypoxia also enhances erythropoietin production by stabilizing newly transcribed erythropoietin mRNA (Goldberg, Gaut & Bunn, 1991).

The production of erythropoietin is tightly controlled at the level of its gene. Although the range for normal plasma erythropoietin levels is wide (4–26 mU/ml), the absolute value in a given individual fluctuates only within the narrow limits of diurnal variation (Wide, Bengtsson & Birgegard, 1989) and even if perturbed by tissue hypoxia, the plasma erythropoietin level returns to its previous baseline promptly with restoration of tissue oxygenation (Embury et al., 1984). Both erythropoietin production and metabolism are independent of its plasma level and marrow cellularity (Fried & Barone-Varelas, 1984; Spivak & Hogans, 1989; Piroso et al., 1991). Normally, as the haemoglobin level declines, plasma erythropoietin increases. However, this relationship does not obtain within the normal range of haemoglobin values and only when the haemoglobin level falls below 10.5 gm/dl does the plasma erythropoietin level rise unequivocally outside the normal range (Spivak & Hogans, 1987). This tight regulation of erythropoietin production presumably reflects the potency of this protein, which is active at the picomolar level and stimulates the erythroid progenitor cell population to expand in exponential fashion (Wagemaker & Visser, 1980).

Since erythropoietin behaves like a hormone, measurements of plasma erythropoietin should be useful in determining when a hormone-deficient state exists. This has proved to be the case because, as mentioned above, erythropoietin production is regulated at the level of its gene and is not subject to feedback regulation by its plasma concentration, nor is its plasma clearance influenced by its plasma level. Furthermore, there are no preformed stores of erythropoietin in the kidneys or the liver, and since genomic and circulating erythropoietin differ only by a single amino acid (Recny, Scoble & Kim, 1987) and since immunoreactive erythropoietin is equivalent to biologically active erythropoietin (Egrie et al., 1987), plasma erythropoietin provides a direct reflection of erythropoietin production at the level of the gene. Interpretation of the erythropoietin assay is further simplified because neither age nor gender influence erythropoietin production under normal circumstances (Spivak & Hogans, 1987).

Plasma erythropoietin is, however, influenced by certain disorders or their treatment in highly specific ways. For example, plasma erythropoietin production may increase in anaemic patients with hepatocellular injury due to either infection or toxins (Simon et al., 1980). Thus, during the regeneration phase of viral hepatitis, plasma erythropoietin may be increased, particularly in the renoprival state (Klassen & Spivak, 1990), and following bone marrow transplantation when the bilirubin is greater than 2 mg%, inappropriate elevations of plasma erythropoietin have been observed (Zahurak, 1992). Furthermore, by an unknown mechanism, the conditioning regimens employed for bone marrow transplantation (Birgegard, Wide & Simonsson, 1989; Schapira et al., 1990) can elevate plasma erythropoietin as can treatment with zidovidine in anaemic AIDS patients (Spivak et al., 1989). Since, in the postnatal period, erythropoietin is produced primarily in the kidneys, renal disease has a significant impact on plasma erythropoietin. Thus, once the creatinine rises above 1.5 mg/dl, the expected inverse linear relationship between plasma erythropoietin and haemoglobin is lost (Spivak & Hogans, 1987). Furthermore, the normally tight control of erythropoietin production is also lost and the plasma erythropoietin level can vary markedly in a given patient. As a general rule, in the absence of other causes, when anaemia is associated with a creatinine of greater than 1.5 mg%, it is usually the consequence of a lack of erythropoietin, and since there is no correlation between plasma erythropoietin and haemoglobin under these circumstances, assay of plasma erythropoietin is unnecessary. The anaemia associated with diabetes mellitus is an example of how the endocrine function of the kidneys is lost more quickly than its exocrine function. All of this, however, is not meant to imply that patients with renal disease lack the capacity to produce adequate quantities of erythropoietin. Rather, they require a greater hypoxic stimulus and lack the capacity to sustain a level of hormone production appropriate to their degree of anaemia. Thus, with sufficient tissue hypoxia, anaemic patients with end-stage renal disease can make substantial quantities of erythropoietin, presumably in their liver. But when the hypoxia is corrected, even though anaemia persists, erythropoietin production is promptly down-regulated to its basal level (Chandra, Clemons & McVicar, 1988).

A similar pattern is seen in many anaemic patients with cancer. In these patients, even in the absence of intrinsic renal disease, the expected inverse relationship between plasma erythropoietin and haemoglobin is essentially lost (Figure 13.1) (Miller et al., 1990). However, just like patients with chronic renal failure, with sufficient tissue hypoxia, anaemic cancer patients can synthesize erythropoietin appropriately. Thus, anaemic patients with cancer appear to have an increased threshold with respect to the degree of hypoxia required to stimulate erythropoietin production. Less extreme examples of this type of behaviour occur in patients with chronic inflammatory or infectious disorders. For example, in anaemic patients with rheumatoid arthritis, the expected inverse relationship between plasma eryth-

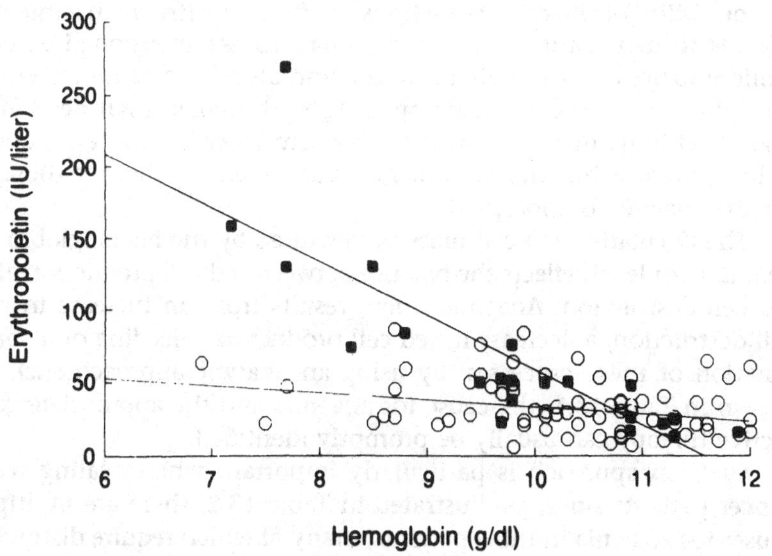

Figure 13.1 Erythropoietin–haemoglobin relationship in 74 anaemic cancer patients (o) compared to iron deficiency controls [■]. (From Miller et al., 1990. Used by permission.)

ropoietin and the haemoglobin level is present but blunted in comparison to what is observed in uncomplicated iron deficiency anaemia (Hochberg et al., 1988). A similar situation is observed in anaemic AIDS patients, since in each instance, plasma erythropoietin is still higher than normal but low in relationship to the degree of anaemia present (Spivak et al., 1989). Since anaemia is present in spite of an increase in erythropoietin production, additional factors causing marrow suppression appear to be operative in both of these situations. In vitro studies indicate that inflammatory cytokines such as γ-interferon, IL-1 and TNF can suppress erythropoietin production and, independently, erythropoiesis (Jelkmann, Wolff & Fandrey, 1990; Faquin, Schneider & Goldberg, 1992). Thus, it is likely that these cytokines are involved in the suppression of erythropoiesis in chronic inflammatory or infectious disorders.

THE INVESTIGATION OF ANAEMIA

The advent of recombinant human erythropoietin has proved an important new means for the correction of anaemia, and the immunoassay for this protein can identify those patients who are hormone deficient. In spite of the remarkable therapeutic promise of recombinant human erythropoietin, it is important to remember that anaemia is always the consequence of some other disorder, and the first responsibility of the clinician who is confronted with an anaemic patient is to define the cause for the anaemia. As mentioned earlier, while impaired erythropoietin production alone can cause anaemia, not infrequently, the disorder impairing erythropoietin synthesis may also affect bone marrow function adversely as well. Thus, evaluation of bone marrow function may be necessary to ensure that the therapy for the anaemia is appropriate.

The circulating red cell mass as measured by the haemoglobin or haematocrit level reflects the balance between red cell production and red cell destruction. Anaemia, then, results from an increase in red cell destruction, a decrease in red cell production, bleeding or a combination of these processes. By using an analytic approach such as shown in Table 13.1, the cause for anaemia and the appropriate corrective therapy can usually be promptly identified.

Such an approach is particularly important when dealing with cancer patients since, as illustrated in Table 13.2, there are multiple causes for anaemia in these patients, many of which require distinctly different therapeutic approaches. In this regard, it is important to remember that there is no correlation between the severity of an anaemia and the disorder causing it.

Table 13.1. Evaluation of Anaemia

Test	Significance
History of prior blood counts[a]	Defines duration and course
History of drug or toxin exposure[a]	Indicates potential causes for red cell destruction or marrow suppression
Reticulocyte count[a]	Defines erythropoietic activity
Blood smear[a]	Evidence for haemolytic, metabolic or nutritional defects
MCV[a]	Evidence for nutritional or maturation defects
Search for blood loss[a]	The site of blood loss and its cause must be identified
Serum creatinine	Defines renal function
Endocrine studies	Defines metabolic status
Bone marrow aspiration	Defines anatomic, nutritional or maturation abnormalities
Iron, folate, B_{12} assays	Defines nutritional status
ESR, serum protein analysis	Evidence for systemic disease
Erythropoietin assay	Evidence for marrow stimulation
Physical examination[a]	Evidence of jaundice, organomegaly or hyperviscosity

[a]Mandatory.

As indicated in Table 13.1, the first order of business is to define, if possible, the duration of anaemia by obtaining prior blood counts. At the same time, the patient's medication history and family history should be reviewed, since each of these may provide clues as to the cause of the anaemia. A reticulocyte count is mandatory, since this will define the status of erythropoiesis. A high reticulocyte count in an anaemic patient suggests a haemolytic process or recovery from recent blood loss. A low reticulocyte count suggests impaired marrow function for which there are many possibilities depending on the underlying tumour.

Review of a peripheral blood smear can further narrow the list of possibilities. For example, as listed in Table 13.2, haemolysis in patients with solid tumours or lymphomas can occur on an autoimmune basis (Spira & Lynch, 1979; Jones, 1973), while metastatic tumour is associated with a microangiopathic form of haemolysis

Table 13.2. Causes of Anaemia Associated With Malignancy

Blood loss
Extrinsic
Iatrogenic
Nutritional deficiencies
Iron
Folic acid
Vitamin B_{12}
Malnutrition
Inflammation[a]
Infection[a]
Drugs and toxins
Autoimmune disorders
Hemolysis
Red cell aplasia
Myelofibrosis
Marrow necrosis
Tumor metastatic to the marrow
Hypersplenism
Myelodysplasia
Haematophagocytosis
Haemodilution
Microangiopathy
Tumor
Intravascular coagulation
Drugs

[a]Usually associated with erythropoietin lack.

(Antman et al., 1979). In some instances, this is due to intravascular coagulation (Schafer, 1985). Certain chemotherapeutic agents can also cause a microangiopathic type of haemolysis (Jackson et al., 1984), and the changes in red cell morphology are sufficiently distinctive that a diagnosis can be made immediately.

The red cell mean corpuscular volume (MCV) and red cell distribution width (RDW) provide a substantial amount of information concerning erythropoiesis. A high MCV suggests the possibility of folate or vitamin B_{12} deficiency but can also be seen with haemolysis, hypothyroidism and dyserythropoiesis. A low MCV is usually associated with iron deficiency, but can be seen in iron-replete, anaemic cancer patients. In general, a high RDW is usually associated with a nutritional deficiency state or haemolysis, and any abnormality in the red cell indices is an indication to scrutinize a peripheral blood smear.

The peripheral blood smear can be valuable in other ways. The presence of nucleated red cells and myelocytes in the blood of a cancer patient is an important clue to the possibility of tumour metastatic to the bone marrow and mandates a bone marrow aspirate and biopsy. Rouleau formation by the red cells indicates the presence of hyperglobulinemia which, if clonal, also mandates examination of the marrow. Red cell aggregates are seen with cold agglutinins.

The physical examination may also provide some assistance with regard to diagnosis. Engorged conjunctival vessels are a clue to hyperviscosity due to hyperglobulinaemia, and this alone can be associated with low erythropoietin production (Singh et al., 1993). Splenomegaly may occur with chronic haemolysis, myeloid metaplasia or portal hypertension. Cachexia suggests the presence of malnutrition or malignancy.

Bone marrow examination is generally mandatory in anaemic cancer patients or in those patients suspected of having cancer. The bone marrow aspirate can provide evidence for nutritional deficiencies of iron, folic acid or vitamin B_{12}; serous fat atrophy; marrow necrosis; haematophagocytosis; red cell aplasia; myelodysplasia; a plasma cell dyscrasia; lymphoma; leukaemia or myelodysplasia. Bone marrow biopsy is useful in detecting myelofibrosis, tumour metastatic to the marrow and in staging lymphomas.

In many anaemic cancer patients, however, in whom erythropoiesis is depressed as indicated by a low reticulocyte count, no cause for anaemia is evident. In some patients, haemodilution may be the cause (Berlin et al., 1955). In others, a normochromic, normocytic anaemia is present with normal marrow morphology. Characteristic biochemical abnormalities are, however, present in this situation and they include a low serum iron and iron-binding capacity, an increased serum ferritin and red cell zinc protoprophyrin and an inappropriately low serum erythropoietin level for the degree of anaemia. Occasionally, the red cell MCV will be low but marrow iron stores are always normal or increased. The serum creatinine is normal as is the level of circulating thyroid hormone.

The anaemia in this situation has been designated as the anaemia of chronic disease (Cartwright, 1966) and, as might be expected from such a designation, the characteristics of this type of anaemia are not specific for cancer patients but can be seen in patients suffering from chronic infections or inflammatory disorders. What is central in each of these situations is that the anaemia is a consequence of the underlying chronic disorder, and correction of that disorder will alleviate the anaemia. The mechanisms for the anaemia associated with chronic diseases are probably multiple and include the elaboration of inflammatory cytokines such as IL-I, TNF, interferon, lactoferrin, prostaglandins and various haematopoietic growth factors that may themselves enhance the secretion of other cytokines. These cytokines may be directly inhibitory to erythropoiesis or activate cells that inhibit erythropoiesis (Johnson et al., 1984; Mamus, Beck-Schroeder & Zanjani, 1985; Schooley, Kullgren & Allison, 1987). Additionally, lactoferrin can compete effectively with transferrin for iron (Malmquist, Hansen & Karlen, 1978; Van Snick & Masson, 1976) and inflammatory cytokines can also suppress erythropoietin production (Faquin, Schneider & Goldberg, 1992; Jelkmann, Wolff & Fandrey, 1990). Thus, multiple mechanisms exist for impairing red cell production while at the same time a shortening of red cell survival has also been documented (Cavill, Ricketts & Napier, 1977). Additionally, it has been postulated that altered thyroid hormone metabolism may reduce tissue oxygen requirements and thus reduce the rate of erythropoietin production (Caro et al., 1981; Utiger, 1990).

ANAEMIA IN MALIGNANCY

Impairment of erythropoietin production in the presence of cancer has been documented in both animal and human studies. Rodents bearing a solid tumour have an impaired production of erythropoietin in response to hypoxia (DeGowin & Gibson, 1979) while anaemic cancer patients have a lower serum erythropoietin level for any degree of anaemia than patients with uncomplicated iron deficiency anaemia (Chandra, Clemons & McVicar, 1988). Furthermore, the erythropoietin response of anaemic cancer patients to anaemia is extremely blunted as determined by the erythropoietin haemoglobin relationship (Figure 13.1), although if tissue hypoxia is extreme, they are capable of substantial erythropoietin production.

It thus appears that anaemic cancer patients not only require a greater hypoxic signal to increase erythropoietin production but probably lack the capacity to sustain a high level of erythropoietin production. In this regard, they appear to behave much like anaemic patients with end-stage renal disease. This is of more than theoretical interest, since anaemic patients with end-stage renal disease respond well to recombinant erythropoietin. The impaired erythropoietin response to anaemia was seen in patients who were not on chemotherapy, but worsened with chemotherapy. The type of chemotherapy (cisplatin versus non–cisplatin-based chemotherapy) did not affect erythropoietin response to anaemia. In this regard, it has been demonstrated that in cancer patients, the marrow complement of erythroid progenitor cells is not only normal but also normally responsive in vitro to erythropoietin (Dainiak et al., 1983). This suggests that the anaemia associated with cancer should be responsive to therapy with recombinant erythropoietin. This contention is supported by early studies of the effects of androgenic steroids in patients with breast cancer (Kennedy & Gilbertsen, 1957). In these studies, a common feature was an increase in the haematocrit. Additionally, it was shown in rodents given sufficient busulfan to reduce their stem cell pool that erythropoietin could increase erythropoiesis, suggesting that recombinant erythropoietin might be effective in alleviating or preventing anaemia in patients receiving chemotherapy (Reissman & Udupa, 1972).

THE TREATMENT OF ANAEMIA OF MALIGNANCY

The data presented above suggest that the anaemia associated with cancer and chemotherapy is at least in part related to a relative erythropoietin deficiency. Recombinant human erythropoietin (HuEPO) has been effective in the treatment of anaemias of other chronic diseases that are associated with erythropoietin deficiency including the anaemia associated with renal failure (Casati et al., 1987; Eschbach et al., 1989a, 1989b; Etlenger, Mark & Grimm, 1991), rheumatoid arthritis (Birgegard et al., 1991; Pincus et al., 1990) and HIV infection (Fischl et al., 1990).

rHuEPO has also been shown to be effective in the treatment of anaemia related to cancer. Oster et al. (1990) treated six transfusion-dependent patients with neoplastic bone marrow infiltration related to low-grade lymphoma or multiple myeloma. rHuEPO treatment was instituted with escalating doses (150 units/kg, 300 units/kg, 450 units/kg) of rHuEPO given twice weekly intravenously. Four of six patients did not require transfusion during rHuEPO therapy, and there was a significant increase in haemoglobin over baseline during the study period. This pilot trial was the first to demonstrate activity of rHuEPO in patients with the anaemia of malignancy.

Ludwig et al. (1990) described the treatment with rHuEPO of 13 patients with anaemia associated with multiple myeloma. rHuEPO was given at a dose of 150 units/kg three times a week subcutaneously with dose escalation by 50 units/kg every three weeks if an adequate response was not seen for a total of six months. Eleven patients responded with at least a 2-gm/dl increase in haemoglobin at a median of five weeks of treatment. A marked increase in corrected reticulocyte count was seen with a median change of 370% above baseline in the 11 responders. This study looked at the effect of rHuEPO on different haematopoietic subsets due to concern that expansion of the erythroid progenitor cell pool may occur at the expense of myeloid progenitors. The erythroid progenitor cell population as measured by bone marrow BFU-E increased significantly; however, there was no significant change in marrow granulocyte progenitors (CFU-G) suggesting that there was no reduction in myelopoiesis. There was also no change in tumour markers such as percent plasma cells or the serum M component, suggesting that the rHuEPO had little effect on the tumour cell burden. These studies suggested that rHuEPO may be useful in patients with anaemia associated with cancer and neoplastic bone marrow infiltration. As in the other studies of rHuEPO in non-dialysis patients, rHuEPO was tolerated well without significant side effects.

In a study of 124 cancer patients with anaemia not related to chemotherapy (Abels et al., 1991) patients were randomized to placebo or rHuEPO (100 units/kg three times a week for eight weeks). There was a significant increase in haematocrit over this time period related to rHuEPO therapy but no effect was seen on percentage of patients requiring transfusion. This may have been due to the short treatment period in this study and the lag time between treatment with rHuEPO and clinical effect. In this study, 40% of the patients had a greater than 6% increase in haematocrit over the study period. In these patients, quality of life measures were improved; however, there was no statistically significant improvement in the quality of life in the group as a whole. This suggests that correcting anaemia in cancer patients does improve their quality of life. Studies of rHuEPO in selected patient populations such as patients with chronic lymphocytic leukaemia are underway.

Patients with chemotherapy-induced anaemia have shown responses to treatment with rHuEPO. In a phase I/II trial of rHuEPO in chemotherapy-induced anaemia (Miller, 1991; Miller et al., 1992; Plantanias et al., 1991), 49 patients were treated with escalating doses (25, 50, 100, 200 and 300 units/kg) of rHuEPO given intravenously five times a week for four weeks. Patients were grouped according to whether cisplatin was part of their chemotherapeutic regimen. Maximal responses were seen in both arms of the study at the 100- and 200-units/kg dose levels, with 70% of the patients treated at these doses responding with increase in haemoglobin of greater than 1 gm/dl over the four weeks without transfusion. The haemoglobin change from baseline is shown in Figure 13.2. These patients continued on their chemotherapeutic regimes during the rHuEPO therapy, and the increase in the haemoglobin seen in the responders was not related to marrow recovery from chemotherapy. Patients tolerated rHuEPO

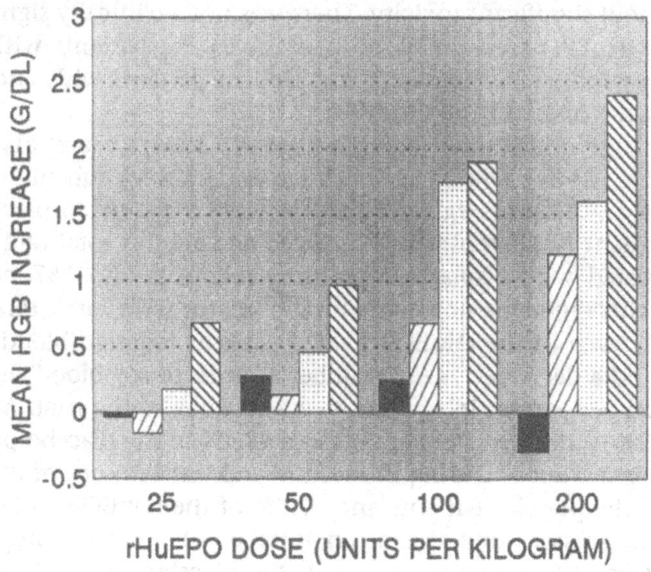

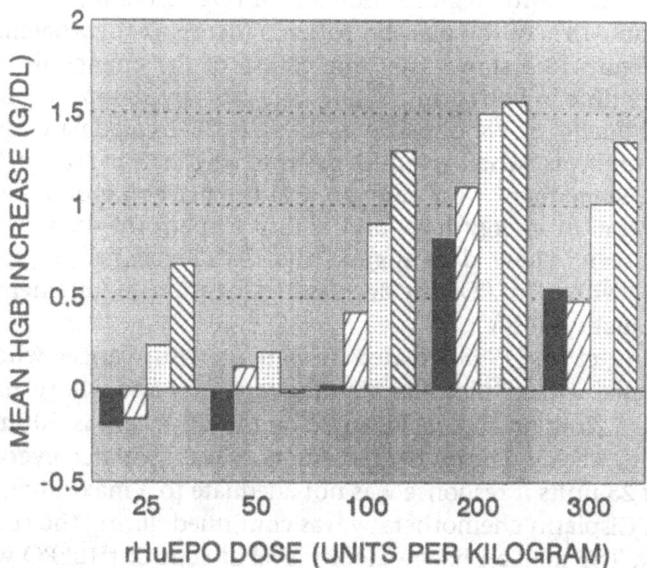

Figure 13.2 Haemoglobin dose response to rHuEPO in anaemic cancer patients receiving chemotherapy. (A) Patients receiving cisplatin as part of their chemotherapeutic regimen. (B) Patients receiving chemotherapy not containing cisplatin.

well without significant toxicity. There was not a clinically significant effect of rHuEPO seen on blood pressure in the patients with chemotherapy-induced anaemia as was seen in patients with end-stage renal disease treated with rHuEPO.

In a large multicenter trial (Abels et al., 1991; Case et al., 1993; Henry et al., 1989), rHuEPO given three times a week subcutaneously at a dose of 150 units/kg for 12 weeks was compared to placebo in the treatment of chemotherapy-induced anaemia. A total of 132 patients treated with cisplatin-containing regimens and 157 patients treated with regimens not containing cisplatin were randomized. In this trial, fewer of the rHuEPO-treated patients required blood transfusions and a decreased mean number of units of red blood cells was transfused per patient in months two and three of the trial. At baseline, 44.7% of the rHuEPO patients and 48.4% of the placebo patients required transfusion. During the second and third month of the trial, 45.5% of the placebo patients and 27.8% of the rHuEPO patients required transfusion, and the mean number of units transfused decreased from 1.8 units per patient in the placebo arm to 1.04 units per patient in the rHuEPO. In the cisplatin-treated patients, 48% of the rHuEPO-treated patients responded with a haematocrit increase of greater than 6% compared to 6.6% of the placebo patients. In the patients treated with regimes not containing cisplatin, 58% of the rHuEPO and 13% of the placebo patients increased their haematocrit by 6%. Figure 13.3 shows the time course of the change in haematocrit over time in both arms. While a statistically significant increase in overall quality of life was seen in the rHuEPO-treated patients compared to controls, when rHuEPO patients who had at least a 6% increase in haematocrit were compared to the placebo group, a significant increase in energy level and ability to perform daily activities was also seen. These data suggest that in chemotherapy patients, treatment with rHuEPO can decrease transfusion requirements and increase quality of life.

Cascinu et al. (1993) treated 20 patients with cancer who were being treated with cisplatin-containing regimens and whose anaemia was related to their chemotherapy. The initial dose was 50 units/kg three times weekly. The erythropoietin dose was escalated every three weeks by 25 units if response was not adequate to a maximum of 100 units/kg. Cisplatin chemotherapy was continued during the course of the study. The median haemoglobin level at start of rHuEPO was 8.6 gm/dl. rHuEPO was well tolerated, with only two patients reporting facial flushing and headache thought possibly related to rHuEPO. Fifteen patients responded with at least a 1-gm/dl increase in haemoglobin over the initial three weeks. The median increase in haemoglobin

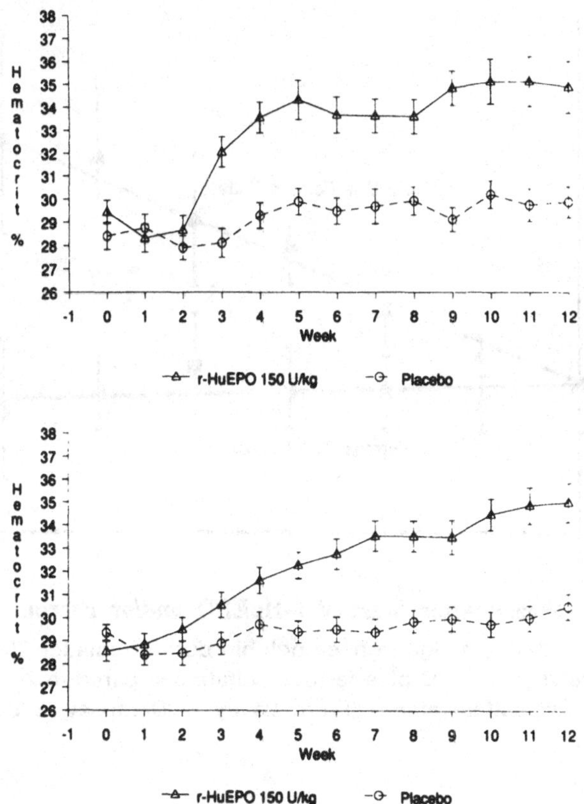

Figure 13.3 Mean weekly haematocrits in rHuEPO-treated patients compared to placebo. rHuEPO was given at a dose of 150 units/kg three times a week for 12 weeks. (A) Patients receiving cisplatin as part of their chemotherapeutic regimen. (B) Patients receiving chemotherapy not containing cisplatin. (From Abels et al., 1991. Used by permission.)

in these responders was 1.9 gm/dl. In the five patients who did not respond to the initial dose, one was not re-treated, two did not respond to any dose and one patient each responded to the 75- and 100-units/kg dose level. There was no significant correlation between the pretreatment erythropoietin level and the response to rHuEPO. This small study again offers support that rHuEPO is efficacious in treating cisplatin-associated anaemia.

Markman et al. (1993) used rHuEPO to prevent or lessen anaemia associated with carboplatin chemotherapy. This study was designed to determine if rHuEPO could be used in a prophylactic setting in patients who had a high risk of developing anaemia. Forty patients

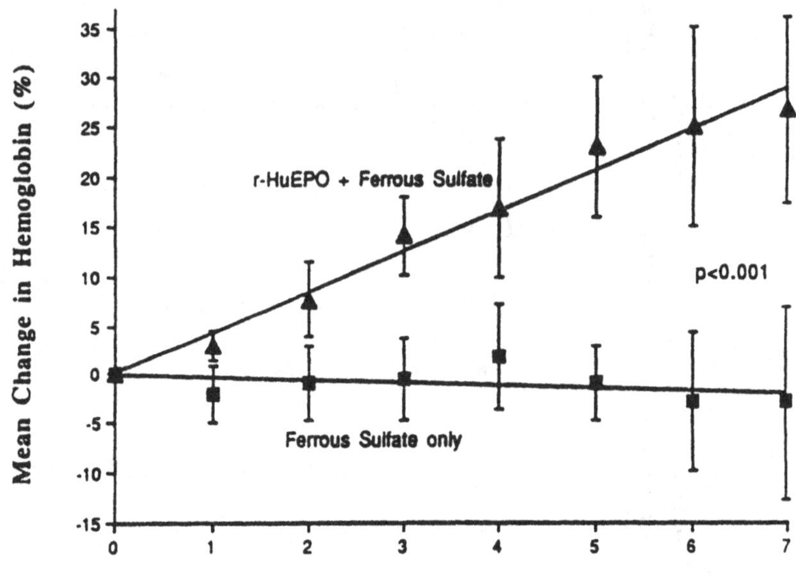

Figure 13.4 Mean change in haemoglobin during radiation therapy in 20 patients receiving rHuEPO plus ferrous sulfate compared to 20 patients receiving ferrous sulfate alone. (From Lavey & Dempsey, 1993. Used by permission.)

who completed at least one cycle of high-dose intraperitoneal carboplatin and etoposide without rHuEPO were used as historical controls. Seventeen patients were treated with rHuEPO before the study was closed because of a patent dispute. Sixteen patients completed at least one cycle of chemotherapy and were considered evaluable. There was no difference in baseline characteristics including age, previous treatment and pretreatment haemoglobin and creatine between the patients and historical controls. rHuEPO was given at a dose of 100 units/kg subcutaneously for a total of nine doses (day −6, −4, −2, +2, +4, +6, +8, +10, +12). The carboplatin dose was 200 mg/m^2 and etoposide dose was 100 mg/m^2 given intraperitoneally monthly. The amount of carboplatin and etoposide delivered was not different in the two patient groups; 60% of the historical controls and 13% of the rHuEPO patients had a nadir haemoglobin of less than 9 gm/dl ($p<.005$). Severe anaemia (haemoglobin <8 gm/dl) occurred in 23% of controls versus 6% of the rHuEPO-treated patients ($p<.05$). Transfusion requirement appeared less in the rHuEPO-treated patients (6% versus 23%); however, statistical significance was not achieved.

A prophylactic trial of rHuEPO in patients with sarcoma receiving intensive chemotherapy in a neoadjuvant and postoperative setting has not yet been completed; however, a preliminary interim analysis is available (Barlogie & Beck, 1993). Patients were randomly assigned to rHuEPO (600 units/kg, eight patients) or placebo (nine patients). The study drug was started when the haemoglobin level fell below 11.5 gm/dl and was given subcutaneously twice a week until the haemoglobin increased to greater than 13.5 gm/dl. The mean duration of rHuEPO therapy was 17.5 weeks. The study drug was well tolerated. rHuEPO-treated patients required a mean of 4.25 units of red blood cells over the course (including surgery) versus 8.7 units in the placebo patients ($p<.01$). Despite the decreased transfusion requirement, the mean haemoglobin was higher in the rHuEPO-treated patients (11.1 gm/dl) compared to controls (10.6 gm/dl). Formal analysis including quality of life is ongoing. This study supports a role for rHuEPO in lessening the severity of anaemia in patients treated with intensive chemotherapy, especially preoperatively.

CONCLUSIONS

Studies are ongoing to better define the role of rHuEPO in the treatment of the anaemia associated with chemotherapy and cancer. Questions that remain to be answered include the timing of therapy (i.e., prevention versus treatment), dose and patient selection. Timing is especially important, as there is at least a two-week lag time from starting drug to seeing a clinical effect. Therefore, if prevention of transfusion is the clinical end point, it may be important to start the drug in patients before they are severely anaemic. Another potential use of rHuEPO in this patient population is in the preparation for cancer surgery by either allowing the patient to bank autologous units or elevation of the pretransplant haematocrit to potentially avoid allogeneic blood transfusion. While controversial, there have been studies that suggest that there is an increase in the relapse rate in patients with cancer who receive allogeneic blood during surgery (Blumberg & Heal, 1987; Burrows & Tartter, 1982; Singh et al., 1987). This has been postulated to be related to immunosuppression from the allogeneic blood; however, this has yet to be proven (Hirose et al., 1993). rHuEPO has been shown to be effective in improving the ability to bank adequate autologous blood preoperatively (Goodnough et al., 1984). rHuEPO may be especially important in preoperative blood banking in patients with cancer, as these patients may be anaemic at the start of a blood banking process and have already been shown to have an inadequate erythropoietin response to anaemia (Clemens &

Spivak, in press). Another major question has been the role of the pretreatment erythropoietin level in predicting response to rHuEPO. The FDA-approved package insert recommends its use in patients with endogenous erythropoietin levels less than 200 mU/ml. There are however, no data to support this cutoff. There has been no correlation in any of the studies discussed above between the baseline serum erythropoietin level and the response to therapy. However, the majority of patients in the studies where data are available have erythropoietin levels less than 200 mU/ml (Abels, 1992; Cascinu et al., 1993; Case et al., 1993; Miller et al., 1992; Plantanias et al., 1991). This is in contrast to patients with HIV infection and anaemia related to zidovudine therapy where an erythropoietin level greater than 500 mU/ml predicted an extremely poor response to therapy (Fischl et al., 1990). Therefore, there is no evidence that an erythropoietin level of 200 mU/ml in patients with cancer has any clinical relevance. However, it may have an impact on the approval of drug reimbursement.

As with any supportive care issue in patients with cancer, it will be important to determine whether the intervention could increase the tumour growth. While there has not been adequate clinical follow-up to rule out that possibility, there are no preclinical data to suggest that erythropoietin would have an effect on tumour cells. Erythropoietin receptors are lineage restricted and with the exception of erythroleukaemia cell lines, there has been no evidence of tumour-associated receptors. As well, tumour growth in vitro does not appear to be stimulated by rHuEPO (Berdel et al., 1991). Preliminary data from the randomized trial showed no increase in tumour progression in the rHuEPO-treated patients compared with placebo; however, longer follow-up is needed.

Finally, is there any role for rHuEPO in improving the therapeutic intent in cancer patients? A novel way to use rHuEPO for a potential therapeutic intent is in patients with cancer receiving radiation therapy. The efficacy of radiation therapy depends on adequate oxygen available at the site of the tumour (Dische, 1991; Girinski et al., 1989). Therefore, anaemia may prevent optimal tumour response to a therapeutic dose of radiation therapy. rHuEPO can correct the anaemia in patients undergoing radiation therapy (Tsukuda et al., 1993; Vijayakuma et al., 1993). In a randomized, open-label trial of rHuEPO in 26 patients who had either breast, lung, cervix or prostate cancer undergoing intensive radiation therapy, patients were assigned to a treatment group (rHuEPO 200 units/kg five times a week subcutaneously) or a control group. In the control group, mean weekly haemoglobin decline was 0.035 gm/dl versus a 0.43-gm/dl haemoglobin increase in the rHuEPO-treated patients. There was no effect on the white blood count or platelet count in the two groups. Subjective improvement in the ability to tolerate radiation therapy was seen in the rHuEPO-treated patients. Whether or not an improvement in disease-free survival would result from the increase in haematocrit could not be answered with this study.

Lavey studied the response to rHuEPO and iron supplementation of 20 patients with localized cancer who were scheduled to receive five to eight weeks of radiation therapy targeted above the diaphragm (Lavey & Demsey, 1993). rHuEPO patients were compared to concurrently treated control patients who received iron supplementation only. rHuEPO was given subcutaneously at a dose of 300 units/kg for three doses followed by 150 units/kg three times a week until the completion of radiation therapy. Baseline characteristics were not different between the two groups. Mean baseline haemoglobin was 11.9 gm/dl in the rHuEPO group and 11.8 gm/dl in the control group. Haemoglobin concentration in the rHuEPO-treated patients rose to a mean of 15.1 gm/dl at the end of radiation therapy, while there was no increase in the haemoglobin in the control group. The rate of increase in the rHuEPO-treated patients was 5% a week (Figure 13.4); 80% of the rHuEPO patients achieved a haemoglobin of greater than 14 gm/dl during radiation therapy compared to 5% of the controls. rHuEPO was well tolerated in this patient population. This study confirmed that rHuEPO can be given safely during radiation therapy and a higher haemoglobin can be achieved. Again, this study was not designed to address whether disease-free survival can be improved with a higher haemoglobin. The Southwest Oncology Group will investigate in a pilot trial whether rHuEPO can maintain or improve haematocrit in patients who receive concurrent cisplatin and radiation therapy for carcinoma of the cervix. A randomized trial will be required to evaluate the effect on disease control.

In conclusion, rHuEPO is an important drug in patients with cancer that can increase the haematocrit and improve quality of life. The optimal dose and timing are still being evaluated.

REFERENCES

Abels R.I. (1992) Use of recombinant human erythropoietin in the treatment of anemia in patients who have cancer. *Seminars in Oncology*, **3**(8), 29–35.

Abels R.I., Larholt K.M., Krantz K.D. & Bryant E.C. (1991) Recombinant human erythropoietin (r-HuEPO) for the treatment of the anemia of cancer. In M.J. Murphy, Jr. (Ed.) *Blood cell growth factors: their present and future use in hematology and oncology*, pp. 121–141. Alpha Med Press, City.

Adamson J.W. et al. (1980) Polycythemia vera: further in vitro studies of hematopoietic regulation. *Journal of Clinical Investigation*, **66**, 1363–8.

Antman K.H., Skarin A.T., Mayer R.J. et al. (1979) Microangiopathic hemolytic anemia and cancer. A review. *Medicine*, **58**, 377.

Antony A.C., Bruno E., Briddell R.A. et al. (1987) Effect of perturbation of specific folate receptors during in vitro erythropoiesis. *Journal of Clinical Investigation*, **80**, 1618–23.

Axelrad A.A., McLeod D.L., Shreeve M.M. et al. (1900) Properties of cells that produce erythrocytic colonies in vitro. In W.A. Robinson (Ed.) *Proceedings of the second international workshop on hemopoiesis in culture*, pp. 226–34. U.S. Government Printing Office, Washington, D.C.

Barlogie B. & Beck T. (1993) Recombinant human erythropoietin and the anemia of multiple myeloma. *Stem Cells*, **11**, 88–94.

Becker A.J., McCulloch E.A., Siminovitch L. et al. (1965) The effect of differing demands for blood cell production on DNA synthesis by hemopoietic colony-forming cells of mice. *Blood*, **26**, 296–308.

Berdel W.E., Oberberg D., Reufi B. et al. (1991) Studies on the role of recombinant human erythropoietin in the growth regulation of human nonhematopoietic tumor cells in vitro. *Annals of Hematology*, **63**(1), 5–8.

Berlin N.I., Hyde G.M., Parsons R.J. et al. (1955) The blood volume in cancer. *Cancer*, **8**, 796–801.

Birgegard G., Gudbjronsson B., Hallgren R. & Wide L. (1991) Anemia of chronic inflammatory arthritides: treatment with recombinant human erythropoietin. In H.J. Gurland, J. Moran, W. Samtleben, P. Scigalla & L. Wieczorek (Eds.) *Erythropoietin in renal and non-renal anemias*, pp. 295–305. Karger, New York.

Birgegard G., Wide L. & Simonsson B. (1989) Marked erythropoietin increase before fall in Hb after treatment with cytostatic drugs suggests mechanism other than anaemia for stimulation. *British Journal of Haematology*, **72**, 462–6.

Blumberg N. & Heal J.M. (1987) Perioperative blood transfusion and solid tumour recurrence. *Blood Reviews*, **1**, 19–229.

Burrows L. & Tartter P. (1982) Effect of blood transfusion on colonic malignancy recurrence rate. *Lancet*, **i**, 662.

Caro J., Silver R., Erslev A.J. et al. (1981) Erythropoietin production in fasted rats. *Journal of Laboratory and Clinical Medicine*, **98**, 860.

Cartwright G.E. (1966) The anemia of chronic disorders. *Seminars in Hematology*, **3**, 351–75.

Casati S., Passerini P., Campise M.R. et al. (1987) Benefits and risks of protracted treatment with human recombinant erythropoietin in patients having haemodialysis. *British Medical Journal*, **295**, 1017–20.

Cascinu S., Fedeli A., Fedeli S.L. et al. (1993) Cisplatin-associated anaemia treated with subcutaneous erythropoietin. A pilot study. *British Journal of Cancer*, **67**, 156–8.

Case D.C., Bukowski R.M., Carey R.W. et al. (1993) Recombinant human erythropoietin therapy for anemic cancer patients on combination therapy. *Journal of the National Cancer Institute*, **85**(10), 801–6.

Cavill I., Ricketts C. & Napier J.A.F. (1977) Erythropoiesis in the anaemia of chronic disease. *Scandinavian Journal of Haematology*, **19**, 509–12.

Chandra M., Clemons G.K. & McVicar M.I. (1988) Relation of serum erythropoietin levels to renal excretory function: evidence for lowered set point for erythropoietin production in chronic renal failure. *Journal of Pediatrics*, **113**, 1015–21.

Dainiak N., Kulkarni V., Howard D. et al. (1983) Mechanisms of abnormal erythropoiesis in malignancy. *Cancer,* **51**, 1101–06.

DeGowin R.L. & Gibson D.P. (1979) Erythropoietin and the anemia of mice bearing extramedullary tumor. *Journal of Laboratory and Clinical Medicine,* **94**, 303–11.

Dische S. (1991) Radiotherapy and anaemia – the clinical experience. *Radiotherapy and Oncology,* **20** (Suppl.), 35–40.

Egrie J.C., Cotes P.M., Lane J. et al. (1987) Development of radioimmunoassays for human erythropoietin using recombinant erythropoietin as tracer and immunogen. *Journal of Immunological Methods,* **99**, 235–41.

Embury S.H., Garcia J.F., Mohandas N., Pennathur-Das R., Clark M.R. et al. (1984) Effects of oxygen inhalation on endogenous erythropoietin kinetics, erythropoiesis, and properties of blood cells in sickle-cell anemia. *New England Journal of Medicine,* **311**, 291–5.

Eschbach J.W., Abdulhadi M.H., Browne J.K. et al. (1989a) Recombinant human erythropoietin in anemic patients with end-stage renal disease. *Annals of Internal Medicine,* **111**, 992–1000.

Eschbach J.W., Kelly M.R., Haley N.R. et al. (1989b) Treatment of the anemia of progressive renal failure with recombinant human erythropoietin. *New England Journal of Medicine,* **321**, 158–61.

Ettenger R.B., Marik J. & Grimm P. (1991) The impact of recombinant human erythropoietin therapy on renal transplantation. *American Journal of Kidney Disease,* **28**(4)1, 57–61.

Faquin W.C., Schneider T.J. & Goldberg M.A. (1992) Effect of inflammatory cytokines on hypoxia-induced erythropoietin production. *Blood,* **79**, 1987–94.

Fischl M., Galpin J.E., Levine J.D. et al. (1990) Recombinant human erythropoietin for patients with AIDS treated with zidovudine. *New England Journal of Medicine,* **322**, 1488–93.

Fried W. & Barone-Varelas J. (1984) Regulation of the plasma erythropoietin level in hypoxic rats. *Experimental Hematology,* **12**, 706–11.

Girinski T., Pejovic-Lenfant M.H., Bourhis J. et al. (1989) Prognostic value of hemoglobin concentrations and blood transfusions in advanced carcinoma of the cervix treated by radiation therapy: results of a retrospective study of 386 patients. *International Journal of Radiation Oncology, Biology, Physics,* **16**, 37–42.

Goldberg M.A., Dunning S.P. & Bunn H.F. (1988) Regulation of the erythropoietin gene: evidence that the oxygen sensor is a heme protein. *Science,* **242**, 1412–14.

Goldberg M.A., Gaut C.C. & Bunn H.F. (1991) Erythropoietin mRNA levels are governed by both the rate of gene transcription and posttranscriptional events. *Blood,* **77**, 271–7.

Goodnough L.T., Rudnick S., Price T.H. et al. (1989) Increased preoperative collection of autologous blood with recombinant human erythropoietin therapy. *New England Journal of Medicine,* **322**(16), 1157–9.

Henry D.H., Rudnick S.A., Bryant E. et al. (1989) Preliminary report of two double blind, placebo controlled studies using recombinant human erythropoietin in the anemia associated with cancer (Abstr.). *Blood,* **73**(Suppl.), 6.

Hirose T., Pepkowitz S., Jacobs A. et al. (1993) The effects of red blood cell transfusion on host immune function. In C. Bauer, K.M. Koch, P. Scigalla

& L. Wieczorek (Eds.) *Erythropoietin: molecular physiology and clinical applications*, pp. 277–90. Marcel Dekker, New York.

Hochberg M.C., Arnold C.M., Hogans B.B. et al. (1988) Serum immunoreactive erythropoietin in rheumatoid arthritis: impaired response to anaemia. *Arthritis and Rheumatism*, **31**, 1318–21.

Iscove N.N. (1977) The role of erythropoietin in regulation of population size and cell cycling of early and late erythroid precursors in mouse bone marrow. *Cell Tissue Kinetics*, **10**, 323–34.

Iscove N.N. (1978) Erythropoietin-independent stimulation of early erythropoiesis in adult marrow cultures by conditioned medium from lectin-stimulated mouse spleen cells. *ICN-UCLA Symposium on Hematopoietic Cell Differentiation*, **10**, 37–52.

Jackson A.M., Rose B.D., Graff L.G. et al. (1984) Thrombotic microangiopathy and renal failure associated with antineoplastic chemotherapy. *Annals of Internal Medicine*, **101**, 41–4.

Jelkmann W., Wolff M. & Fandrey J. (1990) Modulation of the production of erythropoietin by cytokines: in vitro studies and their clinical implications. *Contributions in Nephrology*, **87**, 68–77.

Johnson R.A., Waddelow T.A., Caro J. et al. (1989) Chronic exposure to tumor necrosis factor in vivo preferentially inhibits erythropoiesis in nude mice. *Blood*, **74**, 130–8.

Jones S.E. (1973) Autoimmune disorders and malignant lymphoma. *Cancer*, **31**, 1092–8.

Kennedy B.J. & Gilbertsen A.S. (1957) Increased erythropoiesis induced by androgenic-hormone therapy. *New England Journal of Medicine*, **256**, 719–26.

Kimura H., Finch C.A. & Adamson J.W. (1986) Hematopoiesis in the rat: quantitation of hematopoietic progenitors and the response to iron deficiency anemia. *Journal of Cellular Physiology*, **126**, 298–306.

Klassen D.K. & Spivak J.L. (1990) Hepatitis-related hepatic erythropoietin production. *American Journal of Medicine*, **89**, 684–6.

Kost T.A. et al. (1979) Target cells for Friend virus-induced erythroid bursts in vitro. *Cell*, **18**, 145–52.

Koury M.J. & Bondurant M.C. (1990) A survival model of erythropoietin action. *Science*, **248**, 378–81.

Koury S.T., Bondurant M.C. & Koury M.J. (1988) Localization of erythropoietin synthesizing cells in murine kidneys by in situ hybridization. *Blood*, **71**, 524–7.

Koury S.T., Bondurant M.C., Koury M.J. & Semenza G.L. (1991) Localization of cells producing erythropoietin in murine liver by *in situ* hybridization. *Blood*, **77**, 2497–503.

Koury S.T., Koury M.J., Bondurant M.C., Caro J. & Graber S.E. (1989) Quantitation of erythropoietin-producing cells in kidneys of mice by in situ hybridization: correlation with hematocrit, renal erythropoietin mRNA, and serum erythropoietin concentration. *Blood*, **74**, 645–51.

Lacombe C., DaSilva L., Bruneval P., Fournier J.-G., Wendling F. et al. (1988) Peritubular cells are the site of erythropoietin synthesis in the murine hypoxic kidney. *Journal of Clinical Investigation*, **81**, 620–3.

Lavey R.S. & Dempsey W.H. (1993) Erythropoietin increases hemoglobin in cancer patients during radiation therapy. *International Journal of Radiation Oncology, Biology, Physics*, **27**, 1147–52.

Leary A.G. et al. (1992) Growth factor requirements for survival in GO and entry into the cell cycle of primitive human hemopoietic progenitors. *Proceedings of the National Academy of Sciences of the United States of America*, **89**, 4013–17.

Ludwig H., Fritz E., Kotzmann H. et al. (1990) Erythropoietin treatment of anemia associated with multiple myeloma. *New England Journal of Medicine*, **322**, 1693–9.

Malmquist J., Hansen N.E. & Karle H. (1978) Lactoferrin in haematology. *Scandinavian Journal of Haematology*, **21**, 5–8.

Mamus S.W., Beck-Schroeder S.K. & Zanjani E.D. (1985) Suppression of normal human erythropoietin by gamma interferon in vitro. *Journal of Clinical Investigation*, **75**, 1496–503.

Markman M., Reichman B., Hakes T. et al. (1993) The use of recombinant human erythropoietin to prevent carboplatin-induced anemia. *Gynecologic Oncology*, **49**, 172–6.

Merchav S., Tatarsky I. & Hochberg Z. (1988) Enhancement of erythropoiesis in vitro by human growth hormone is mediated by insulin-like growth factor I. *British Journal of Haematology*, **70**, 267–71.

Metcalf D., Johnson G.R. & Burgess A.W. (1980) Direct stimulation by purified GM-CSF of the proliferation of multipotential and erythroid precursor cells. *Blood*, **55**, 138–47.

Miller C.B. (1991) Erythropoietin in renal and non-renal anemias. Contributions to nephrology. In H.J. Gurland, J. Moran, W. Samtleben, P. Scigalla & L. Wieczorek (Eds.) *Chemotherapy-induced anemia*, pp. 248–51. Karger, Basel.

Miller C.B., Jones R.J., Piantadosi S., Abeloff M.D. & Spivak J.L. (1990) Decreased erythropoietin response in patients with the anemia of cancer. *New England Journal of Medicine*, **322**, 1689–92.

Miller C.B., Plantanias L.C., Ratain M.J. et al. (1992) A phase I/II trial of erythropoietin in the treatment of chemotherapy-induced anemia in patients with cancer. *Journal of the National Cancer Institute*, **84**(2), 98–103.

Nakahata T., Gross A.J. & Ogawa M. (1982) A stochastic model of self-renewal and commitment to differentiation of the primitive hemopoietic stem cells in culture. *Journal of Cellular Physiology*, **113**, 455–8.

Nicola N.A. (1989) Hemopoietic cell growth factors and their receptors. *Annual Review of Biochemistry*, **58**, 45–77.

Ogawa M., Porter P.N. & Nakahata T. (1983). Renewal and commitment to differentiation of hemopoietic stem cells: an interpretive review. *Blood*, **61**, 823–9.

Oster W., Herrmann F., Gamm H. et al. (1990) Erythropoietin for the treatment of anemia of malignancy associated with neoplastic bone marrow infiltration. *Journal of Clinical Oncology*, **8**, 956–61.

Pincus T., Olsen N.J., Russell I.J., et al. (1990) Multicenter study of recombinant human erythropoietin in correction of anemia in rheumatoid arthritis. *American Journal of Medicine*, **89**, 161–8.

Piroso E., Erslev A.J., Flaharty K. & Caro J. (1991) Erythropoietin life span in rats with hypoplastic and hyperplastic bone marrows. *American Journal of Hematology*, **36**, 105–10.

Plantanias L.C., Miller C.B., Mick R. et al. (1991) Treatment of chemotherapy-induced anemia in cancer patients with recombinant human erythropoietin. *Journal of Clinical Oncology*, **9**(11), 2021–6.

Recny M.A., Scoble H.A. & Kim Y. (1987) Structural characterization of natural human urinary and recombinant DNA-derived erythropoietin. *Journal of Biological Chemistry*, **262**, 17156–63.

Reissman K.R. & Udupa K.B. (1972) Effect of erythropoietin on proliferation of erythropoietin-responsive cells. *Cell Tissue Kinetics*, **5**, 481–9.

Sawada K., Krantz S.B., Dai C.-H. et al. (1990) Purification of human blood burst-forming units-erythroid and demonstration of the evolution of erythropoietin receptors. *Journal of Cellular Physiology*, **142**, 219–30.

Schafer A.I. (1985) The hypercoagulable states. *Annals of Internal Medicine*, **102**, 814–28.

Schapira L., Antin J.H., Ransil B.J. et al. (1990) Serum erythropoietin levels in patients receiving intensive chemotherapy and radiotherapy. *Blood*, **76**, 2354–9.

Schooley J.C., Kullgren B. & Allison A.C. (1987) Inhibition by interleukin-1 of the action of erythropoietin on erythroid precursors and its possible role in the pathogenesis of hypoplastic anaemia. *British Journal of Haematology*, **67**, 11–17.

Simon P., Meyrier A., Tanquerel T. et al. (1980) Improvement of anaemia in haemodialysed patients after viral or toxic hepatic cytolysis. *British Medical Journal*, **1**, 892–4.

Singh A., Eckardt K.U., Zimmermann A. et al. (1993) Increased plasma viscosity as a reason for inappropriate erythropoietin formation. *Journal of Clinical Investigation*, **91**, 251–6.

Singh S.K., Marquet R.L., Westbroek D.L. et al. (1987) Enhanced growth of artificial tumor metastases following blood transfusion: the effect of erythrocytes, leukocytes and plasma transfusion. *European Journal of Cancer and Clinical Oncology*, **23**(10), 1537–40.

Spivak J.L. (1992) The mechanism of action of erythropoietin: erythroid cell response. In J.W. Fisher (Ed.) *Handbook of experimental pharmacology*, biochemical pharmacology of blood and bloodforming organs, Vol. 101, pp. 49–114. Springer-Verlag, Berlin Heidelberg.

Spivak J.L., Barnes D.C., Fuchs E. et al. (1989) Serum immunoreactive erythropoietin in HIV-infected patients. *Journal of the American Medical Association*, **261**, 3104–7.

Spivak J.L. & Hogans B.B. (1987) Clinical evaluation of a radioimmunoassay for serum erythropoietin using reagents derived from recombinant erythropoietin. *Blood*, **70**, 143a.

Spivak J.L. & Hogans B.B. (1989) The in vivo metabolism of recombinant human erythropoietin in the rat. *Blood*, **73**, 90–9.

Spivak J.L., Pham T.H., Isaacs M.A. & Hankins W.D. (1991) Erythropoietin is both a mitogen and a survival factor. *Blood*, **77**, 1228–33.

Spira M.A. & Lynch E.C. (1979) Autoimmune hemolytic anemia and carcinoma: an unusual association. *American Journal of Medicine*, **67**, 753–8.

Stephenson J.R. & Axelrad A.A. (1971) Separation of erythropoietin-sensitive cells from hemopoietic spleen colony-forming stem cells of mouse fetal liver by unit gravity sedimentation. *Blood*, **37**, 427.

Suda T., Suda J. & Ogawa M. (1983) Proliferative kinetics and differentiation of murine blast cell colonies in culture: evidence for variable G0 periods and constant doubling rates of early pluripotent hemopoietic progenitors. *Journal of Cellular Physiology*, **117**, 308–18.

Tsukuda M., Mochimatsu I., Nagahara T. et al. (1993) Clinical application of recombinant human erythropoietin for treatments in patients with head and neck cancer. *Cancer Immunology Immunotherapy*, **36**, 52–6.

Udupa K.B. & Reissmann K.R. (1977) In vivo and in vitro effect of bacterial endotoxin on erythroid precursors (CFU-e and ERG) in the bone marrow of mice. *Journal of Laboratory and Clinical Medicine*, **89**, 278–84.

Utiger R.D. (1990) Decreased extrathyroidal triiodothyronine production in nonthyroidal illness: benefit or harm? *American Journal of Medicine*, **69**, 807–10.

Van Snick J.L. & Masson P.L. (1976) The binding of human lactoferrin to mouse peritoneal cells. *Journal of Experimental Medicine*, **144**, 1568–80.

Vijayakuma S., Roach M., Wara W. et al. (1993) Effect of subcutaneous recombinant human erythropoietin in cancer patients receiving radiotherapy: preliminary results of a randomized, open-labeled, phase II trial. *International Journal of Radiation Oncology, Biology, Physics*, **26**, 721–9.

Wagemaker G. & Visser, T.P. (1980). Erythropoietin-independent regeneration of erythroid progenitor cells following multiple injections of hydroxyurea. *Cell Tissue Kinetics*, **13**, 505–17.

Walker F., Nicola N.A., Metcalf D. et al. (1985) Hierarchical down-modulation of hemopoietic growth factor receptors. *Cell*, **43**, 269–76.

Wide L., Bengtsson C. & Birgegard G. (1989) Circadian rhythm of erythropoietin in human serum. *British Journal of Haematology*, **72**, 85–90.

Zahurak M., Santos G.W. et al. (1992) Impaired erythropoietin response after bone marrow transplantation. *Blood*, **80**, 2677–82.

Index